看護・医学
略語・用語
ガイドブック

監修/**飯田恭子**
日本医療科学大学保健医療学部学部長

サイオ出版

監修

飯田恭子

首都大学東京名誉教授

日本医療科学大学保健医療学部 学部長

編集/制作

編集協力　　：天野　修司
　　　　　　　日本医療科学大学保健医療学部 助教

はじめに

　看護は非常に専門性の高い分野です。それだけに使われる専門用語も数多くあり、またそこには一つひとつの言葉の正確な理解と使い方も求められます。

　こうした専門用語も、見て、聞いて、パッとすぐに何のことかわかれば問題はないのですが、略語で表されたり、カルテのように英独語で表記されたりしていると、そうもいきません。数もまた膨大です。

　そこで、知らない単語や、忘れてしまった略語・用語に出くわしたときに、その意味を正確かつ迅速に引ける本が必要になってきます。

　本書はそうしたニーズに応えるべく生まれました。第1章では英独の略語・用語を、第2章では臨床現場で頻用されるカタカナ用語を、第3章では難読漢字・難読病名を扱っています。

　あらゆる看護・医療用語やカルテ用語をカバーできるよう約6,500語を収載し、分からない略語・用語をすぐに引けるように構成しました。第4章は和文から略語を調べられる逆引きになっています。

　初版の発行から3年半。読者の方々に好評いただき、今回で2回目の改訂・増補になります。第1章に対義語、関連用語、併せて参照しておきたい用語を盛り込みました。

　1つの略語を引いた時に、これら対義語や関連用語などを同時に押さえることで、より知識の定着や理解が深まればと思います。

　引き続き、本書が皆さんの学習や看護実践のうえで助けになれば幸いです。

2015年10月

飯田恭子

凡　例

【第1章】
1．略語・用語は、アラビア数字、ローマ数字、ABC、和文順に配列した。
2．略語は略語・原語・和文の順に、用語は用語・和文の順に配列した。
3．同じ意味の略語は別々に掲載したが、近接する時は「、」で区切って併記した。別々に掲載した場合には、和文に「＝」をもって他方の略語を示した。
4．用語と略語が同じ意味の場合は、それぞれの和文の末尾に「＝」をもって他方の用語、略語を示した。
5．原語に〔　〕を付したものは、〔　〕内の文字を省略したものも通常使用されていることを示す。

【第2章】
1．同じ意味の語句は、「、」で区切って併記した。
2．和文における（　）の意味は、①（　）の前の語句の略語または欧文原語を示す、②（　）内の文字を省略したものも通常使用する、③（　）内の文字をその前の一部の文字と置き換えることができる、④全文を（　）内の文字で置き換えることができる、⑤（　）の前の語句の解説を示す、の4つである。
3．日常的会話文は「　」をもって示した。

【第3章】
1．難読漢字、難読病名は、漢字→読み方の順に配列した。
2．語句の先頭漢字の画数順に並べた。
3．読み方は国語辞典と異なる読みでも、医学用語として慣用されている読みに従った。

【第4章】
1．和文・略語の順に配列した。
2．数字、欧文（ギリシャ文字、ABC順）、和文の五十音順に配列した。

対：対義語　　**関連**：関連する略語・用語　　**参照**：併せて参照してほしい略語・用語

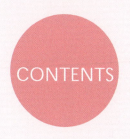

はじめに …………………………………………… 3

第1章
略語・用語（英独語⇒日本語） …………………… 7

第2章
頻用カタカナ用語 ………………………………… 251

第3章
難読漢字・難読病名 ……………………………… 281

第4章
逆引き（和文⇒略語） …………………………… 297

略語・用語
英独語⇒日本語

・a・

数字

2DE(two dimensional echocardiogram)	断層心エコー図
2R(2nd intercostal space right sternal border)	第2肋間胸骨右縁
3L/3LSB (3rd intercostal space left sternal border)	第3肋間胸骨左縁
47XXYsyndrome(Klinefelter syndrome)	クラインフェルター症候群
4L/4LSB (4th intercostal space left sternal border)	第4肋間胸骨左縁
5-FU(5-fluorouracil)	5-フルオロウラシル
10 RM(10 repetition maximum)	漸増抵抗運動(10段階)
^{131}I-PVP test	^{131}I標識ポリビニルピロリドン試験
17-OHCS(17-hydroxycorticosteroid)	17-ヒドロキシコルチコステロイド

A

a(arterial blood)	動脈血　◀対▶静脈血：V
a(assessment)	アセスメント
A(alcoholic psychosis)	アルコール精神病
A(allergy)	アレルギー
A(anterior segment)	右葉前区域(肝)
A(artery)	動脈　◀対▶静脈：V
A(ascending colon)	上行結腸　◀関連▶横行結腸：T　下行結腸：D　S状結腸：S
a0-3	食道癌の組織学的外膜癌浸潤程度を示す記号
A1/3(lower third of the stomach)	胃下1/3
A2(aortic second sound)	第2大動脈音
A領域	前庭部領域(胃下部1/3)
A-Ⅱ(angiotensinⅡ)	アンギオテンシンⅡ

AB

AA(acupuncture analgesia)	鍼麻酔
AA(alcoholics anonymous)	匿名断酒会
AA(alopecia areata)	円形脱毛症
AA(amyloid angiopathy)	アミロイドアンギオパチー
AA(aplastic anemia)	再生不良性貧血
AA(arbeitsangina)	労作性狭心症
	◀関連▶ 安定性狭心症：SA
AA(artificial abortion)	人工流産
AA(ascending aorta)	上行大動脈＝AAA
AA(ascorbic acid)	アスコルビン酸
AA(atlantoaxial)	環軸椎の
AAA(abdominal aortic aneurysm)	腹部大動脈瘤
AAA(acute anxiety attack)	急性不安大発作
AAA(aneurysm of ascending aorta)	上行大動脈瘤＝AA
AAD(antibiotic-associated diarrhea)	抗生物質随伴下痢症
AAD(α_1−antitrypsin deficiency)	α_1−アンチトリプシン欠損症
A-A dislocation(atlantoaxial dislocation)	環軸椎脱臼
a-ADN$_2$ (arterial alveolar nitrogen pressure difference)	動脈血肺胞気窒素ガス分圧差
A-aDO$_2$ (alveolar arterial oxygen pressure difference)	肺胞気動脈血酸素分圧差
AAE(active assistive exercise)	積極的介助運動
AAE(acute allergic encephalitis)	急性アレルギー性脳炎
AAE(annuloaortic ectasia)	大動脈弁輪拡張症
AAFB(atypical acid-fast bacilli)	非定型抗酸菌
AAH(atypical adenomatous hyperplasia)	異型腺腫過形成
AAI(atrium atrium inhibit pacing)	心房抑制型心房ペーシング
AAL(anterior axillary line)	前腋窩線
AAMI(aged associated memory impairment)	老年性記憶障害
AAR(antigen antibody reaction)	抗原抗体反応
AAS(aortic arch syndrome)	大動脈弓症候群、大動脈炎症候群
AAS(atlantoaxial subluxation)	環軸椎亜脱臼
AB gap(air bone gap)	気導骨導差

◆AB◆

AB(abortion)	流産
Ab(antibody)	抗体
ab(antigen-binding capacity)	抗原結合能
AB(asthmatic bronchitis)	喘息性気管支炎
abasia	歩行不能
A bile(gallduct bile)	胆管胆汁
ABC(airway breathing circulation)	気道確保、人工呼吸、閉胸式心マッサージ
ABC(aneurysmal bone cyst)	動脈瘤様骨嚢腫、動脈瘤様骨腫
ABC(aspiration biopsy cytodiagnosis)	吸引生検細胞診
abd resp(abdominal respiration)	腹式呼吸
	◀関連▶胸式呼吸:cost resp
abd(abdomen)	腹部
ABD(aged, blind, disabled)	高齢者、眼の見えない人、障害者
ABD(average body dose)	平均身体投与量
ABD(abductor)	外転筋
	◀対▶内転筋:Add
ABD, Abd(abduction)	外転
	◀対▶内転:ADD, Add
abd.(abdominal)	腹部の
abdominal breathing	腹式呼吸
abdominal distention	腹部膨隆
abdominal pain	腹痛
abdominocentesis	腹腔穿刺
abducens N	外転神経
ABE(acute bacterial endocarditis)	急性細菌性心内膜炎
ABF(anti-bleeding factor)	抗出血因子
ABG(arterial blood gas)	動脈血ガス
ABL(abetalipoproteinemia)	無βリポ蛋白症
ABLB test (alternate binaural loudness balance test)	両耳音の大きさバランス検査、両耳閾聴力バランス検査
ABO(ABO blood group system)	ABO式血液型

AC

ABP(acute bacterial prostatitis)	急性細菌性前立腺炎 ◀関連▶慢性細菌性前立腺炎：CBP
ABP(arterial blood pressure)	動脈圧＝AP, PA ◀対▶静脈圧：VP
ABPA (allergic broncho-pulmonary aspergillosis)	アレルギー性気管支肺アスペルギルス症
ABPM(allergic broncho-pulmonary mycosis)	アレルギー性気管支肺真菌症
ABPM (ambulatory blood pressure monitoring)	携帯型自動血圧計、24時間血圧測定
ABR(auditory brainstem response)	聴性脳幹反応（聴覚脳幹反応）＝BEAR
abrasion	すり傷
ABS(acute brain syndrome)	急性脳症候群
ABS(amniotic band syndrome)	羊膜索症候群
abscess	膿瘍
ABSCT(autologous peripheral blood stem cell transplantation)	自家末梢血幹細胞移植＝auto-PBSCT
ABSI(abbreviated burn severity index)	簡易式熱傷重傷度指数
abstinence symptom	禁断症状
ABU(asymptomatic bacteriuria)	無症候性細菌尿
ABVD(adriamycin, bleomycin, vinblastine, dacarbazine)	アドリアマイシン、ブレオマイシン、ビンブラスチン、ダカルバジンの併用療法（ホジキン病の治療）
AC, ac(abdominal circumference)	腹囲
AC(adenocarcinoma)	腺癌、アデノカルチノーマ＝ad-ca
AC(adrenal cortex)	副腎皮質＝ADC ◀関連▶副腎髄質：ADM
AC(adult children)	アダルト・チルドレン
AC(air conduction)	気導、気導聴力
AC(anterior chamber)	前房、前眼房
AC(anticoagulant)	抗凝固薬
AC(arm circumference)	上腕囲

AC

AC (asymptomatic carrier)	無症候性キャリア
AC (alveolar-capillary) block syndrome	肺胞毛細管ブロック症候群
A-C bypass (aorto-coronary artery bypass procedure)	大動脈冠動脈バイパス術
a.c. (ante cibum)	食前 参照 食後：p.c.
AC-IOL (anterior chamber intraocular lens)	前房内レンズ
ACA (anterior cerebral artery)	前大脳動脈 対 後大脳動脈：PCA
ACA (anterior communicating artery)	前交通動脈＝Acom 対 後交通動脈：PC, Pcom
acalculia	失算
ACB (antibody coated bacteria)	抗体被覆細菌
ACBE (air contrast barium enema)	空気注腸造影
ACBG (aortocoronary bypass graft)	大動脈冠動脈バイパス移植術＝CABG, CABS, AC bypass
ACC (acinic cell carcinoma)	腺房細胞癌
ACC (adenoid cystic carcinoma)	腺様嚢胞癌
ACC (adrenocortical carcinoma)	副腎皮質癌
ACC (alveolar cell carcinoma)	肺胞上皮癌
ACC (aplasia cutis congenita)	先天性皮膚欠損症
ACC (articular chondrocalcinosis)	関節軟骨石灰化症
acceleration	一過性頻脈
accessory N (nerve)	副神経
ACCS (alternating convergent comitant strabismus)	交代性共同性内斜視
ACD (alcoholic cerebellar degeneration)	アルコール中毒性小脳変性
ACD (allergic contact dermatitis)	アレルギー性接触性皮膚炎
ACD (anterior chest diameter)	前胸部横径
ACDK (acquired cystic disease of the kidney)	多嚢胞化萎縮腎
ACE (angiotensin-converting enzyme)	アンギオテンシン変換酵素
ACEI (angiotensin converting enzyme inhibitor)	アンギオテンシン変換酵素阻害薬

AC

ACF(abnormal colposcopic findings)	腟鏡的異常所見
ACF(accessory clinical findings)	付随的臨床所見
ACF(adriamycin, chloroethyl, 5-fluorouracil)	アドリアマイシン、クロロマイセチン、フルオロウラシル併用療法
ACG(angiocardiography)	心血管造影法
ACG(aortocoronary graft)	大動脈冠動脈移植術
ACG(apex cardiogram)	心尖拍動図
ACh(acetylcholine)	アセチルコリン
ACH(active chronic hepatitis)	活動性慢性肝炎
ACH(amyotrophic cerebellar hypoplasia)	筋萎縮性小脳形成不全
achalasia	アカラシア（噴門痙攣）
achillobursitis	アキレス腱滑液包炎
achillodynia	アキレス腱痛
achillorrhaphy	アキレス腱縫合術
ACI(acute coronary infarction)	急性冠動脈梗塞
ACI(acute coronary insufficiency)	急性冠動脈不全
ACI(adrenocortical insufficiency)	副腎皮質機能不全
acidosis	アシドーシス 対 アルカローシス：alkalosis
ACJ(acromioclavicular joint)	肩峰鎖骨関節
AC joint(acromioclavicular joint)	肩峰鎖骨関節
ACKD(acquired cystic kidney disease)	後天性嚢胞腎
ACL(anterior contact lens)	前房コンタクトレンズ
ACL(anterior cruciate ligament)	前十字靱帯
ACLE(acute cutaneous lupus erythematosus)	急性皮膚エリテマトーデス
ACLS(advanced cardiac life support)	二次循環救急処置 参照 ACLSI(ACLS instructor)：二次循環救命処置指導者
ACM(adriamycin, cyclophosphamide, medroxyprogesterone)	アドリアマイシン、シクロホスファミド、メドロキシプロゲステロン併用療法
ACM(adriamycin, cyclophosphamide, methotrexate)	アドリアマイシン、シクロホスファミド、メトトレキセート併用療法

AC

ACMP (adriamycin, cylocide, 6-mercaptopurine, predonine)	アドリアマイシン、キロサイド、6-メルカプトプリン、プレドニン併用療法
ACN (amyloidosis cutis nodularis)	結節性皮膚アミロイドーシス
ACNA (amyloidosis cutis nodularis atrophicans)	萎縮性結節性皮膚アミロイドーシス
acne	挫瘡
ACO (acute coronary occlusion)	急性冠動脈閉塞症
A com (anterior communicating artery aneurysm)	前交通動脈瘤
A com (anterior communicating artery)	前交通動脈 対 後交通動脈：Pcom
acoustic aid	補聴器
acquired	後天性の 対 先天性の：congenital 遺伝性の：genetic
acromegaly	先端巨大症
acrophobia	高所恐怖
ACS (acute confusional state)	急性錯乱状態
ACS (acute coronary syndrome)	急性冠動脈症候群
ACS (alternating convergent strabismus)	交代性内斜視
ACT (adriamycin, cyclophosphamide, tamoxifen)	アドリマイシン、シクロホスファミド、タモキシフェン併用療法
ACT (atropine coma therapy)	アトロピン昏睡療法
ACT (activated coagulation time)	活性化凝固時間
ACTH (adrenocorticotrophic hormone)	副腎皮質刺激ホルモン
ACUP (adenocarcinoma of unknown primary tumor site)	原発巣不明腺癌
acupressure	指圧
acupuncture	鍼治療
acute alcohol intoxication	急性アルコール中毒
acute infantile hemiplegia	急性乳児片麻痺
acute nephritic syndrome	急性腎炎症候群
acute otitis media	急性中耳炎

acute poststreptococcal glomerulonephritis	溶連菌感染後急性糸球体腎炎
ACV(acyclovir)	アシクロビル（ゾビラックス）
ACVD(atherosclerotic cardiovascular disease)	アテローム硬化性心血管疾患
ACW(anterior chest wall)	前胸壁
AD(addict)	常用者、常習者
Ad(adnexa)	付属器
AD(adrenaline)	アドレナリン
AD(Aleutian disease)	アリューシャン病
AD(Alzheimer dementia)	アルツハイマー型認知症
AD(Alzheimer disease)	アルツハイマー病
AD(atopic dermatitis)	アトピー性皮膚炎
AD(auris dextra／right ear)	右耳　対 左耳：AS
AD(autosomal dominant inheritance)	常染色体優性遺伝
A&D(admission and discharge)	入院と退院
Adam's apple	咽頭隆起、のどぼとけ
AD-CA, ad-ca(adenocarcinoma)	腺癌、アデノカルチノーマ＝AC
ADCMC(antibody-dependent cell-mediated cytotoxicity)	抗体依存性細胞媒介性細胞傷害作用
ad.feb.(adstante febre)	有熱時
ADC(adrenal cortex)	副腎皮質
	◀関連▶ 副腎髄質：AdM
ADCC(antibody-dependent cell-mediated cytotoxicity)	抗体依存性細胞障害
ADD, Add(adduction)	内転、内反
	対 外転：ABD, Abd
Add(adductor)	内転筋
	対 外転筋：ABD
ADD(attention deficit disorder)	注意欠陥障害
adductor reflex	内転筋反射
ADE(acute disseminated encephalomyelitis)	急性播種性脳脊髄膜炎
ADEM (acute disseminated encephalomyelitis)	急性散在性脳脊髄膜炎
ademonia	精神障害

·AD

ADEN (acute disseminated epidermal necrosis)	急性播種性表皮壊死
adenoid	アデノイド
adenoidectomy	アデノイド切除術
adenotonsillectomy	扁桃腺アデノイド切除術
ADH(adhesion)	癒着
ADH(antidiuretic hormone)	抗利尿ホルモン
ADH(atypical ductal hyperplasia)	異型乳管過形成
AD-HD (attention deficit hyperactivity disorder)	注意欠陥多動障害
ADI(acceptable daily intake)	許容摂取量
ADI(atlanto-dental interval)	環椎歯突起間距離
ADL(activities of daily living)	日常生活動作
ADM(abductor digiti minimi)	小指外転筋=ADQ
Adm(admission)	入院
	参照 退院：Disc、DS
AdM(adrenal medulla)	副腎髄質
	関連 副腎皮質：ADC, AC
admission by legal control	措置入院
ADML(acute duodenal mucosal lesion)	急性十二指腸粘膜病変
adolescence	思春期
ADP(abductor pollicis)	母指外転筋
ADPKD(autosomal dominant polycystic kidney disease)	常染色体優性遺伝型多発性囊胞腎
ADQ(abductor digiti quinti)	小指外転筋=ADM
adrenal cortex	副腎皮質=ADC
adrenal gland	副腎
adrenal medulla	副腎髄質
adrenalectomy	副腎摘出術
adrenarche	副腎皮質徴候発現
Adrex(adrenalectomized)	副腎を摘出した
ADS(antidiuretic substance)	抗利尿性物質
ADS(alternative divergent strabismus)	交代性外斜視
ADS(anatomical dead space)	解剖学的死腔=Vdan

ADS(antibody deficiency syndrome)	抗体不全症候群、抗体欠損症候群
Ad-St(Adams-Stokes syndrome)	アダムス・ストークス症候群
ad.us.ext.(ad usum externum)	外用
ad.us.int.(ad usum internum)	内用
AdVP(adriamycin, vincristine, prednisolone)	アドリアマイシン、ビンクリスチン、プレドニゾロン併用療法
adynamic ileus	麻痺性イレウス
AE amp(above-elbow amputation)	上腕切断
AE(active exercise)	自動運動 **対** 他動運動：passive exercise exercise：自動運動、他動運動
AECD(allergic eczematous contact dermatitis)	アレルギー性湿疹状接触皮膚炎
AED(antiepileptic drug)	抗てんかん薬
AED(automated external defibrillator)	自動体外除細動器
AEDH(acute epidural hematoma)	急性硬膜外血腫
AEP(auditory evoked potential)	聴覚誘発電位
AER(auditory evoked response)	聴覚誘発反応
AES(aortic ejection sound)	大動脈駆出音
AF(abdominal flap)	腹部皮弁
AF(amniotic fluid)	羊水
AF(anteflexio)	前屈
AF(anterior fontanel)	大泉門 **関連** 小泉門：posterior fontanel
AF(ascitic fluid)	腹水
Af(atrial fibrillation)	心房細動
AF(atrial flutter)	心房粗動
AFB(acid-fast bacillus)	抗酸菌
AFB(aorta femoral bypass)	大動脈大腿動脈バイパス術
AFC(antibody forming cell)	抗体産生細胞
AFCE(acute focal cerebral edema)	急性局所性脳浮腫

AF

AFD(appropriate-for-dates) infant	適性発育児／相当体重児
AFE(amniotic fluid embolism)	羊水塞栓症
affect	情動
afferent arteriole	輸入細動脈
AFI(amaurotic familial idiocy)	黒内障性家族性白痴
AFO(ankle-foot orthesis)	短下肢装具＝SLB
AFP(α-fetoprotein)	αフェトプロテイン(胎児性蛋白)
AFRD(acute febrile respiratory disease)	急性熱性呼吸器疾患
Afta(Kunstafter)	人工肛門
AFV(amniotic fluid volume)	羊水量
AG(abdominal girth)	腹囲
AG(angina pectoris)	狭心症＝AP 参照 安定性狭心症：SA 不安定性狭心症：UA
AG(angiography)	血管造影
Ag(antigen)	抗原
AG(arteriography)	動脈造影
AGA(allergic granulomatous angiitis)	アレルギー性肉芽腫性血管炎
AGA (appropriate for gestational age〔infant〕)	在胎期間に比して適当な大きさの児(適性発育児)
AGC(advanced gastric cancer)	末期胃癌 ◀関連▶ 早期胃癌：EGC
AGC(automatic gain control)	自動音量調節
AGD(anogenital distance)	肛門性器間距離
AGE(acute gastroenteritis)	急性胃腸炎
agenesis of corpus callosum	脳梁欠損症
AGG(agammaglobulinemia)	無γグロブリン血症
agitation	不穏
AGL(acute granulocytic leukemia)	急性顆粒球性白血病
AGML(acute gastric mucosal lesion)	急性胃粘膜病変
AGN(acute glomerulonephritis)	急性糸球体腎炎 ◀関連▶ 慢性糸球体腎炎：CGN
AGN(agnosia)	失認

AI

agnosia	失認＝AGN
agoraphobia	広場恐怖
agraphia	失書
A/G ratio(albumin-globulin ratio)	アルブミン／グロブリン比
AGS(adrenogenital syndrome)	副腎性器症候群
AGS(amenorrhea-galactorrhea syndrome)	乳汁漏出・無月経症候群
AGTT(abnormal glucose tolerance test)	異常糖負荷試験
AH interval(atrio-His bundle interval)	心房－ヒス束時間
AH(abdominal hysterectomy)	腹式子宮摘出術
AH(acute hepatitis)	急性肝炎
	◀関連▶慢性肝炎：CH
AH(alcoholic hepatitis)	アルコール性肝炎
AHA(acquired hemolytic anemia)	後天性溶血性貧血
AHA(antihemophilic factor A)	抗血友病A因子
AHA(autoimmune hemolytic anemia)	自己免疫性溶血性貧血＝AIHA
AHC(acute hemorrhagic colitis)	急性出血性腸炎
AHC(acute hemorrhagic conjunctivitis)	急性出血性結膜炎
AHD(acquired heart disease)	後天性心疾患
AHD(acute heart disease)	急性心疾患
AHD(arteriosclerotic heart disease)	動脈硬化性心疾患＝ASHD
AHD(autoimmune hemolytic disease)	自己免疫性溶血性疾患
AHF(acute heart failure)	急性心不全
	◀関連▶慢性心不全：CHF
AHF(antihemophilic factor)	抗血友病因子、血液凝固Ⅷ因子
AHI(acromiohumeral interval)	肩峰骨頭距離
AHO(Albright hereditary osteodystrophy)	アルブライト遺伝性骨形成異常症
AHP(acute hemorrhagic pancreatitis)	急性出血性膵炎、劇症膵炎
AI(acetabular index)	臼蓋指数
AI(aortic insufficiency)	大動脈弁閉鎖不全症＝AR
AI(apnea index)	無呼吸指数
AI(artificial insemination)	人工授精

● AI ●

AIA(aspirin-induced asthma)	アスピリン誘発喘息
AICA(anterior inferior cerebellar artery)	前下小脳動脈
AICD(Automatic implantable cardioverter-defibrillator)	植込み型除細動器＝ICD
AICF(autoimmune complement fixation)	自己免疫補体結合反応
aichmophobia	尖鋭恐怖（症）
AID(acute infectious disease)	急性伝染病
AID(artificial insemination with donor's semen)	非配偶者間人工授精　対 配偶者間人工授精：AIH
AID(autoimmune disease)	自己免疫疾患
AIDP(acute inflammatory demyelinating polyradicuropathy)	ギラン・バレー症候群（急性炎症性多発ニューロパチー）
AIDS(acquired immunodeficiency syndrome)	後天性免疫不全症候群
AIE(acute infectious endocarditis)	急性感染性心内膜炎
AIH(artificial insemination with husband's semen)	配偶者間人工授精　対 非配偶者間人工授精：AID
AIH(autoimmune hepatitis)	自己免疫性肝炎
AIHA(autoimmune hemolytic anemia)	自己免疫性溶血性貧血
AIIS(anterior inferior iliac spine)	下前腸骨棘
AIM(abnormal involuntary movement)	異常不随意運動
AIMD(abnormal involuntary movement disorder)	異常不随意運動疾患
AIMP(acute immune-mediated polyneuritis)	急性免疫性多発神経炎
AIN(acute interstitial nephritis)	急性間質性腎炎
AIN(autoimmune neutropenia)	自己免疫性好中球減少症
AIOD(aortoiliac occlusive disease)	大動脈腸骨動脈閉塞症
AION(anterior ischemic optic neuropathy)	前部虚血性視神経症
AIP(acute idiopathic pericarditis)	急性特発性心膜炎
AIP(acute inflammatory polyneuropathy)	急性炎症性多発ニューロパチー
AIP(acute intermittent porphyria)	急性間欠性ポルフィリン症

AL

AIP(acute interstitial pneumonia)	急性間質性肺炎
AIP(alcohol induced pancreatitis)	アルコール性膵炎
AIPD (anterior inferior pancreatic duodenal artery)	前下膵十二指腸動脈
AIPD(autoimmune progesterone dermatitis)	自己免疫性プロゲステロン皮膚炎
AIS(abbreviated injury scale)	簡易式外傷指数
AJ(ankle jerk)	アキレス腱反射
a. j.(ante jentaculum)	朝食前 ◆参照◆ 夕食前：a.p.
AK(actinic keratosis)	日光角化症
AK(artificial kidney)	人工腎臓
AK(astigmatic keratotomy)	乱視矯正角膜切開（術）
AK amp(above-knee amputation)	大腿切断
AKBR(arterial ketone body ratio)	動脈血中ケトン体比
AL(acute leukemia)	急性白血病
	◀関連▶ 慢性白血病：CL
ALA(antilymphocyte antibody)	抗リンパ球抗体
alar	鼻翼
ALbL(acute lymphoblastic leukemia)	急性リンパ芽球性白血病
albuminuria	アルブミン尿
alc(alcoholism)	アルコール依存症
alcoholic amnestic disorder	アルコール健忘症
alcoholic dementia	アルコール性痴呆
alcoholic epilepsy	アルコールてんかん
alcoholic hallucinosis	アルコール幻覚症
alcoholism	アルコール中毒
ALD(adreno-leukodystrophy)	副腎白質ジストロフィ
ALD(alcoholic liver disease)	アルコール性肝障害
ALD(anterior latissimus dorsi)	前広背筋
aldosterone	アルドステロン
alert	意識清明
alexia	失読
ALF(acute liver failure)	急性肝不全
ALG(antilymphocyte globulin)	抗リンパ球グロブリン

·al·

algolagnia	疼痛嗜愛
ALI(acute lung injury)	急性肺障(傷)害
alkalosis	アルカローシス
	対 アシドーシス：acidosis
ALL(acute lymphocytic leukemia)	急性リンパ性白血病
	関連 慢性リンパ性白血病：CLL
ALL(anterior longitudinal ligament)	前縦靱帯
allele	対立遺伝子
allo(allogenic)	同種の
allo-BMT(allogeneic bone marrow transplantation)	同種骨髄移植
allo-PBSCT(allogeneic peripheral blood stem cell transplantation)	同種末梢血幹細胞移植
allo-SCT (allogeneic stem cell transplantation)	同種造血幹細胞移植
ALM(acral lentiginous melanoma)	末／先端部黒子型黒色腫
alopecia areata	円形脱毛症＝AA
ALP, AP(alkaline phosphatase)	アルカリホスファターゼ
Alport's syndrome	アルポート症候群
ALS(advanced life support)	二次救命処置
	参照 一次救命処置：BLS
ALS(amyotrophic lateral sclerosis)	筋萎縮性側索硬化症
ALS(antilymphocyte serum)	抗リンパ球血清
ALS(artificial liver support)	人工的肝機能補助
ALT(alanine aminotransferase)	アラニンアミノトランスフェラーゼ＝GPT
ALTE(apparent life threatening event)	乳幼児突発性危急事態
alveolus	肺胞
Alzheimer disease	アルツハイマー病
am(ante meridiem／before noon)	午前 参照 午後：pm
AM(amygdala)	扁桃腺、小脳扁桃
AM(atypical mycobacteriosis)	非定型抗酸菌症
AMA(antimyocardial antibody)	抗心筋抗体

Am

ambivalence	両価性
amblyopia	弱視
AMC(arthrogryposis multiplex congenita)	先天性多発性関節拘縮症
AMD, ARMD (age-related macular degeneration)	加齢性黄斑変性
AME(amebic meningoencephalitis)	アメーバ性髄膜脳炎
amenorrhea-galactorrhea syndrome	無月経・乳汁分泌症候群
AMI(acute myocardial infarction)	急性心筋梗塞 参照 周術期心筋梗塞(症)：PMI(perioperative myocardial infarction) 後壁心筋梗塞(症)：PMI(posterior myocardial infarction)
AMI(anterior myocardial infarction)	前壁心筋梗塞
aminoaciduria	アミノ酸尿
AML(acute monocytic leukemia)	急性単球性白血病＝AMOL ◀関連▶慢性単球性白血病：CMoL
AML(acute myeloblastic leukemia)	急性骨髄芽球性白血病
AML(acute myelocytic leukemia)	急性骨髄性白血病 ◀関連▶慢性骨髄性白血病：CML
AML(angiomyolipoma)	血管筋脂肪腫
AML(anterior mitral leaflet)	僧帽弁前尖
AMMoL(acute myelomonocytic leukemia)	急性骨髄単球性白血病
AMN(adrenomyeloneuropathy)	副腎脊髄神経障害
amnesia	健忘症
amnestic syndrome	健忘症候群
amniocentesis	羊水穿刺
amnion	羊膜
AMOL(acute monocytic leukemia)	急性単球性白血病＝AMoL, AML
Amp(amputation)	切断

AM

AMV(assist mechanical ventilation)	補助機械換気
amyloidosis	アミロイドーシス
amyotonia	筋無緊張症
amyotrophy	筋萎縮症
Amytal interview	アミタール面接
AN(acanthosis nigricans)	黒色表皮症、黒色表皮腫
AN(acoustic neuroma)	聴神経腫
AN(Angstneurose)	不安神経症
AN(anorexia nervosa)	神経性食思不振症
AN(aseptic necrosis)	無菌性壊死
ANA(antinuclear antibody)	抗核抗体
anal atresia	鎖肛
analgesic	鎮痛剤
anaphylactoid purpura nephritis	アナフィラクトイド紫斑病性腎炎
anasarca	全身性浮腫
	◀関連▶ 浮腫：edema
ANC(absolute neutrophil count)	好中球絶対数
androgen	アンドロゲン
ANE(angioneurotic edema)	血管運動神経性浮腫
anencephaly	無脳症
anesthesia	知覚脱失
ANF(antinuclear factor)	抗核因子
ANF(avascular necrosis of the femoral head)	無血管性大腿骨頭壊死症
anginal pain	狭心痛
Angio(angiography)	血管造影
	参照 CAG：coronary angiography（冠動脈造影法）、cerebral angiograply（脳血管造影法）
angioma	血管腫
angioplasty	血管形成
angiotensin	アンギオテンシン
anisocoria	瞳孔不同
ankle joint	足関節

ankylosis	強直
ANLL(acute non-lymphocytic leukemia)	急性非リンパ性白血病
annular ligament	輪状靱帯
anorexia	食欲不振
anorexia nervosa	神経性食思不振症
anoxic encephalopathy	無酸素性脳症
ANP(acute necrotizing pancreatitis)	急性壊死性膵炎
ANP(atrial natriuretic peptide)	心房性ナトリウム利尿ペプチド
ANS(anterior nasal spine)	前鼻棘
ANS(autonomic nervous system)	自律神経系
	参照 中枢神経系：CNS
	末梢神経系：PNS
ANSD (autonomic nervous system dysfunction)	自律神経機能障害
anterior pituitary	下垂体前葉
anthropophobia	対人恐怖
anti-GBM nephritis	抗糸球体基底膜腎炎
antiacid	消化剤
antibiotic	抗生物質
anticipatory anxiety	予期不安
anticoagulant therapy	抗凝固療法
antidepressant	抗抑うつ薬
antimitochondrial antibody	抗ミトコンドリア抗体
antisocial personality disorder	反社会性人格障害
Anton's syndrome	アントン症候群
anuria	無尿
anxiety	不安
anxiety attack	不安発作
anxiolytic	抗不安薬
Ao(aorta)	大動脈　対 大静脈：VC
AoAW(anterior wall of aorta)	大動脈前壁
AOC(acute obstructive cholangitis)	急性閉塞性胆管炎
AOD(adult-onset diabetes)	成人発症型糖尿病
AOD(arterial occlusive disease)	動脈閉塞性疾患

AO

AOG(auditory electro-oculomotogram)	聴覚性電気眼球運動図
AOM(acute otitis media)	急性中耳炎
AoPW(posterior wall of aorta)	大動脈後壁
AOSC(acute obstructive suppurative cholangitis)	急性閉塞性化膿性胆管炎
AoV(aortic valve)	大動脈弁＝AV
AP(acute phase)	急性期　参照 慢性期：CP
AP(acute pneumonia)	急性肺炎
AP(anaphylactoid purpura)	アナフィラキシー性紫斑病
AP(angina pectoris)	狭心症＝AG 参照 労作性狭心症：AA, EA 異型狭心症：VAP
AP(appendectomy)	虫垂切除術
AP(appendix)	虫垂
AP(arterial pressure)	動脈圧＝ABP, PA 対 静脈圧：VP
AP(artificial pneumothorax)	人工気胸
A&P(auscultation and percussion)	聴診と打診
A-P(anteroposterior)	前後方向、背腹方向
a.p.(ante prandium)	夕食前 参照 朝食前：a.j.
AP window(aorticopulmonary window)	大動脈肺動脈窓
APA(aldosterone-producing adenoma)	副腎皮質腺腫、アルドステロン産生腫瘍
apallic syndrome	失外套症候群
apathy	感情鈍麻
APB(abductor pollicis brevis muscle)	短母指外転筋
APB(atrial premature beat)	心房性期外収縮＝PAC
APBD(anomalous arrangement of pancreaticobiliary ducts)	膵管胆道合流異常
APC(atrial premature contraction)	心房性期外収縮＝PAC
APCD(adult polycystic disease)	成人型多嚢胞症
APD(anteroposterior diameter)	腹部前後径
APD(automated peritoneal dialysis)	自動腹膜灌流

AP

ape hand	猿手
apex of the lung	肺尖
APGAR score(appearance-pulse-grimace-activity-respiration score)	アプガー・スコア
APH(anterior pituitary hormone)	下垂体前葉ホルモン
APH(aphasia)	失語症
APH(apical hypertrophy)	心尖部肥大型心筋症
aphasia	失語症＝APH
APKD(adult-onset polycystic kidney disease)	成人発症型多嚢胞腎
APL(abductor pollicis longus muscle)	長母指外転筋
APL(acute promyelocytic leukemia)	急性前骨髄性白血病
aplastic anemia	再生不良性貧血＝Aplas
APMPPE(acute posterior multifocal placoid pigment epitheliopathy)	急性後極部多発性鱗状網膜色素上皮症
APN(acute pyelonephritis)	急性腎盂腎炎　◀関連▶慢性腎盂腎炎：CPN、CP
apnea	無呼吸
apneic breathing	無呼吸
Apo(apoplexia cerebri)	脳卒中
apophyseal joint	椎間関節
app(appendicitis)	虫垂炎
appetite	食欲
APR(abdominoperineal resection)	腹会陰式直腸切除術
APR(auropalpebral reflex)	耳性眼瞼反射
AProL(acute promyelocytic leukemia)	急性前骨髄性白血病＝APL
APRV(airway pressure release ventilation)	気道圧開放換気
APS(antiphospholipid syndrome)	抗リン脂質抗体症候群
APS(atrial premature systole)	心房性早期収縮
APSD(aorticopulmonary septal defect)	大動脈肺動脈中隔欠損症
APSGN(acute poststreptococcal glomerulonephritis)	急性溶連菌感染後糸球体腎炎
APTT(activated partial thromboplastin time)	活性化部分トロンボプラスチン時間

AP

APVC (anomalous pulmonary venous connection)	肺静脈還流異常
APW (aortic pulmonary window)	大動脈肺動脈中隔欠損
aq. (aqua)	水
AR (allergic rhinitis)	アレルギー性鼻炎
AR (anterior resection)	前方切除術
AR (aortic regurgitation)	大動脈弁閉鎖不全症
AR (assisted respiration)	補助呼吸法
AR (atrophic rhinitis)	萎縮性鼻炎
AR (autosomal recessive inheritance)	常染色体劣性遺伝
arachnoid cyst	クモ膜嚢腫
arachnoid membrane	クモ膜
ARC (AIDS related complex)	エイズ関連症候群
ARC (automatic recruitment control)	自動明聴調節
arch support	足底挿板
ARD (acute respiratory disease)	急性呼吸器疾患 ◀関連▶慢性呼吸器疾患：CRD
ARDS (adult respiratory distress syndrome)	成人呼吸窮迫症候群
ARE (active resistance exercise)	能動抵抗運動
ARF (acute renal failure)	急性腎不全 ◀関連▶慢性腎不全：CRF
ARF (acute respiratory failure)	急性呼吸不全 ◀関連▶慢性呼吸不全：CRF
ARF (acute rheumatic fever)	急性リウマチ熱
arm span	指端距離
ARM (artificial rupture of membrane)	人工破膜
ARMD (age-related macular degeneration)	加齢性黄斑変性
ARN (acute retinal necrosis)	急性網膜壊死
ARPKD (autosomal recessive polycystic kidney disease)	常染色体劣性多発性嚢胞腎
arrhythmia	不整脈 参照 VT：心室性頻拍 Vf：心室細動

ARS (acute radiation syndrome)	急性放射線症候群
arthralgia	関節痛
arthritis	関節炎
arthrodesis	関節固定術
arthrography	関節造影
arthroplasty	関節形成術
arthroscopy	関節鏡検査
arthrosis deformans	変形性関節症
articular cartilage	関節軟骨
artificial	人工の
artificial feeding	人工栄養
artificial insemination	人工授精
artificial pacemaker	人工ペースメーカー
ARZ (Achilles sehnenreflexzeit)	アキレス腱反射時間
AS (ankylosing spondylitis)	強直性脊椎炎
AS (aortic stenosis)	大動脈弁狭窄症
AS (arteriosclerosis)	動脈硬化症
As (astigmatism)	乱視
	◀対▶ 正(常)視：emmetropia
AS (auris sinistra／left ear)	左耳　◀対▶ 右耳：AD
ASB (assisted spontaneous breathing)	自発呼吸補助換気
ASC (arteria subclavia)	鎖骨下動脈
ASC (asymptomatic carrier)	無症候性キャリア
ascites	腹水
ASCVD (arteriosclerotic cardiovascular disease)	動脈硬化性心血管疾患
ASD (academic skills disorders)	学習能力障害
ASD (acute stress disorder)	急性ストレス障害
ASD (Alzheimer senile dementia)	アルツハイマー型老年痴呆
ASD (atrial septal defect)	心房中隔欠損症
ASDH (acute subdural hematoma)	急性硬膜下血腫
	◀関連▶ 慢性硬膜下血腫：CSH、CSDH
aseptic meningitis	無菌性髄膜炎
aseptic necrosis	無菌性壊死

AS

ASF (anterior spinal fusion)	脊髄前方固定
ASH (ankylosing spinal hyperostosis)	強直性脊椎骨増殖症
ASH (asymmetric septal hypertrophy)	非対称性心室中隔肥大
ASHD (arteriosclerotic heart disease)	動脈硬化性心疾患
ASI (aortic steno-insufficiency)	大動脈弁狭窄および閉鎖不全症
ASIS (anterior superior iliac spine)	上前腸骨棘＝ASS
ASK (antistreptokinase)	抗ストレプトキナーゼ
ASLE (acute systemic lupus erythematosus)	急性全身性エリテマトーデス
ASLO (antistreptolysin)	アスロー
ASM (atrial systolic murmur)	心房収縮期雑音
ASN (arteriosclerotic nephritis)	動脈硬化性腎炎
ASO (arteriosclerosis obliterans)	閉塞性動脈硬化症
Aspergillus	アスペルギルス
asplenia syndrome	無脾症候群
ASR (achilles-sehnen reflex)	アキレス腱反射
ASR (aortic stenosis & regurgitation)	大動脈弁狭窄および閉鎖不全症
ASS (anterior superior iliac spine)	上前腸骨棘＝ASIS
AST (aspartase aminotransferase)	アスパラギン酸アミノトランスフェラーゼ＝GOT
AST (astrocytoma)	星細胞腫
Asth (asthenopia)	眼精疲労
asthmatic breathing	喘息性呼吸音
asthmatic bronchitis	喘息様気管支炎
asymptomatic bacteriuria	無症候性細菌尿
asymptomatic hematuria	無症候性血尿
asymptomatic proteinuria	無症候性蛋白尿
AT (acoustic tumor)	聴神経腫瘍
AT (activity therapy)	活動療法
AT (aortic triangle)	大動脈三角
AT (art therapy)	芸術療法
AT (arterial thrombosis)	動脈血栓症

AT(ataxia telangiectasia)	毛細血管拡張性運動失調
AT(atypical transformation zone)	異型移行形
AT(autogenous training)	自律訓練
AT(doxorubicin, taxotere)	ドキソルビシン、タキソテール併用療法
A&T(adenoidectomy and tonsillectomy)	アデノイド切除・扁桃摘出術
AT-Ⅲ(antithrombin Ⅲ)	アンチトロンビンⅢ
ataxia	運動失調
ataxic breathing	失調性呼吸
ATD(Alzheimer type dementia)	アルツハイマー型認知症
atelectasis	無気肺
ATG(antithymocyte globulin)	抗胸腺細胞グロブリン
ATH(abdominal total hysterectomy)	腹式子宮単純全摘術
athetoid syndrome	アテトーゼ症候群
ATL(adult T-cell leukemia)	成人T細胞白血病
ATL(adult T-cell lymphoma)	成人T細胞リンパ腫
ATL(anterior tricuspid leaflet)	三尖弁前尖
ATLA(adult T cell leukemia antigen)	成人T細胞白血病関連抗原
atlantoaxial joint	環軸関節
atlantoaxial subluxation	環軸関節亜脱臼
ATLL(adult T-cell leukemia lymphoma)	成人T細胞白血病(リンパ腫)
ATLV(adult T cell leukemia virus)	成人T細胞白血病ウイルス
ATM(acute transverse myelopathy)	急性横断性ミエロパチー
ATN(acute tubular necrosis)	急性尿細管壊死
ATN(acute tubulointerstitial nephritis)	急性尿細管間質性腎炎
ATNR(asymmetrical tonic neck reflex)	非対称性緊張性頚反射
ATP(adenosine triphosphate)	アデノシン三リン酸
ATP(atypical epithelium)	異型上皮
ATP(atypical psychosis)	非定型精神病
ATP (autoimmune thrombocytopenic purpura)	自己免疫性血小板減少性紫斑病
ATR(Achilles tendon reflex)	アキレス腱反射
Atr(atrophic changes)	萎縮
atrophy	萎縮、無栄養症

・AT

ATS(abdominal traumatic score)	腹部外傷スコア
ATS(antitetanic serum)	抗破傷風血清
attitude	態度
auditory hallucination	幻聴
auditory N	聴神経
AUL(acute unclassified leukemia)	急性非分類型白血病
Aus(Auskratzung)	人工妊娠中絶(搔爬術)
auscultation	聴診
autism	自閉症
auto(autologous)	自己(自家)
auto-BMT(autologous bone marrow transplantation)	自家骨髄移植＝ABMT
auto-PBSCT(autologous peripheral blood stem cell transplantation)	自家末梢血幹細胞移植＝ABSCT
auto-SCT(autologous stem cell transplantation)	自家造血幹細胞移植
AV(aortic valve)	大動脈弁＝AoV
AV(atrioventricular)	房室
aV(atypical vessel)	異型血管
A-V(arteriovenous)	動静脈の
A-V(azygos vein)	奇静脈
AVA(arteriovenous anastomosis)	動静脈吻合
AVB(atrioventricular block)	房室ブロック、A-V block
AVC(automatic volume control)	自動音量調節
AVCD(atrioventricular canal defect)	房室管孔欠損
AVD(aortic valve disease)	大動脈弁疾患
AVF(arterio-venous fistula)	動静脈瘻
AVH(acute viral hepatitis)	急性ウイルス性肝炎
AVIP(adriamycin, vincristine, iphosphamide, prednisolone)	アドリアマイシン、ビンクリスチン、イホスファミド、プレドニゾロン併用療法
AVM(arteriovenous malformation)	動静脈奇形
AVN(atrioventricular node)	房室結節
AV node(atrioventricular node)	房室結節

avoidant personality disorder	回避性人格障害
AVP(aortic valvuloplasty)	大動脈弁形成術
AVR(aortic valve replacement)	大動脈弁置換術
AVRT(atrioventricular reentrant tachycardia)	房室回帰性頻拍
avulsion fracture	裂離骨折
AVV(atrioventricular valve)	房室弁　参照 僧帽弁：MV　三尖弁：TV
AW(＋),(－)(anal wedge ＋, －)	肉眼的肛門側断端癌浸潤の有無
AW(airway)	気道、エアウェイ
awake	覚醒している
AWO(airway obstruction)	気道閉塞
azotemia	高窒素血症

B

B(blood)	血液
B(bronchiole)	細気管支
B-Ⅰ(Billroth Ⅰ)	ビルロートⅠ法
B-Ⅱ(Billroth Ⅱ)	ビルロートⅡ法
BA top(basilar top aneurysm)	脳底動脈頂点動脈瘤
Ba(barium)	バリウム
BA(basilar artery)	脳底動脈
BA(biliary atresia)	胆道閉鎖(症)
BA(bone age)	骨年齢
BA(brachial artery)	上腕動脈
BA(bronchial asthma)	気管支喘息
BAC(basal acid concentration)	基礎分泌最高酸濃度
BAC(blood alcohol concentration)	血中アルコール濃度＝BAL
bacterial meningitis	細菌性髄膜炎
bacteriuria	細菌尿
BAE(bronchial artery embolism)	気管支動脈閉塞症
BAE(bronchial artery embolization)	気管支動脈塞栓術
BAG(bronchial arteriography)	気管支動脈造影
BAI(bronchial artery infusion)	気管支動脈注入
BAL(blood alcohol concentration)	血中アルコール濃度＝BAC
BAL(bronchoalveolar lavage)	気管支肺胞洗浄
balance traction	つりあい牽引
Balint syndrome	バリント症候群
BALL(B-cell acute lymphoblastic leukemia)	B細胞急性リンパ芽球性白血病
ballottement of patella	膝蓋跳動
balneotherapy	温泉療法
BALT(bronchus-associated lymphoid tissue)	気管支関連リンパ組織
BAO(basal acid output)	基礎酸分泌量
Bartter's syndrome	バーター症候群
BAS(balloon atrioseptostomy)	バルーン心房中隔裂開術

Bas(basophil)	好塩基球
	参照 好中球：Neutro
	好酸球：Eo, Eos
Basedow disease	バセドウ病
BB(bed bath)	床上浴
BB(beta blocker)	β遮断薬
BB(breast biopsy)	乳房生検
BB(buffer base)	緩衝塩基
BBB(blood brain barrier)	血液脳関門
BBB(bundle branch block)	脚ブロック
	参照 右脚ブロック：RBBB
	左脚ブロック：LBBB
BBBB(bilateral bundle branch block)	両脚ブロック
BBD(benign breast disease)	良性乳房疾患
B bile(gallbladder bile)	胆嚢胆汁
BBO(broncho bronchiolitis obliterans)	閉塞性気管支細気管支炎
BBT(basal body temperature)	基礎体温曲線
BC(biliary colic)	胆石仙痛
BC(blastic crisis)	急性転化
BC(blood culture)	血液培養＝BLC
BC(bone conduction)	骨導
BC(bronchial carcinoma)	気管支癌
BCAA(branched-chain amino acid)	分枝鎖アミノ酸
BCC(basal cell carcinoma)	基底細胞癌
BCD(bleomycin, cyclophosphamide, actinomycin-D)	ブレオマイシン、シクロホスファミド、アクチノマイシンD併用療法
BCE(basal cell epithelioma)	基底細胞上皮腫
BCECT(benign childhood epilepsy with centro temporal spike)	中心・側頭部に棘波を伴う良性小児てんかん
B-cell(bone marrow derived cell)	骨髄由来細胞
B-CLL (B cell chronic lymphocytic leukemia)	B細胞慢性リンパ性白血病

BC

BCLS(basic cardiac life support)	一次循環救命処置
	参照 **ACLS**:二次循環救命処置
BCO(blood carbon monoxide)	血液一酸化炭素
BCO2(blood carbon dioxide)	血液二酸化炭素
BCP(birth control pill)	経口避妊薬＝OC
BCPP(BCNU, cyclophosphamide, naturan, prednisolone)	BCNU、シクロホスファミド、ナツラン、プレドニゾロン併用療法
BCS(battered child syndrome)	被虐待児症候群
BCU(burn care unit)	熱傷集中治療室
BD(base deficit)	塩基欠乏
BD(behavior disorder)	行動異常
BD(brain death)	脳死
BD(bronchodilator)	気管支拡張薬
b.d.(bis die)	１日２回
	参照 １日３回：t.i.d.
	１日４回：q.i.d.
BDAE (Boston diagnostic aphasia examination)	ボストン失語診断検査
BDH(bullous dermatosis of hemodialysis)	血液透析性水疱症
BDR(Bauchdecken reflex)	腹壁反射
BE amp(below-elbow amputation)	前腕切断
BE(bacterial endocarditis)	細菌性心内膜炎
BE(barium enema)	バリウム注腸検査
BE(base excess)	塩基過剰
BE(bronchiectasis)	気管支拡張症
BEAR(brainstem evoked auditory response)	聴性脳幹反応
Beck depression inventory	ベック法
bedsore	褥瘡
BEE(basal energy expenditure)	基礎エネルギー消費量
Behcet's disease	ベーチェット病
behavior	ふるまい
behavioral therapy	行動療法
BEL(Beckenendlage)	骨盤位

belch	げっぷ
Bell's palsy	ベル麻痺
Bender-Gestalt test	ベンダー・ゲシュタルト法
bends	潜函病＝caisson disease
BENP(bleomycin, endoxan, 6-MP, prednin)	ブレオマイシン、エンドキサン、6−MP、プレドニン併用療法
Benton visual retention test	ベントン視覚記銘力検査
BEP(cisplatin, etoposide, bleomycin)	シスプラチン、エトポシド、ブレオマイシン併用療法
BER(brain stem evoked response)	(聴性)脳幹反応
BET(benign〔auditory〕epithelial tumor)	良性上皮腫瘍
BFHR(basal fetal heart rate)	基礎胎児心拍数
BFO(balanced forearm orthosis)	肩関節動的装具
BFP(R)(biological false positive〔reaction〕)	生物学的偽陽性(反応)
BFS(bronchofiberscope)	気管支ファイバースコープ
BG(bronchography)	気管支造影
BGA(blood gas analysis)	血液ガス分析
BGTT(borderline glucose tolerance test)	境界型ブドウ糖負荷試験
BHL(bilateral hilar lymphadenitis)	両側肺門リンパ節腫脹
BI(biischial diameter)	骨盤出口横径
BI(burn index)	熱傷指数
bicycle ergometer	自転車エルゴメーター
big(bigemini)	二段脈 参照 三段脈：trigeminal pulse
BIH(benign intracranial hypertension)	良性頭蓋内圧亢進
Bil(bilateral)	両側＝bil
Bile-duct drainage	胆管ドレナージ
bilirubinuria	ビリルビン尿
Binet-Simon scale	ビネー・シモン法
biopsy	生検
BIP(bleomycin, ifosfamide, cisplatin)	ブレオマイシン、イホスファミド、シスプラチン併用療法

BI

BIP(bronchiolar interstitial pneumonia)	細気管支性間質性肺炎
BiPAP(bi-levels of positive airway pressures)	バイパップ、二相性陽圧呼吸
bipolar endoprothesis	双極機能体内プロステーシス
birth asphyxia	出生時仮死
birth injury	出生時外傷
birth palsy	分娩麻痺
birthmark	母斑
Bishop's pelvic score	ビショップ・スコア
BJ(biceps jerk)	上腕二頭筋反射
B&J(bone and joint)	骨と関節
BJP(Bence Jones protein)	ベンス・ジョーンズ蛋白
BJP(Bence Jones proteinuria)	ベンス・ジョーンズ蛋白尿
BK amp(below-knee amputation)	下腿切断
BK(below knee)	膝下（下腿）
BL(bronchial lavage)	気管支洗浄＝TBL
blackout	意識喪失
bladder	膀胱
bladder stone	膀胱結石
BLC(blood culture)	血液培養＝BC
bleeder's disease	血友病
blepharoptosis	眼瞼下垂
blind loop syndrome	ブラインドループ症候群
blister	水疱、疱疹、水ぶくれ
blood clot	血栓、凝血
blood gas	血液ガス
bloody expectoration	喀血
bloody sputum	血痰
bloody stool	血便
BLS(basic life support)	一次救命処置
	参照 二次救命処置：ALS
BM(basal medium)	基礎培地
Bm(betamethasone)	ベタメサゾン
BM(bone marrow)	骨髄
BM(bowel movement)	排便、便通

Bo

BMD (Becker type progressive muscular dystrophy)	ベッカー型進行性筋ジストロフィー
BMG(benign monoclonal gammopathy)	良性単クローン性免疫グロブリン症
BME(biomedical engineering)	医用生体工学
BMI(body mass index)	肥満指数
BMM(bone marrow metastasis)	骨髄転移
BMR(basal metabolic rate)	基礎代謝率
BMT(bone marrow transplantation)	骨髄移植
BNB(blood-nerve barrier)	血液神経関門
BNC(bladder neck contracture)	膀胱頚部狭窄症
BO(bronchiolitis obliterans)	閉塞性細気管支炎
BOAI(balloon-occluded arterial infusion)	バルーン閉塞下動注法
BOD(biochemical oxygen demand)	生物(化)学的酸素要求量
BOHA(balloon-occluded hepatic arteriography)	バルーンカテーテル閉塞下肝動脈造影
BOMP(bleomycin, vincristine, mitomycin-C, cisplatin)	ブレオマイシン、ビンクリスチン、マイトマイシンC、シスプラチン併用療法
bone age	骨年齢
bone graft	骨移植
bone union	骨癒合
BONP(bleomycin, oncovin, naturan, prednisolone)	ブレオマイシン、オンコビン、ナツラン、プレドニゾロン併用療法
bony ankylosis	骨性強直
BOOP(bronchiolitis obliterans-organizing pneumonia)	閉塞性細気管支炎器質化肺炎
BOPA(balloon-occluded pulmonary angiography)	バルーンカテーテル閉塞下肺血管造影
BOR(bowel open regular)	便通正常
borderline case	境界例
Borr Ⅰ~Ⅳ(Borrmann classification)	ボールマンの胃癌分類

bo

bowleg	O脚
	関連 X脚：knock-knee
Bowman's capsule	ボウマン嚢
Bp(blood pressure)	血圧
BP(Bell palsy)	ベル麻痺
BP(blastic phase)	急性期
BP(blood pressure)	血圧
BP(bullous pemphigoid)	水疱性類天疱瘡
BPD(biparietal diameter)	(児頭)大横径
BPD(borderline personality disorder)	境界性人格障害
BPD(broncho pulmonary dysplasia)	気管支肺異形成
BPH(benign prostatic hyperplasia)	前立腺肥大症
BPM, bpm(beats per minute)	毎分心拍数
BPM, bpm(breaths per minute)	毎分呼吸数
BPN(brachial plexus neuropathy)	上腕神経叢神経症
BPO(base pepsin output)	基礎ペプシン分泌量
BPPV(benign paroxysmal positional vertigo)	良性発作性体位性眩暈
BR(bed rest)	床上安静
	関連 絶対床上安静：CBR
br(breath)	呼吸
BR(breathing reserve)	換気予備量
br(bronchus)	気管支
BRA(brain metastasis)	脳転移
BrA(bronchial artery)	気管支動脈
brachial plexus palsy	腕神経叢麻痺
brady	緩徐、徐脈
bradycardia	徐脈
	対 頻脈：tachycardia
bradypnea	呼吸緩徐
brain	脳
BRD(benign respiratory distress)	良性呼吸窮迫症
breast feeding	母乳栄養
breast preserving procedure	乳房温存法
breast reconstruction	乳房再建

breath holding spells	ひきつけ啼泣
breathing difficulty	呼吸不全, 呼吸困難
Breech (breech delivery)	骨盤位分娩
Bright's disease	糸球体腎炎
BRO (bronchoscopy)	気管支鏡検査
Broca's aphasia	運動性失語
bromism	ブローム中毒
bronchial breathing	気管支呼吸音
bronchiectasis	気管支拡張症
bronchitis	気管支炎
bronchography	気管支造影
bronchoplasty	気管支形成術
bronchopleural fistula	気管支瘻
BRP (bathroom privileges)	入浴(トイレ)歩行可
bruise	打撲傷
BRVO (branch retinal vein occlusion)	網膜静脈分枝閉塞症
BS (blood serum)	血清＝S
BS (blood sugar)	血糖＝BG
BS (bowel sound)	腸雑音
BS (breath sound)	呼吸音
BSA (body surface area)	体表面積
BSA (burn surface area)	熱傷面積
BSB (body surface burned)	体表熱傷
BSE (bovine spongiform encephalopathies)	牛海綿状脳症(狂牛病)
BSE (breast self-examination)	乳房自己検診
BSO (bilateral salpingo-oophorectomy)	両側卵管卵巣摘出術
BSP test (bromsulphalein test)	ブロムサルファレイン試験
BSV (basal secretion volume)	基礎分泌量
BT (balloon tube)	膀胱留置カテーテル
BT (behavior therapy)	行動療法
BT (bladder tumor)	膀胱腫瘍
BT (bleeding time)	出血時間
BT (blood transfusion)	輸血＝BTF
BT (blood type)	血液型

BT

BT(body temperature)	体温
BT(brain tumor)	脳腫瘍
BT(breast tumor)	乳房腫瘍
BT(bronchial toilet)	気管支洗浄
BTF(blood transfusion)	輸血＝BT
BTL(bilateral tubal ligation)	両卵管結紮術
BTP(brain tissue pressure)	脳組織圧
BTR(biceps tendon reflex)	二頭筋腱反射
BTS(bradycardia-tachycardia syndrome)	徐頻脈症候群
B-T shunt(Blalock-Taussig shunt)	ブラロック・タウシッヒ短絡術
bU(benign ulcer)	良性潰瘍
bubbling rale	水泡音
	参照 乾性ラ音：dry rale
	湿性ラ音：moist rale
	捻髪音：crepitant rale
buffalo hump	水牛様脂肪沈着
bulimia	食欲亢進、過食症
bulimia nervosa	神経性過食症
bull's eye	ブルズアイ表示、同心円表示
bulla	水疱
BUN(blood urea nitrogen)	血液尿素窒素
BUO(bleeding of undetermined origin)	部位不明出血
burn	熱傷
bursa	滑液包
bursitis	滑液包炎
burst fracture	破裂骨折
buttonhole deformity	ボタン穴変形
BV(binocular vision)	両眼視力
BV(blood vessel)	血管
BV(blood volume)	血液量
bV(smooth branching vessels)	樹枝状血管
BVCP(bleomycin, vincristine, cyclophosphamide, prednisolone)	ブレオマイシン、ビンクリスチン、シクロホスファミド、プレドニゾロン併用療法

BVH(biventricular hypertrophy)	両室肥大
BW(Brustwirbel)	胸椎
BW(birth weight)	出生時体重
BWG(Bland White Garland syndrome)	ブランド・ホワイト・ガーランド症候群
BWS syndrome (Beckwith-Wiedemann syndrome)	ベックウィズ・ウィーデマン症候群
Bx(biopsy)	生検

C

c(capillary blood)	毛細血管
C(cardia of stomach)	噴門部
C(cecum)	盲腸
C(cervical)	頚椎の、頚髄の
C(cervical spine)	頚椎
C(columnar epithelium)	円柱上皮
C(complement)	補体
C(costa)	肋骨
C(upper third)	胃上部
C/kcal(calorie)	カロリー
C領域	噴門部領域(胃上部1／3)
C1〜7(1〜7 cervical vertebra)	第1〜7頚椎
Ca(calcium)	カルシウム
CA(carcinoma, cancer)	癌腫
CA(cardiac arrest)	心停止
CA(cardiac arrhythmia)	不整脈
CA(catecholamine)	カテコールアミン
CA(celiac artery)	腹腔動脈
CA(chorea acanthocytosis)	舞踏病−有棘赤血球症
CA(chronological age)	歴年齢
CA(coarctation of the aorta)	大動脈縮窄症
CA(coronary artery)	冠動脈
	◀関連▶ 右冠状動脈：RCA
	左冠状動脈：LCA
	左回旋枝：LCX
CA(cystic artery)	胆嚢動脈
Ca-P(carcinoma of prostate)	前立腺癌
ca.(cancer)	癌
CA19-9(carbohydrate antigen 19-9)	糖鎖抗原19-9
CAB(coronary artery bypass)	冠動脈バイパス
CABB(complete atrioventricular block)	完全房室ブロック＝CHB
CABG(coronary artery bypass grafting)	冠動脈バイパス術

CABS (coronary artery bypass surgery)	冠動脈バイパス手術
CAD (chronic actinic dermatitis)	慢性光線皮膚炎
CAD (computer assisted diagnosis)	コンピュータ（補助）診断システム
CAD (congenital alveolar dysplasia)	先天性肺胞異形成
CAD (coronary artery disease)	冠動脈疾患 **参照** 狭心症：AP, AG 　　　心筋梗塞：MI
cadaveric kidney	死体腎
CAE (cyclophosphamide, adriamycin, cisplatin)	シクロホスファミド、アドリアマイシン、シスプラチン併用療法
CAF (cyclophosphamide, adriamycin, 5-FU)	シクロホスファミド、アドリアマイシン、フルオロウラシル併用療法
CAG (cardioangiography)	心血管造影法
CAG (carotid angiography)	頸動脈造影法
CAG (cerebral angiography)	脳血管造影法
CAG (chronic atrophic gastritis)	慢性萎縮性胃炎
CAG (coronary angiography)	冠動脈造影法
CAGS (congenital adrenogenital syndrome)	先天性副腎性器症候群
CAH (chronic active hepatitis)	慢性活動性肝炎
CAH (congenital adrenal hyperplasia)	先天性副腎過形成
CAHD (coronary arteriosclerotic heart disease)	冠動脈硬化性心疾患
caisson disease	潜函病＝bends
CAL (coracoacromial ligament)	烏口肩峰靭帯
calcification	石灰化
calcinosis	石灰沈着
calcitonin	カルシトニン
calcium antagonist	カルシウム拮抗薬
calculus	結石
CALD (chronic active liver disease)	慢性活動性肝疾患
calf cramps	こむら返り

CA

CALL (common acute lymphocytic leukemia)	共通性急性リンパ球性白血病
callosity	皮膚肥厚
calyx	腎杯
CAM(cell adhesion molecule)	細胞接着分子
CAM(chorioamnionitis)	絨毛羊膜炎
CAM (complementary and alternative medicine)	代替補完医療
cAMP(cyclic adenosine monophosphate)	サイクリックAMP
CAO(chronic airway obstruction)	慢性気道閉塞
CAO(chronic arterial obstruction)	慢性動脈閉塞
CAO(coronary artery obstruction)	冠動脈閉塞
CAOD(coronary artery occlusive disease)	冠動脈閉塞性疾患
Cap	カプセル
CAP(central arterial pressure)	中心動脈圧 対 中心静脈圧:CVP
CAP(chronic alcoholic pancreatitis)	慢性アルコール性膵炎
CAP (cyclophosphamide, adriamycin, cisplatin)	シクロホスファミド、アドリアマイシン、シスプラチン併用療法
CAP (cyclophosphamide, doxorubicin, cisplatin)	シクロホスファミド、ドキソルビシン、シスプラチン併用療法
CAPD (continuous ambulatory peritoneal dialysis)	持続式携帯腹膜透析
CAPRCA (chronic acquired pure red cell aplasia)	慢性後天性真性赤血球系無形成症
caput succedaneum	産瘤
Car, CAP(carotid pulse wave〔pulse〕)	頸動脈波
cardiotonic	強心剤=cardiotonicum
carina	気管分岐部
carpal joint	手関節
carpal tunnel	手根管
carrying angle	肘外偏角
cast	円柱、ギプス包帯
cast syndrome	ギプス症候群

castration anxiety	去勢不安
casual blood pressure	座位随時血圧値
Cat(cataract)	白内障
	◀関連▶緑内障：GL, Gla
CAT(cellular atypia)	細胞異型度
CAT(children's apperception test)	小児統覚テスト
catalepsy	強直症
catatonic excitement	緊張病興奮
catatonic syndrome	緊張症候群
catatonic type	緊張型(統合失調症)
catheter ablation	心筋焼灼術
Cattel anxiety scale	キャテル不安検査
cauda equina	馬尾
caudal block	仙骨ブロック
CAV(cyclophosphamide, adriamycin, vincristine)	シクロホスファミド、アドリアマイシン、ビンクリスチン併用療法
CAVC(common arterioventricular canal)	共通房室弁口
CAVH (continuos arterio-venous hemofiltration)	持続的動静脈血液濾過法
cavity	空洞
CB(chronic bronchitis)	慢性気管支炎
CB(ciliary body)	毛様体
CB(croupous bronchitis)	クループ性気管支炎
CBA(congenital biliary atresia)	先天性胆道閉鎖症
CBC(complete blood count)	全血球計算
CBD(common bile duct)	総胆管
CBD(congenital biliary dilatation)	先天性胆道拡張症
CBDC (chronic bullous dermatosis of childhood)	小児慢性水疱症
CBDS(common bile duct stone)	総胆管結石
CBE(chronic bacterial endocarditis)	慢性感染性心内膜炎
CBF(cerebral blood flow)	脳血流量
CBF(coronary blood flow)	冠動脈血流量

Cb

C bile(hepatic bile)	肝内胆汁
CBP(chronic bacterial prostatitis)	慢性細菌性前立腺炎
CBR(complete bed rest)	絶対床上安静
CBS(chronic bed rest)	長期床上安静
CBS(chronic brain syndrome)	慢性脳症候群
CBSCT (cord blood stem cell transplantation)	臍帯血幹細胞移植
CBT(cognitive behavioral therapy)	認知行動療法
CBV(cerebral blood volume)	脳血液量
CBV(circulating blood volume)	循環血液量
CBV(cisplatin, bleomycin, vincristine)	シスプラチン、ブレオマイシン、ビンクリスチン併用療法
CC(cancer of the cervix)	子宮頚癌
CC(cardiac catheterization)	心臓カテーテル法
CC(chief complaint)	主訴
CC(cholangiocarcinoma)	胆管癌
CC(choriocarcinoma)	絨毛癌
CC(clinical conference)	臨床検討会
CC(common cold)	感冒
CC(corpus callosum)	脳梁
CC(critical condition)	危篤状態
Cca(colon carcinoma)	結腸癌
CCA(common carotid artery)	総頚動脈
CCC(cholangiocellular carcinoma)	胆管細胞癌
CCC(chronic calculous cholecystitis)	慢性有結石胆嚢炎
CCCC(closed chest cardiac compression)	非開胸心マッサージ＝CCM
CCF(carotid-cavernous fistula)	頚動脈－海綿静脈洞瘻
CCF(congenital club foot)	先天性内反足
CCF(congestive cardiac failure)	うっ血性心不全
C-C fistula(carotid cavernous fistula)	頚動脈海綿静脈洞瘻＝CCF
CCHD(cyanotic congenital heart disease)	チアノーゼ性先天性心疾患
CCI(chronic coronary insufficiency)	慢性冠動脈不全
CCI(craniocerebral injuries)	外傷性脳障害

CCK-PZ(cholecystokinin-pancreozymin)	コレシストキニン・パンクレオザイミン
CCLE (chronic cutaneous lupus erythematosus)	慢性皮膚エリテマトーデス
CCM(closed chest cardiac compression)	非開胸心マッサージ＝CCCC
CCM(congestive cardiomyopathy)	うっ血型心筋症＝COCM
CCM(critical care medicine)	重症管理医学／集中治療医学
CCMPADRI-V(cyclophosphamide, vincristine, methotrexate, melphalan)	シクロホスファミド、ビンクリスチン、メトトレキサート、メルファラン併用療法
CCP(chronic cor pulmonale)	慢性肺性心
CCP(critical closing pressure)	臨界閉鎖圧
CCPD(continuous cyclic peritoneal dialysis)	持続的循環式腹膜透析
CCPP(cyclophosphamide, vincristine, procarbazine, prednisolone)	シクロホスファミド、ビンクリスチン、プロカルバジン、プレドニゾロン併用療法＝C-MOPP
CCPR (cerebro cardio pulmonary resuscitation)	心肺脳蘇生法＝CPCR ◀関連▶心肺蘇生法：CPR
Ccr(creatinine clearance)	クレアチニン・クリアランス
CCSK(clear cell sarcoma of the kidney)	腎明細胞肉腫
CCU(coronary care unit)	冠疾患集中治療室
CCU(critical care unit)	緊急集中治療室
CCVD(chronic cerebrovascular disease)	慢性脳血管疾患
CD(Cesarean delivery)	帝王切開による出産
CD(character disorder)	性格障害
CD(choroidal detachment)	脈絡膜剥離
CD(cluster of differentiation)	白血球分類
CD(collagen disease)	膠原病
CD(contact dermatitis)	接触皮膚炎
CD(convulsive disorder)	痙攣性疾患
CD(Crohn's disease)	クローン病
CDA(congenital dyserythropoietic anemia)	先天性赤血球産生異常性貧血

CD

CDAI(Crohn disease active index)	クローン病活動指数
CDC(calculated date of confinement)	分娩予定日
CDH(cervical disc herniation)	頚椎椎間板ヘルニア
CDH(congenital diaphragmatic hernia)	先天性横隔膜ヘルニア
CDH(congenital dislocation of hip)	先天性股関節脱臼
CDI(central diabetes insipidus)	中枢性尿崩症
CDI(childhood depression inventory)	小児うつ病特性尺度
CDLE(chronic discoid lupus erythematosus)	慢性円板状エリテマトーデス
CDR(clinical dementia rating)	臨床痴呆評価尺度
CDS(cervical dry smear)	子宮頚管乾燥スミア
CDV(cisplatin, dacarbazine, vindesine)	シスプラチン、ダカルバジン、ビンデシン併用療法
CDW(compulsive water drinking)	心因性多飲症
CE(centrilobular emphysema)	小葉中心性肺気腫
CE(cerebral embolism)	脳閉塞症
Ce(cervical esophagus)	頚部食道
CEA(carcinoembryonic antigen)	癌胎児性抗原
central hyperventilation	中枢性過呼吸
central obesity	中心性肥満
CEP(cerebral evoked potential)	大脳誘発電位
CEP(congenital erythropoietic porphyria)	先天性骨髄性ポルフィリン症
cephalo-hematoma	頭血腫
CEPP(cyclophosphamide, etoposide, procarbazine, prednisolone)	シクロホスファミド、エトポシド、プロカルバジン、プレドニゾロン併用療法
cerebellar astrocytoma	小脳星細胞腫
cerebellum	小脳
cerebral hemisphere	大脳半球
cerebrum	大脳
cervical myelopathy	頚髄症
CES(central excitatory state)	中枢興奮状態
CET(controlled environment treatment)	調節環境治療法
CF(cardiac failure)	心不全

CF(cisplatin, fluorouracil)	シスプラチン、フルオロウラシル併用療法
CF(complement fixation)	補体結合反応
CF(cystic fibrosis)	嚢胞性線維症
CF, CFS(colonofiberscope)	大腸ファイバースコープ
CFIDS(chronic fatigue and immune dysfunction syndrome)	慢性疲労免疫異常症候群
CFR(complement fixation reaction)	補体結合反応
CFS(cerebrospinal fluid)	脳脊髄液
CFS(chronic fatigue syndrome)	慢性疲労症候群
CG(chronic glomerulonephritis)	慢性糸球体腎炎＝CGN ◀関連▶ 急性糸球体腎炎：AGN
CG(cystography)	膀胱造影
CGD(chronic granulomatous disease)	慢性肉芽腫症
CGD(congestive heart disease)	うっ血型心疾患
CGL(chronic granulocytic leukemia)	慢性顆粒球性白血病
CGN(chronic glomerulonephritis)	慢性糸球体腎炎＝CG
CGS(cardiogenic shock)	心原性ショック＝CS
CGTT(cortisone glucose tolerance test)	コルチゾンブドウ糖負荷試験
CH(chronic hepatitis)	慢性肝炎 ◀関連▶ 急性肝炎：AH
CHA(chronic hemolytic anemia)	慢性溶血性貧血
CHA(common hepatic artery)	総肝動脈
CHA(congenital hypoplastic anemia)	先天性再生不良性貧血
CHAI(continuous hepatic arterial infusion)	肝動脈持続動注療法
chalasia	噴門弛緩症
character	性格
CHB(chronic hepatitis B)	B型慢性肝炎
CHB(complete heart block)	完全房室ブロック
CHC(chronic hepatitis C)	C型慢性肝炎
CHCP(cyclophosphamide, doxorubicin, vincristine, prednisolone)	シクロホスファミド、ドキソルビシン、ビンクリスチン、プレドニゾロン併用療法

CH

CHD (chronic hemodialysis)	長期血液透析
CHD (common hepatic duct)	総胆管
CHD (congenital heart disease)	先天性心疾患
CHD (continuous hemodialysis)	持続血液透析
CHD (coronary heart disease)	冠動脈性心疾患
CHD (cyanotic heart disease)	チアノーゼ性心疾患
CHDF (continuous hemodiafiltration)	持続血液濾過透析
ChE (cholinesterase)	コリンエステラーゼ
CHE (chronic hepatic encephalopathy)	慢性肝性脳症
chemotherapy	化学療法
chest pain	胸痛
Cheyne-Stokes' breathing	チェーン・ストークス呼吸
CHF (chronic heart failure)	慢性心不全 ◀関連▶ 急性心不全：AHF
CHF (congenital hepatic fibrosis)	先天性肝線維症
CHF (congestive heart failure)	うっ血性心不全
CHF (continuous hemofiltration)	持続的血液濾過
chickenpox	水痘
child abuse	児童虐待
child schizophrenia	児童統合失調症
childhood experience	幼児体験
Chinese herbal medicine	漢方薬
CHMOL (chronic myelomonocytic leukemia)	慢性骨髄単球性白血病
choked disc	うっ血乳頭
cholesterol	コレステロール
chondromalacia patellae	膝蓋軟骨軟化症
CHOP (cyclophosphamide, doxorubicin, oncovin, prednisolone)	シクロホスファミド、ドキソルビシン、オンコビン、プレドニゾロン併用療法
CHOP (cyclophosphamide, adriamycin, vincristine, prednisolone)	シクロホスファミド、アドリアマイシン、ビンクリスチン、プレドニゾロン併用療法
Chopart joint	横足根関節
choreic syndrome	舞踏病症候群

chorio(chorionepithelioma)	絨毛上皮癌
CHP(cranial hypertrophic pachymeningitis)	肥大型硬髄膜炎
CHPP(continuous hyperthermic peritoneal perfusion)	持続温熱腹膜灌流
chpx(chickenpox)	水痘
chr(chronic)	慢性の
	対 急性の：acute
chromosome aberration	染色体異常
chronic alcoholism	慢性アルコール中毒
chronic nephritic syndrome	慢性腎炎症候群
chronic suppurative otitis media	慢性化膿性中耳炎
chronic thyroiditis	慢性甲状腺炎
CHRS(cerebrohepatorenal syndrome)	脳肝腎症候群
CHS(chronic hypersensitivity syndrome)	慢性過敏性症候群
chylothorax	乳糜胸
CI(cardiac index)	心係数
CI(cellular immunity)	細胞性免疫
CI(cerebral infarction)	脳梗塞
CI(color index)	色素指数
CIA(common iliac artery)	総腸骨動脈
cicatricial contracture	瘢痕拘縮
CICU(cardiac intensive care unit)	心臓集中治療室
CID(combined immunodeficiency)	複合免疫不全
CIDP(chronic inflammatory demyelinating polyneuropathy)	慢性炎症性脱髄性多発根神経炎
CIDS (cellular immunity deficiency syndrome)	細胞性免疫不全症候群
CIDS (congenital immunity deficiency syndrome)	先天性免疫不全症候群
CIH(chronic inactive hepatitis)	慢性非活動性肝炎
CIII(continuous intravenous insulin infusion)	持続静脈内インスリン注入療法
CIIP(chronic idiopathic intestinal pseudo-obstruction)	慢性特発性腸管仮性閉塞症

Cl

CIN(cervical intraepithelial neoplasia)	子宮頚部上皮内新生物
circumstantiality	迂遠
CIRPN(chronic idiopathic relapsing polyneuropathy)	慢性特発性再発性多発神経症
CIS(carcinoma in situ)	上皮内癌
CISCA(cisplatin, cyclophosphamide, adriamycin)	シスプラチン、シクロホスファミド、アドリアマイシン併用療法
cisternal puncture	大槽穿刺
CJD(Creutzfeldt-Jakob disease)	クロイツフェルト・ヤコブ病
C-J stomy(choledocho-jejunostomy)	総胆管空腸吻合
CK(Colon Krebs)	大腸癌
CK(creatine kinase)	クレアチンキナーゼ
Cl(chlorine)	塩素
CL(chronic leukemia)	慢性白血病
	◀関連▶急性白血球：AL
CL(cleft lip)	唇裂
CL(contact lens)	コンタクトレンズ
claustrophobia	閉所恐怖
claw finger	かぎ爪指
claw hand	鷲手
CLBBB(complete left bundle branch block)	完全左脚ブロック
	◀関連▶完全右脚ブロック：CRBBB
CLD(chronic liver disease)	慢性肝疾患
CLD(chronic lung disease)	慢性肺疾患
CLE(cutaneous lupus erythematosus)	皮膚エリテマトーデス
cleft palate	口蓋裂＝CP
click sign	クリック徴候
client centered psychotherapy	クライアント中心精神療法
CLL(chronic lymphocytic leukemia)	慢性リンパ性白血病
	◀関連▶急性リンパ性白病：ALL
CLN(cervical lymph node)	頚部リンパ節
closed fracture	皮下骨折

clouded consciousness	意識混濁
clouding of consciousness	意識混濁
CLP(cleft lip palate)	口唇口蓋裂
CLT(clotting time)	血液凝固時間
club foot	内反足
clubbed finger	ばち状指
CM(cardiomyopathy)	心筋症
CM(carpometacarpal)	手根中手骨の
CM(congenital malformation)	先天奇形
CM(contrast medium)	造影剤
CM(T)(cervical mucus〔test〕)	(子宮)頚管粘液(検査)
CMA(chronic metabolic acidosis)	慢性代謝性アシドーシス
CMC(carpometacarpal)	手根中手間関節＝CMJ
CMC(closed mitral commissurotomy)	非直視下僧帽弁交連切開術
CMCC(chronic mucocutaneous candidiasis)	慢性皮膚粘膜カンジダ症
CMD(congenital muscular dystrophy)	先天性筋ジストロフィー症
CME(cystoid macular edema)	嚢胞様黄斑浮腫
CMF(cyclophosphamide, methotrexate, fluorouracil)	シクロホスファミド、メソトレキセート、フルオロウラシル併用療法
CMG(cystometrography)	膀胱内圧測定
CMH(congenital malformation of heart)	先天性心臓奇形
CMI(cell-mediated immunity)	細胞性免疫
CMI(Cornell medical index)	コーネル健康調査法
CMID(cytomegalic inclusion 〔body〕 disease)	巨細胞性封入体病
CMJ(carpometacarpal joint)	手根中手間関節
CMK(congenital multicystic kidney)	先天性多嚢胞性腎
CML(chronic myelocytic leukemia)	慢性骨髄性白血病 ◀関連▶急性骨髄性白血病：AML
CMML(chronic myelomonocytic leukemia)	慢性骨髄単球性白血病＝CMMoL
CMMoL(chronic myelomonocytic leukemia)	慢性骨髄単球性白血病

CM

CMoL(chronic monocytic leukemia)	慢性単球性白血病
C-MOPP(cyclophosphamide + vincristine, procarbazine, prednisolone)	シクロホスファミド+ビンクリスチン、プロカルバジン、プレドニゾロン併用療法
CMP(chondromalacia patellae)	膝蓋軟骨軟化症
CMPD(chronic myeloproliferative disease)	慢性骨髄増殖性疾患
CMR(cerebral metabolic rate)	脳代謝率
CMR glu(cerebral metabolic rate of glucose)	脳ブドウ糖代謝率
CMRO$_2$(cerebral metabolic rate of oxygen)	脳酸素代謝率
CMS(chronic myelodysplastic syndrome)	骨髄異形成症候群=MDS
CMT(cervical mucus test)	神経性子宮頸管粘液検査
CMT(Charcot-Marie-Tooth disease)	シャルコー・マリー・ツース病
CMV(cisplatin, methotrexate, vinblastine)	シスプラチン、メソトレキセート、ビンブラスチン併用療法
CMV(continuous mandatory ventilation)	持続的強制換気
CMV(controlled mechanical ventilation)	調節機械換気
CMV(cytomegalo virus)	サイトメガロウイルス
CMV(cytomegalo virus infection)	サイトメガロウイルス感染症
CN(cranial nerve)	脳神経
CNI(olfactory nerve)	嗅神経
CNL(chronic neutrophic leukemia)	慢性好中球性白血病
CNM(congenital nonprogressive myopathy)	先天性非進行性ミオパシー
CNP(chronic nonbacterial prostatitis)	慢性非細菌性前立腺炎
CNP(continuous negative pressure)	持続陰圧呼吸
CNS(central nervous system)	中枢神経系 参照 末梢神経系:PNS 自律神経系:ANS
CNS(clinical nurse specialist)	専門看護師
CNS-leukemia(central nervous system leukemia)	中枢神経系白血病
CNSDC(chronic nonsuppurative destructive cholangitis)	慢性非化膿性破壊性胆管炎
CNSLD(chronic nonspecific lung disease)	慢性非特異的肺疾患
CNT(connecting tubule)	接合尿細管

CO (carbon monoxide)	一酸化炭素
CO (cardiac output)	心拍出量
C/O (complain of)	症状の訴え
COA, CoA (coarctation of aorta)	大動脈縮窄(症)
COAC (coarctation of aorta complex)	大動脈縮窄複合
COAD (chronic obstructive airway disease)	慢性閉塞性気道疾患
coarse rale	大水泡性ラ音
COB (chronic obstructive bronchitis)	慢性閉塞性気管支炎
COBS (chronic organic brain syndrome)	慢性器質性脳症候群
COBT (chronic obstruction of biliary tract)	慢性胆道閉塞症
cocainism	コカイン中毒
COCM (congestive cardiomyopathy)	うっ血型心筋症＝CCM
COD (cause of death)	死因
COD (chemical oxygen demand)	化学的酸素必要量
CODE (cisplatin, vincristine, adriamycin, etoposide)	シスプラチン、ビンクリスチン、アドリアマイシン、エトポシド併用療法
cognitive therapy	認知療法
coin lesion	銭形陰影
cold intolerance	寒がり
	対 暑がり：heat intolerance
cold sweat	冷汗
COLD (chronic obstructive lung disease)	慢性閉塞性肺疾患
collagen disease	膠原病
collapse therapy	虚脱療法
collecting duct	集合管
collective unconscious	集団的無意識
Colon-Ca (colon-carcinoma)	大腸癌
colostrum	初乳
coma	昏睡
comminuted fracture	粉砕骨折
COMPARDR (cyclophosphamide, vincristine, methotrexate, melphalan, doxorubicin)	シクロホスファミド、ビンクリスチン、メソトレキセート、メルファラン、ドキソルビシン併用療法

CO

complete ECD (complete endocardial cushion defect)	完全型心内膜床欠損症
compound fracture	複雑骨折
comprehension	領識
compression fracture	圧迫骨折
compulsion	強迫行為
compulsive personality disorder	強迫性人格障害
compulsive polydipsia	心因性多飲症
compulsiveness	強迫観念
Con A (concanavalin A)	コンカナバリンA
Con (condyloma)	コンジローマ
conduct disorder	行動障害
conduction deafness	伝音性難聴
conduction velocity	伝導速度
congenital	先天性の 対 後天性／獲得性の：acquired 遺伝性：genetic
congenital diaphragmatic hernia	先天性横隔膜ヘルニア
congenital dislocation	先天性脱臼
congenital esophageal atresia	先天性食道閉鎖症
congenital hypertrophic pyloric stenosis	先天性肥厚性幽門狭窄症
congenital hypothyroidism	先天性甲状腺機能低下症
congenital malformation	先天奇形
congenital nephrosis	先天性ネフローゼ
congenital toxoplasmosis	先天性トキソプラズマ症
congested papilla	うっ血乳頭
cons (consciousness)	意識
constipation	便秘 参照 下痢：diarrhea
continuous traction	持続牽引
conversion disorder	転換症
convulsion	痙攣

COP(capillary osmotic pressure)	毛細管浸透圧
COP(cyclophosphamide, oncovin, prednisolone)	シクロホスファミド、オンコビン、プレドニゾロン併用療法
COP(cyclophosphamide, vincristine, prednisolone)	シクロホスファミド、ビンクリスチン、プレドニゾロン併用療法
COP-BLAM(cyclophosphamide, adriamycin, vincristine, procarbazine, prednisolone)	シクロホスファミド、アドリアマイシン、ビンクリスチン、プロカルバジン、プレドニゾロン、ブレオマイシン併用療法
COPD(chronic obstructive pulmonary disease)	慢性閉塞性肺疾患
COPDD(childhood onset pervasive developmental disorder)	小児期発症型広範性発達障害
COPP(cyclophosphamide, oncovin, procarbazine, prednisolone)	シクロホスファミド、オンコビン、プロカルバジン、プレドニゾロン併用療法
cord around neck	臍帯頸部巻絡
cord sign	脊髄徴候
corneal ulcer	角膜潰瘍
coronary spasm	冠れん縮
coronary stent	冠動脈ステント
corrective cast	矯正ギプス包帯
cortical necrosis	腎皮質壊死
cost resp(costal respiration)	胸式呼吸
	◀関連▶腹式呼吸：abd resp
cough	咳嗽
Cox-V(Coxsackie virus)	コクサッキーウイルス
coxarthrosis	変形性股関節症
CP angle(cerebello-pontine angle)	小脳橋角部
CP(canal paresis)	半規管機能低下
CP(cerebral palsy)	脳性麻痺
CP(cerebral poliomyelitis)	脳性小児麻痺
CP(chest pain)	胸痛
CP(chronic pancreatitis)	慢性膵炎

・CP・

CP(chronic phase)	慢性期
	参照 急性期：AP
CP(chronic pyelonephritis)	慢性腎盂腎炎＝CPN
CP(cisplatin, peplomycin)	シスプラチン、ペプロマイシン併用療法
CP(cleft palate)	口蓋裂
CP(clinical psychologist)	臨床心理士
CP(cor pulmonale)	肺性心
CP(cyclophosphamide, carboplatin)	シクロホスファミド、カルボプラチン併用療法
CP(cyclophosphamide, cisplatin)	シクロホスファミド、シスプラチン併用療法
CPA(cardiopulmonary arrest)	心肺停止
CPA(cerebello-pontine angle)	小脳橋角部
CPAA(cardiopulmonary arrest immediately after arrival)	到着後心肺停止
CPAOA(cardio-pulmonary arrest on arrival)	到着時心肺停止
CPAP(continuous positive airway pressure)	持続陽圧呼吸
CPB(cardiopulmonary bypass)	人工心肺
CPB(celiac plexus block)	腹腔神経叢ブロック
CPBV(cardiopulmonary blood volume)	心肺血流量
CPC(clinical pathological conference)	臨床病理討論会
CPCR(cardiopulmonary cerebral resuscitation)	心肺脳蘇生法
	関連 心肺蘇生法：CPR
CPD(cephalo-pelvic disproportion)	児頭骨盤不適合(不均衡)
CPD(chronic peritoneal dialysis)	慢性腹膜透析
CPD(chronic photosensitivity dermatitis)	慢性光線過敏性皮膚炎
CPD(contagious pustular dermatitis)	接触性膿疱性皮膚炎
CPD(continuous peritoneal dialysis)	持続腹膜透析
CPE(cardiac pulmonary edema)	心原性肺水腫
CPE(chronic pulmonary emphysema)	慢性肺気腫
CPE(cytopathic effect)	細胞変性効果
CPEO(chronic progressive external ophthalmoplegia)	慢性進行性外眼筋麻痺

CR

CPGN(chronic proliferative glomerulonephritis)	慢性増殖性糸球体腎炎
CPH(chronic persistent hepatitis)	慢性持続性肝炎
CPI(California psychological inventory)	カリフォルニア心理検査
CPIP(chronic pulmonary insufficiency of prematurity)	未熟児慢性肺機能不全
CPK(creatine phosphokinase)	クレアチンリン酸酵素(クレアチンホスホキナーゼ)
CPKD(childhood polycystic kidney disease)	小児型多囊胞腎
CPK-MB(Creatine Phosphokinase muscle and brain)	クレアチンホスホキナーゼMB
CPL(cirrhotic, progressive and lymphatic forms)	CPL(硬性、進行性、リンパ管型癌組織)分類
CPLD(congenital pancreatic lipase deficiency)	先天性リパーゼ欠損症
CPM(central pontine myelinolysis)	橋中心髄鞘崩壊症
CPM(chronic progressive myelopathy)	慢性進行性ミエロパチー
CPM(continuous passive motion)	持続他動運動
CPN(chronic pyelonephritis)	慢性腎盂腎炎=CP
	◀関連▶ 急性腎盂腎炎:APN
CPP(cerebral perfusion pressure)	脳灌流圧
CPPB(continuous positive pressure breathing)	持続陽圧呼吸
CPPV(continuous positive pressure ventilation)	持続陽圧換気法
CPR(C-peptide)	Cペプチド
CPR(cardiopulmonary resuscitation)	心肺蘇生法
CPS(cardiopulmonary supported device)	心肺補助装置
CPS(cavopulmonary shunt)	大静脈肺動脈吻合術
CPS(cholangiopancreatoscopy)	胆膵管鏡
CPS(complex partial seizure)	複雑部分発作
	◀関連▶ 単純部分発作:SPS
CPSE(complex partial status epilepticus)	複雑部分てんかん重積発作
CR(cardiorespiratory)	心臓呼吸性の
CR(closed reduction)	非観血的整復
CR(complete remission)	完全寛解
	◀関連▶ 部分寛解:PR

CR

CR (complement receptor)	補体レセプター
CR (conditioned reflex)	条件反射
CR (controlled respiration)	調節呼吸
CR (cough reflex)	咳嗽反射
Cr (creatine)	クレアチン
	参照 クレアチニン・クリアランス：Ccr
craniectomy	開頭術(骨弁除去)
craniopharyngioma	頭蓋咽頭腫＝CRP
craniosynostosis	頭蓋骨早期融合症
craniotabes	頭蓋癆＝CT
craniotomy	開頭術(骨弁形成)
CRAO (central retinal artery occlusion)	網脈中心動脈閉塞症
CRBBB (complete right bundle branch block)	完全右脚ブロック
	関連 完全左脚ブロック：CLBBB
CRC (colorectal cancer)	大腸直腸癌
CRC (concentrated red cell)	赤血球濃厚液
CRD (chronic renal disease)	慢性腎疾患
CRD (chronic respiratory disease)	慢性呼吸器疾患
	関連 急性呼吸器疾患：ARD
crep (crepitus)	捻髪音
crescentic glomerulonephritis	半月体形成性糸球体腎炎
cretinism	クレチン症
CRF (chronic renal failure)	慢性腎不全
	関連 急性腎不全：ARF
CRF (chronic respiratory failure)	慢性呼吸不全
	関連 急性呼吸不全：ARF
CRH (corticotropin-releasing hormone)	副腎皮質刺激ホルモン放出ホルモン
crisis intervention	危機介入法
CRL (crown-rump length)	頭殿長
CRM (cross reacting material)	交叉反応物質

CRP(C-reactive protein)	C反応性蛋白
CRP(craniopharyngioma)	頭蓋咽頭腫
CRS(catheter related sepsis)	カテーテル肺血症
CRS(congenital rubella syndrome)	先天性風疹症候群
CRT(chemoradiation therapy)	放射線化学療法
crush fracture	圧壊骨折
crust	痂皮
CRVF(congestive right ventricular failure)	うっ血性右心不全
CRVO(central retinal vein occlusion)	網膜中心静脈閉塞症
cryoglobulinemia	クリオグロブリン血症
cryptorchidism	停留精巣
crystal arthritis	結晶性関節炎
CS(cardiogenic shock)	心原性ショック=CGS
CS(cervical spine)	頸椎
CS(cervical spondylosis)	頸部脊椎症
CS(Cesarean section)	帝王切開
CS(chondrosarcoma)	軟骨肉腫
CS(chronic schizophrenia)	慢性統合失調症
CS(chronic sinusitis)	慢性副鼻腔炎
CS(conditioning stimulus)	条件刺激
CS(coronary sclerosis)	冠動脈硬化症
CS(coronary sinus)	冠静脈洞
CS(cystoscope)	膀胱鏡
CSAS(central sleep apnea syndrome)	中枢型睡眠時無呼吸症候群
CSB(Cheyne-Stokes breathing)	チェーン・ストークス呼吸
CSDH(chronic subdural hematoma)	慢性硬膜下血腫=CSH
	◀関連▶ 急性硬膜下血腫：ASDH
CSF(cerebrospinal fluid)	脳脊髄液
CSF(colony-stimulating factor)	コロニー刺激因子
CSF(cyanide-sensitive factor)	青酸感受性因子
CSH(chronic subdural hematoma)	慢性硬膜下血腫=CSDH
CSII(continuous subcutaneous insulin infusion)	持続皮下インスリン注入法

CS

CSM(cerebrospinal meningitis)	脳脊髄膜炎
CSM(cervical spondylotic myelopathy)	頚椎症性脊髄症
CSMA(chronic spinal muscular atrophy)	慢性脊髄性筋萎縮症
CSR(cervical spondylotic myelopathy)	頚部脊椎症性脊髄症
CSR(central supply room)	中央材料室
CST(contraction stress test)	子宮収縮ストレステスト
CST(convulsive shock therapy)	痙攣ショック療法
CSU(catheter specimen of urine)	カテーテル尿
CT(calcitonin)	カルシトニン
CT(cerebral thrombosis)	脳血栓
CT(chemotherapy)	化学療法
CT(cognitive therapy)	認知療法
CT(computerized tomography)	コンピュータ断層撮影 参照 磁気共鳴画像診断装置：MRI
CT(craniotabes)	頭蓋癆
CT(cytotoxic test)	細胞傷害試験
CTCL(cutaneous T cell lymphoma)	皮膚T細胞性リンパ腫
CTD(connective tissue disease)	結合織疾患
CTG(cardio-tocograph)	胎児心拍陣痛図
CTGA(corrected transposition of the great arteries)	修正大血管転位
CTL(cytotoxic T lymphocyte)	細胞障害性Tリンパ球
CTN(chronic tubulointerstitial nephritis)	慢性尿細管間質性腎炎
CTO(cerebral thromboangiitis obliterans)	脳閉塞性血栓血管炎
CTR(cardio thoracic ratio)	心胸郭比
CTS(carpal tunnel syndrome)	手根管症候群
CTx(cardiac transplantation)	心臓移植術
cubital tunnel	肘部管
cubitus valgus	外反肘
cubitus varus	内反肘
CUC(chronic ulcerative colitis)	慢性潰瘍性大腸炎
CUD(cause undetermined)	原因不明
CUG(cystourethrography)	膀胱尿道造影法

curative operation	治癒手術
Cushing disease	クッシング病
CV(central vein)	中心静脈
CV(central venous nutrition)	中心静脈栄養＝IVH, TPN
	対 末梢静脈栄養：PVN
CV(conjugata vera)	真結合線
CVA(cardiovascular accident)	心臓血管障害
CVA(cerebral vascular accident)	脳血管障害
CVC(central venous catheter)	中心静脈カテーテル
CVD(cerebro-vascular disease)	脳血管疾患
CVD(combined valvular disease)	連合弁膜症
CVD(continuous ventricular drainage)	持続脳室ドレナージ
CVG(cerebral venography)	脳静脈造影
CVH(combined ventricular hypertrophy)	両室肥大＝BVH
CVI(check valve index)	呼気閉塞指数
CVO(conjugata vera obstetrica)	産科真結合線
CVP(central venous pressure)	中心静脈圧
	対 末梢静脈圧：PVP
CVP(cyclophosphamide. vincristine, prednisolone)	シクロホスファミド、ビンクリスチン、プレドニゾロン併用療法
CVVH (continuous veno-venous hemofiltration)	持続的静脈－静脈血液濾過
CVVHD (continuous veno-venous hemodialysis)	持続静脈血液透析
CW(crutch walking)	松葉杖歩行
CWD(continuous wave Doppler)	連続波ドプラー
Cx(cervix)	頚部
CX(circumflex)	冠動脈回旋枝
cyanosis	チアノーゼ
cyclic vomiting	周期性嘔吐症
cylinder	円柱
cylinder cast	筒状ギプス包帯
cyst of septi pellucidum	透明中隔嚢腫
cystic kidney	嚢胞腎

cy

cystitis	膀胱炎
cystography	膀胱造影
cystometry	膀胱内圧測定法
cystoscope	膀胱鏡
CYVADIC(cyclophosphamide, vincristine, doxorubicin, dacarbazine)	シクロホスファミド、ビンクリスチン、ドキソルビシン、ダカルバジン併用療法

D(+), d(+)	肛門側不完全切除（肉眼的、組織学的）の記号
D(death)	死亡
D(depression)	うつ病
D(descending colon)	下行結腸 ◀関連▶ 上行結腸：A 横行結腸：T S状結腸：S
D(diagnosis)	診断＝Dx
D(diaphragm)	横隔膜
D(dorsal)	背部の
DA(degenerative arthritis)	変性関節炎
DA(diabetic amyotrophy)	糖尿病性筋萎縮症
DA(dopamine)	ドパミン
DA(ductus arteriosus)	動脈管
DAA(dissecting aortic aneurysm)	解離性大動脈瘤
DAD(diffuse alveolar damage)	びまん性肺胞障害
DAI(diffuse axonal injury)	びまん性軸索損傷
dandruff	ふけ
DAP(draw a person test)	人物画テスト
DAPT(direct agglutination pregnancy)	直接凝集妊娠試験
DAR(death after resuscitation)	蘇生後死亡
DAR(dual asthmatic response)	2相性喘息反応
DART(dementia of AIDS related type)	エイズ関連痴呆
DAT(dementia of Alzheimer)	アルツハイマー型認知症＝AD, ATD
DAV(dacarbazine, nimustine, vincristine)	ダカルバジン、ニムスチン、ビンクリスチン併用療法
DAVP(dacarbazine, nimustine, vincristine, peplomycin)	ダカルバジン、ニムスチン、ビンクリスチン、ペプロマイシン併用療法
dB(decibel)	デシベル

DB

DB(deep burn)	皮下熱傷(第3度)
DB(direct reacting bilirubin)	直接型ビリルビン
DBE(diffuse bronchiectasis)	びまん性気管支拡張症
DBP(diastolic blood pressure)	拡張期血圧
	対 収縮期血圧：SAP
DC(dressing change)	包帯交換
D&C(cervical dilatation and uterine curettage)	子宮頚管拡張および掻爬術
DCA(directional coronary arterectomy)	アテレクトミー、方向性冠状動脈粥腫切除
DCH(delayed cutaneous hypersensitivity)	遅延型皮膚過敏症
DCM(dilatative cardiomyopathy)	拡張型心筋症
DCMP(daunorubicin, cytarabine, mercaptopurine, prednisolone)	ダウノルビシン、シタラビン、メルカプトプリン、プレドニゾロン併用療法
DCP(daunomycin, cylocide, predonine)	ダウノマイシン、サイロサイド、プレドニン併用療法
DC shock(direct current shock)	直流除細動
DD(differential diagnosis)	鑑別診断
DDB(deep dermal burn)	真皮深層熱傷(第2度)
DDH(developmental dislocation of the hip)	発育性股関節脱臼
DDR(diastolic descent rate)	拡張期弁後退速度
DDS(drug delivery system)	ドラッグデリバリーシステム
DdVP(adriamycin, vincristine, prednisolone)	アドリアマイシン、ビンクリスチン、プレドニゾロン併用療法
dead space	死腔
	参照 解剖学的死腔：ADS
deafness	難聴
debridement	病巣清掃術(デブリードマン)
decerebrated posture	除脳硬直姿位
decorticated posture	除皮質硬直姿位
decortication	骨皮質除去術(デコルチカシオン)
decubitus	褥瘡

de

deeply comatose	深昏眠状態
defecation	排便
defense	防衛
defense mechanism	防衛機構
DEG(degeneration)	変性
degloving injury	手袋状剥皮損傷
deglutition	嚥下
	参照 嚥下困難：dysphagia
dehydration	脱水(症)
delayed speech	言語遅滞
delayed union	遷延治癒
delirium	せん妄
deltoid ligament	三角靱帯
delusion	妄想
delusion of belittlement	卑小妄想
delusion of guilt	罪業妄想
delusion of invention	発明妄想
delusion of jealousy	嫉妬妄想
delusion of negation	否定妄想
delusion of persecution	被害妄想
delusion of poisoning	被毒妄想(被害妄想の一種)
delusion of possession	憑きもの妄想
delusion of poverty	貧困妄想
delusional idea	妄想着想
delusional mood	妄想気分
delusional perception	妄想知覚
demand pacemaker	ディマンド(型)ペースメーカー／応需型ペースメーカー
dementia	痴呆
denture	義歯
dependent personality disorder	依存性人格障害
depersonalization	離人症
depersonalization neurosis	離人神経症
depolarization	脱分極

de

deposit	沈着物
depressed mood	抑うつ
depression	うつ病
depressive type	うつ状態
derm(dermatitis)	皮膚炎
descent delusion	血統妄想
desquamation	剥離
dexamethasone suppression test	デキサメサゾン抑制試験
DF(defibrillation)	除細動
	参照 自動体外除細動：AED
DF(depressed fracture)	陥没骨折
DFP(diastolic filling phase)	拡張期充満
DFSP(dermatofibrosarcoma protuberans)	隆起性皮膚線維肉腫
DG(developmental glaucoma)	発育異常緑内障
DG(Duodenalgeschwür)	十二指腸潰瘍
DGN(diffuse glomerulonephritis)	びまん性糸球体腎炎
DGS(diabetic glomerulosclerosis)	糖尿病性糸球体硬化症
DH(delayed hypersensitivity)	遅延型過敏症反応
DHA(dehydroacetic acid)	デヒドロ酢酸
DHAP(dexamethazone, high-dose cytarabine, cisplatin)	デキサメサゾン、高用シタラビン、シスプラチン併用療法
DHP(direct hemoperfusion)	血液吸着
DHT(dihydrotestosterone)	ジヒドロテストステロン
DI(diabetes insipidus)	尿崩症
DI(discomfort index)	不快指数
DI(drip infusion)	点滴
DIAB(diabetic retinopathy)	糖尿病性網膜症＝DMR, DR, RET
diabetic nephropathy	糖尿病性腎症
diabetic retinopathy	糖尿病性網膜症
dialysis	透析
dialysis dysequilibrium syndrome	透析不均衡症候群
dialyzer	透析器
diaper	オムツ

·Di·

diaphragm	横隔膜
diaphysis	骨幹
diarrhea	下痢
	参照 便秘：constipation
DIC(disseminated intravascular coagulation)	播種性血管内凝固症候群
DIC(drip infusion cholangiography)	点滴静注胆管造影法
DIC(drug-induced colitis)	薬剤性大腸炎
DIE(death in emergency)	突然死
diencephalic and mesencephalic syndrome	間脳・中脳症候群
diencephalic syndrome	間脳症候群
diencephalon	間脳
	関連 大脳：cerebrum
	小脳：cerebellum
diet therapy	食事療法
Difficulty in breathing	呼吸困難
diffusion	拡散
DIFP(diffuse interstitial fibrosing pneumonia)	びまん性間質性線維化肺炎
DIHN(drug-induced hypersensitivity nephritis)	薬剤誘発性過敏性腎炎
DILV(double inlet left ventricle)	左心性単心室
diminished superficial reflex	表在反射消失
DIND(delayed ischemic neurologic deficit)	遅発性虚血性神経脱落症状
DIP joint(distal interphalangeal joint)	遠位指(趾)節間関節
DIP(desquamative interstitial pneumonia)	剥離性間質性肺炎
DIP(drip infusion pyelography)	点滴静注腎盂造影法
diplegia	両麻痺
	参照 片麻痺：hemiplegia
dipper	夜間血圧下降例
directive psychotherapy	指示的療法
disarray	錯綜配列
Disc(discharge)	退院＝ENT
	参照 入院：Adm

di

disc herniation	椎間板ヘルニア
discography	椎間板造影
DIS(dislocation)	脱臼
disorganized type	解体型／破瓜型(統合失調症)
disorientation	失見当識
dissociative disorder	分離症
distal tubular acidosis	遠位尿細管性アシドーシス
distortion	捻挫
distortion of recognition	再認障害
disturbance of affect	感情障害
disturbance of consciousness	意識障害
disturbance of development	発育障害
disturbance of impression	記銘障害
disturbance of intelligence	知能障害
disturbance of memory	記憶障害
disturbance of recall	想起障害
disturbance of thinking	思考障害
disturbance of consciousness	意識障害
disturbed level of consciousness	意識レベル低下
diurnal variation	日内変動
DIV(drip infusion of vein)	点滴静脈内注射
DIVP(drip-infusion pyelography)	点滴静注腎盂造影＝DIP
dizziness	めまい
DJD(degenerative joint disease)	変形性関節疾患
D-J syndrome (Dubin-Johnson syndrome)	デュビン・ジョンソン症候群
DKA(diabetic ketoacidosis)	糖尿病性ケトアシドーシス
DL(diffusing capacity of lung)	肺拡散能力
DLC(double lumen catheter)	ダブルルーメンカテーテル
D$_{LCO}$ (diffusing capacity for carbon monoxide)	CO拡散能
DLE(discoid lupus erythematosus)	円板状エリテマトーデス
DLT(donor lymphocyte transfusion)	ドナーリンパ球輸注

DLV(differential lung ventilation)	左右肺別換気
DM(dermatomyositis)	皮膚筋炎
DM(diabetes mellitus)	糖尿病
DM(diastolic murmur)	拡張期心雑音
DMD(Duchenne muscular dystrophy)	デュシュンヌ型筋ジストロフィー
DMD(dystonia musculorum deformans)	変形性筋異緊張症
DMIT(dementia of multiinfarct type)	多発性梗塞性痴呆
DMLC(diffuse metastatic leptomeningeal carcinomatosis)	びまん性転移性髄膜癌腫症
DMP(dystrophia musculorum progressiva)	進行性筋ジストロフィー＝PMD
DMP(enocitabine, daunomycin, methylprednisolone, prednisolone)	エノシタビン、ダウノマイシン、メチルプレドニン、プレドニゾロン併用療法
DMPS(dysmyelopoietic syndrome)	骨髄異形成症候群
DMR(diabetic retinopathy)	糖尿病性網膜症＝DR, RET, DIAB
DN(diabetic neuropathy)	糖尿病性神経症
DN(dicrotic notch)	重複切痕
DNA(deoxyribonucleic acid)	デオキシリボ核酸
DNR(Do not resuscitatate)	蘇生せず（臨死の際に無理な蘇生を行わないこと）
DNT (dysembryoplastic neuroepithelial tumor)	肺芽異形性神経上皮腫瘍
do	同じ（処方箋などで前回と同じ内容の場合にdoと書く）
Do(dissolved oxygen)	溶存酸素
DOA(dead on arrival)	来院時心肺停止
DOA(dopamine hydrochloride)	塩酸ドパミン
DOB(dobutamine hydrochloride)	塩酸ドブタミン
DOE(dyspnea on exertion)	労作性呼吸困難
DOL(dignity of life)	生命の尊厳
DOLV(double outlet left ventricle)	両大血管左室起始
dominant hemispheric signs	大脳優位半球症候
doner	ドナー

DO

DOPA(3, 4-dihydroxyphenylalanine)	ドーパ（3，4 -ジヒドロキシフェニルアラニン）
dorsal position	仰臥位 ◀関連▶腹臥位：proneness 側臥位：lateral recumbent position
DORV(double outlet right ventricle)	両大血管右室起始
DOS(dosis)	用量
double lumen catheter	ダブルルーメン・カテーテル
double monster of the uterus	奇形子宮
double personality	二重人格
double ureter	重複尿管
double vision	複視
Down's syndrome	ダウン症候群
DP(dementia precox)	早発性痴呆
DP(distal pancreatectomy)	膵尾部切除術
DP(dorsalis pedis)	足背動脈
DP(taxotere, cisplatin)	タキソテール、シスプラチン併用療法
DPB(diffuse panbronchiolitis)	びまん性汎細気管支炎
DPD(diffuse pulmonary disease)	びまん性肺疾患
DPG(distal partial gastrectomy)	幽門側胃切除
DPGN(diffuse proliferative glomerulonephritis)	びまん性増殖性糸球体腎炎 ジフテリア・百日咳・破傷風
DPL(diagnostic peritoneal lavage)	診断的腹腔洗浄
DPLN(diffuse proliferative lupus nephritis)	びまん性増殖性ループス腎炎
DPT(diphtheria, pertussis, tetanus)	三種混合
DQ(developmental quotient)	発達指数
DR(diabetic retinopathy)	糖尿病性網膜症＝ DIAB, DMR, RET
drawer sign	引き出し徴候
DRG(diagnosis related groups)	診断群別分類
drop foot	下垂足、尖足
drop hand	下垂手

drowsy	ボンヤリしている、傾眠
DRPLA (dentato-rubro-pallido-luysian atrophy)	歯状核赤核淡蒼球ルイ体萎縮症
dry cough	乾咳
dry rale	乾性ラ音 対 湿性ラ音：bubbling rale
DS(Dauerschlafkur)	持続睡眠療法
DS(discharge from hospital)	退院＝Adm
DS(Down syndrome)	ダウン症候群
DS(dumping syndrome)	ダンピング症候群
DSA(destructive spondyloarthropathy)	破壊性脊椎関節症
DSA(digital subtraction angiography)	デジタル減算（サブトラクション）血管造影法
DSD(depression sine depression)	抑うつなきうつ病
DSM(Diagnostic and Statistical Manual of Mental Disorders)	精神障害の診断・統計便覧
DSN(deviatio septi nasi)	鼻中弯曲症
DSO(dermal sutures out)	抜糸＝SR
DSS(double simultaneous stimulation)	2点同時刺激
DST(donor specific transfusion)	生体腎移植
DST(dexamethasone suppression test)	デキサメサゾン抑制試験
DT(diphtheria-tetanus toxoid)	ジフテリア・破傷風トキソイド
DTAA(dissecting thoracic aortic aneurysm)	解離性胸部大動脈瘤
DTH(delayed type hypersensitivity)	遅延型アレルギー
DTICH (delayed traumatic intracerebral hematoma)	遅発性外傷性脳内血腫
DTR(deep tendon reflex)	深部腱反射
DTR(increased deep tendon reflex)	深部腱反射亢進
DTs(delirium tremens)	振戦せん妄
DU(decubitus ulcer)	褥瘡、潰瘍
DU(duodenal ulcer)	十二指腸潰瘍
DUB(dysfunctional uterine bleeding)	不正性器出血
dullness	濁音
dura mater	硬膜

DV

DV(domestic violence)	家庭内暴力
DV(dorsoventral)	背腹方向
DVD(dissociated vertical deviation)	交代性上斜位
DVP (daunomycin, vincristine, prednisolone)	ダウノマイシン、ビンクリスチン、プレドニゾロン併用療法
DVR(double valve replacement)	2弁置換
DVT(deep venous thrombosis)	深部静脈血栓症
DW0-3, dw0-3	胆管癌の十二指腸側胆管断端の癌浸潤(肉眼的、組織学的)の程度を示す記号
dwarfism	小人症
Dx(diagnosis)	診断=D
dysesthesia	しびれ感、感覚異常
dyspepsia	消化不良
dysphagia	嚥下困難 参照 嚥下：deglutition
dysphasia	失語症
dysphoria	不機嫌
dysplastic kidney	異形成腎
dyspnea	呼吸困難
dysuria	排尿困難
DZ(dizygotic twins)	二卵性双生児 参照 一卵性双生児：MZ,（EZ）

E

E(endoscope)	内視鏡
E(enema)	浣腸
E(epinephrine)	エピネフリン
E(erythrocyte)	赤血球＝ER
E1(estrone)	エストロン
E1-4	肝癌占拠率を示す記号
E2(estradiol)	エストラジオール
E3(estriol)	エストリオール
Ea(abdominal esophagus)	腹部食道
EA(effort angina)	労作性狭心症 ◀関連▶安定性狭心症：SA
EAA(essential amino acid)	必須アミノ酸 ◀関連▶非必須アミノ酸：NEAA
EAM(external acoustic meatus)	外耳道＝EAC
EAP(etoposide, adriamycin, cisplatin)	エトポシド、アドリアマイシン、シスプラチン併用療法
ear noises	耳鳴
early deceleration	早発一過性徐脈
eating disorder	摂食障害
EB(epidermal burn)	表皮熱傷
EB(epidermolysis bullosa)	表皮水疱症
EBA(extrahepatic biliary atresia)	肝外胆道閉鎖症
EBD(endoscopic biliary drainage)	内視鏡下胆道ドレナージ
EBM(evidence-based medicine)	証拠に基づいた医療
EBN(evidence-based nursing)	証拠に基づいた看護
EBV(Epstein-Barr virus)	エプスタイン・バー・ウイルス
EC(endocarditis)	心内膜炎
EC(endocervix)	頚管
EC(escherichia coli)	大腸菌
EC,ECa(esophageal carcinoma)	食道癌＝Eca

EC

ECA(external carotid artery)	外頚動脈
	対 内頚動脈：ICA, IC
ECC(embryonal cell carcinoma)	胎児性細胞癌
ECC(emergency cardiac care)	救急心処理、心臓急迫症管理
ECC(external cardiac compression)	胸壁外心〔臓〕圧迫
ECC(extracorporeal circulation)	体外循環
ECCE(extracapsular cataract extraction)	水晶体嚢外摘出術
ECD(endocardial cushion defect)	心内膜床欠損症
ECDUS (endoscopic color doppler ultrasonography)	内視鏡的超音波カラー・ドプラー法
ECF(eosinophil chemotactic factor)	好酸球遊走因子
ECF(extracellular fluid)	細胞外液
ECFE(endocardial fibroelastosis)	心内膜線維弾性症
ECG(electrocardiogram)	心電図
echolalia	反響語
echopraxia	反響動作
EC-IC bypass (extracranial-intracranial bypass)	外頚－内頚動脈バイパス
ECJ(esophagocardial junction)	食道噴門接合部
E-C junction(esophago-cardial junction)	食道噴門接合部
ECLA(extracorporeal lung assist)	体外式肺補助
ECLHA(extracorporeal lung and heart assist)	体外式心肺補助
ECM(external cardiac massage)	体外心マッサージ
ECMO(extracorporeal membrane oxygenation)	体外式膜型人工肺
E coli(*Escherichia coli*)	大腸菌
ECRB(extensor carpi radialis brevis〔muscle〕)	短橈側手根伸筋
ECRL(extensor carpi radialis longus〔muscle〕)	長橈側手根伸筋
ecstasy	恍惚
ECSWL(extracorporeal shock wave lithotripsy)	体外腎砕石術

ECT(electric convulsive therapy)	電撃療法
ECT(emission CT)	エミッションCT
ectopic thyroid	異所性甲状腺
ectrodactyly	指欠損症
ECU(extensor carpi ulnaris〔muscle〕)	尺側手根伸筋
ECUM (extracorporeal ultrafiltration method)	体外限外濾過法
ECV(external cephalic version)	骨盤位外回転術
ED(effective dose)	有効量
ED(elbow disarticulation)	肘関節離断
ED(elemental diet)	成分栄養
ED(emergency department)	救急部
ED(erectile dysfunction)	勃起障害
ED(eye drop)	点眼液
EDA(electrodermal activity)	皮膚電気活動
EDC(expected date of confinement)	分娩予定日
EDC (extensor digitorum communis〔muscle〕)	総指伸筋
edema	浮腫　◀関連▶全身性浮腫：anasarca
EDH(epidermal hematoma)	硬膜外血腫＝EH
EDP(end-diastolic pressure)	拡張末期圧
EDTA (ethylenediaminetetraacetic acid; edetic acid)	エチレンジアミン四酢酸(エデト酸)
EDV(end-diastolic volume)	拡張末期容量
Edward personal preference schedule	エドワード個人嗜好検査
E-E(end-to-end)	端々
EEA(end-to-end inverting anastomosis)	消化管端々吻合
EEG(electroencephalogram)	脳波
EEG audiometry (electroencephalographic audiometry)	脳波聴力検査
EEM(erythema exudativum multiforme)	多形滲出性紅斑
EF(ejection fraction)	駆出率

EF

EF(esophafiberscope)	食道ファイバースコープ
Ef0-3	肺癌治療効果の組織学的判定基準を示す記号
EFBW(estimated fetal body weight)	推定胎児体重
efferent arteriole	輸出細動脈
EFM(electronic fetal monitor)	胎児監視装置
EG(encounter group)	エンカウンターグループ
EGC(early gastric cancer)	早期胃癌 ◀関連▶進行胃癌：AGC
EGF(epidermal growth factor)	上皮成長因子
EGJ(esophagogastric junction)	食道胃接合部
ego	自我
EGTA(esophageal gastric tube airway)	食道胃管式エアウェイ
EH(epidermal hematoma)	硬膜外血腫＝EDH
EH(essential hypertension)	本態性高血圧症
Eh(hemorrhagic pleural effusion)	血性胸水
EHBF(effective hepatic blood flow)	有効肝血流量
EHEC(enterohemorrhagic Escherichia coli)	腸管出血性大腸菌
EHF(epidemic hemorrhagic fever)	流行性出血熱
EHL(extensor hallucis longus)	長母趾伸筋
EHO(extrahepatic portal occulusion)	肝外門脈閉塞症
Ei(lower intrathoracic esophagus)	胸部下部食道
EIA(enzyme immunoassay)	酵素免疫測定法
EIA(exercise-induced asthma)	運動誘発性気管支喘息
EIA(external iliac artery)	外腸骨動脈
EIS(endoscopic injection sclerotherapy)	内視鏡的硬化(薬剤注入)療法
EJ(elbow jerk)	肘反射
EKC(epidemic keratoconjunctivitis)	流行性角結膜炎
EKG(Elektrokardiogramm)	心電図
EL(eosinophilic leukemia)	好酸球性白血病
elation	爽快
elbow joint	肘関節
ELBW(extreme low birth weight)	超未熟児

elective mutism	選択無言症
Ellsworth-Howard test	エルスワース・ハワード試験
ELSS(emergency life support system)	緊急生命維持装置
ELST(emergency life-saving technician)	救急救命士
EM(Eisenmenger syndrome)	アイゼンメンゲル症候群
EM(endometriosis)	子宮内膜症
EM(endometrium)	子宮内膜
EMA-CC(methotrexate, actinomycin D-etoposide, leucovorin)	メソトレキセート、アクチノマイシンD、エトポシド、ロイコボリン併用療法
EMA-CP(etoposide, methotrexate, dactinomycin, cyclophosphamide, vincristine)	エトポシド、メソトレキセート、ダクチノマイシン、シクロホスファミド、ビンクリスチン併用療法
emaciation	るいそう(やせ) 対 肥満(症)：obesity
embryo	胎芽
embryonal carcinoma	胎児性癌
embryopathy	胎芽病
EMCa(endometrial cancer)	子宮内膜癌
EMD(electromechanical dissociation)	伝導収縮解離
emesis	嘔吐
EMF(endomyocardial fibrosis)	心内膜心筋線維症
EMG syndrome(exomphalos macroglossia gigantism syndrome)	臍ヘルニア・巨大舌・巨人症症候群
EMG(electromyogram)	筋電図
EML(extracorporeal micro-explosive lithotripsy)	体外的微小発破砕石術
empathy	感情移入
emphysema	肺気腫＝PE
empy(empyema maxillaris)	上顎洞炎
Empy(empyema paranasalis)	副鼻腔炎(蓄膿症)
empyema	膿胸
EMR(endoscopic mucosal resection)	内視鏡的粘膜切除術
EMS(emergency medical system)	救急医療システム

EM

EMS(endometrial smear)	子宮内膜細胞診
EMU(early morning urine)	早朝尿
EN(enteral nutrition)	経腸栄養
EN(erythema nodosum)	結節性紅斑
ENBD(endoscopic naso-biliary drainage)	内視鏡的経鼻胆管ドレナージ
end-to-end anastomosis	端々吻合
endomyocardial biopsy	心内膜心筋生検
ENG(electronystagmogram)	電気眼振図
ENGBD (endoscopic naso-gallbladder drainage)	内視鏡的経鼻胆嚢ドレナージ
ENPBD (endoscopic naso-pancreaticobiliary drainage)	内視鏡的経鼻膵胆管ドレナージ
ENPD(endoscopic naso-pancreatic drainage)	内視鏡的経鼻膵管ドレナージ
ENT(entlassen)	退院
ENT(ear, nose, throat)	耳、鼻、咽喉
enthesopathy	腱付着部症
entrapment neuropathy	絞扼性神経障害
enuresis	夜尿症
EO(eye ointment)	眼軟膏
Eo, Eos(eosinophile)	好酸球
	◀関連▶ 好中球：N, Neutro 好塩基球：Bas
EOA(esophageal obturator airway)	食道閉鎖式エアウェイ
EOG(electro oculogram)	電気眼位図
EOG(electro olfactogram)	嗅電図
EOM(extra ocular movement)	外眼筋運動
EOM(extraocular muscle)	外眼筋
EOM(eye ocular movement)	眼球運動
EP(ectopic pregnancy)	子宮外妊娠＝EUP, GEU
EP(endocochlear potential)	蝸牛内直流電位
EP(ependymoma)	上衣腫
EP(etoposide, cisplatin)	エトポシド、シスプラチン併用療法
ep(intraepithelium)	粘膜上皮内

ER

Ep, Epi(epilepsy)	てんかん
EPAP(expiratory positive airway pressure)	呼気気道陽圧
EPB(extensor pollicis brevis〔muscle〕)	短母指伸筋
EPBP(endoscopic papillary balloon dilation)	内視鏡的乳頭バルーン拡張
EPC(epilepsia partialis continua)	持続性部分てんかん
EPCG (endoscopic pancreatocholangiography)	内視鏡的膵胆管造影法
EPEC(enteropathogenic Escherichia coli)	病原性大腸菌
EPH(edema, proteinuria, hypertension)	浮腫、蛋白尿、高血圧（妊娠高血圧症候群）
EPH(essential pulmonary hypertension)	特発性肺高血圧症
epicanthus	眼角贅皮
Epid(epidural anesthesia)	硬膜外麻酔
Epidura(epidural hematoma)	硬膜外血腫（エピドラ）
epigastralgia	心窩部痛
epigastric distress	胃部不快感
epileptic seizure	てんかん発作
epiphyseal cartilage	骨端軟骨
epiphysis	骨端
episodic secretion	脈状分泌
EPL(endoscopic pancreatolithotripsy)	内視鏡的膵石破砕術
EPL(extensor pollicis longus〔muscle〕)	長母指伸筋
EPO(erythropoietin)	エリスロポエチン
EPOCH(etoposide, prednisolone, vincristine, cyclophosphamide, doxorubicin)	エトポシド、プレドニゾロン、ビンクリスチン、シクロホスファミド、ドキソルビシン併用療法
EPP(end-plate potential)	終板電位
EPS(extrapyramidal syndrome)	錐体外路症候群
EPSP(excitatory postsynaptic potentials)	興奮性シナプス後電位
EPT(endoscopic papillotomy)	内視鏡的乳頭切開術
ER(emergency room)	救急外来室
ER(endoplasmic reticulum)	小胞体
Er(erosion)	びらん
ER(external rotation)	外旋　対 内旋：IR

ER

ERB(essential renal bleeding)	本態性腎出血
ERBD (endoscopic retrograde biliary drainage)	内視鏡的逆行性胆管ドレナージ
ERBE(endoscopic retrograde biliary endoprosthesis)	内視鏡的逆行性胆管内瘻術
ERBIM(endoscopic retrograde bowel insertion method)	内視鏡的逆行性大腸挿入法
ERC (endoscopic retrograde cholangiography)	内視鏡的逆行性胆管造影
ERCP(endoscopic retrograde cholangio-pancreatography)	内視鏡的逆行性胆管膵管造影
ERG(electroretinogram)	網膜電図
ERGBD (endoscopic retrograde gallbladder and biliary drainage)	内視鏡的逆行性胆嚢胆管ドレナージ
EROM(early rupture of membranes)	早期破水
erosion	びらん＝Er
erotomania	恋愛妄想
ERP(effective refractory period)	有効不応期
ERP(endoscopic retrograde pancreatography)	内視鏡的逆行性膵管造影
ERS(endoscopic retrograde sphincterotomy)	内視鏡的逆行性括約筋切開術
ERT(emergency room thoracotomy)	緊急開胸
erythema	紅斑
erythema infectiosum	伝染性紅斑
erythrophobia	赤面恐怖
ES(electric shock therapy)	電気ショック療法
ES(esophagus)	食道
ES(exanthema subitum)	突発性発疹
E-S(end-to-side)	端側
ESHAP(etoposide, methylprednisolone, high dose cytarabine, cisplatin)	エトポシド、メチルプレドニゾロン、高用量シタラビン、シスプラチン併用療法
ESI(exit site infection)	カテーテル出口部感染

ESM (ejection systolic murmur)	駆出性収縮期雑音
esophageal carcinoma	食道癌
esophageal v arix	食道静脈瘤
esophagus	食道
ESR (erythrocyte sedimentation rate)	赤血球沈降速度
ESRD (end stage renal disease)	末期腎不全＝ESRF
ESRF (end stage renal failure)	末期腎不全＝ESRD
EST (endoscopic sphincterotomy)	内視鏡的乳頭括約筋切開術
estrogen	エストロゲン
ESV (end-systolic volume)	収縮末期容量
ESWL (extra- corporal shock wave lithotripsy)	体外衝撃波結石破砕療法
ET (ejection time)	駆出時間
ET (embryo transfer)	胚移植
ET (endotoxin)	内毒素、エンドトキシン
ET (enterostomal therapist)	ストーマ療法士
ET (esotropia)	内斜視　対　外斜視：XT
ETA (endotracheal airway)	気管内エアウェイ
ETCO2 (end tidal CO2)	呼気終末炭酸ガス濃度
ETS (endoscopic thoracic sympathectomy)	胸腔鏡下交感神経遮断術
ETT (endotracheal tube)	気管内挿管チューブ
ETT (eye tracking test)	視標追跡検査
EUP (extrauterine pregnancy)	子宮外妊娠＝EP, GEU
euphoria	多幸症、上機嫌
EUS (endoscopic ultrasonography)	超音波内視鏡検査法
EVB (etoposide, enocitabine, vindesine)	エトポシド、エノシタビン、ビンデシン併用療法
EVC (expiratory vital capacity)	呼気肺活量
EVL (endoscopic variceal ligation)	内視鏡的静脈瘤結紮術
Evs (endoscopic variceal sclerotherapy)	内視鏡的食道静脈瘤硬化療法
ex (exercise)	運動、訓練
ex (extra)	臨時（臨時処方などの意味で使われる）

ex

exanthema subitum	突発性発疹
exchange transfusion	交換輸血
exercise tolerance test	運動負荷試験
exhibitionism	露出症
existential psychotherapy	現存在分析療法
exophthalmos	眼球突出
Exp(expiration)	呼気
experience of influence	させられ体験
ext(extension)	伸展　対 屈曲：fl
extended operation	拡大手術
extension contracture	伸展拘縮 対 屈曲拘縮：flexion contracture
extrinsic muscle	外因筋
eye strain	眼精疲労
Ez(eczema)	湿疹
EZ(Eineiige Zwillinge)	一卵性双生児＝MZ 参照 二卵性双生児：DZ

F

f(respiratory frequency)	呼吸数＝RR
F(feces)	大便
F(frontal plane)	前額面
F(frontal)	前頭部の
	対 後頭部の：O
F1-3	食道静脈瘤形態の分類記号
fa(family)	家族
FA(femoral artery)	大腿動脈
	対 大腿静脈：FV
FA(fructosamine)	フルクトサミン
FAB(French-American-British cooperative group classification)	FAB分類（急性白血病の分類）
fabella	ファベラ
FABERE(flexion, abduction, external rotation and extension test)	股関節の屈曲、外転、外旋、伸展テスト
FAC(fluorouracil, adriamycin, cyclophosphamide)	フルオロウラシル、アドリアマイシン、シクロホスファミド併用療法
facet joint	椎間軟骨
facial expression	表情
facial N	顔面神経
F_ACO_2(alveolar CO_2 concentration)	肺胞気炭酸ガス濃度
FADIRE(flexion, adduction, internal rotation and extension test)	股関節の屈曲、内転、内旋、伸展テスト
FAG(fluorescein angiography)	蛍光（眼底）血管造影
failure	不全
FAM(fluorouracil, adriamycin, methotrexate)	フルオロウラシル、アドリアマイシン、メソトレキセート併用療法
FAM (fluorouracil, adriamycin, mitomycin-C)	フルオロウラシル、アドリアマイシン、マイトマイシンC併用療法

fa

family therapy	家族療法
FAMT(fluorouracil, cyclophosphamide-A, mitomycin-C, toyomycin)	フルオロウラシル、シクロホスファミドA、マイトマイシンC、トヨマイシン併用療法
F_AO_2(alveolar O_2 concentration)	肺胞気酸素濃度
FAP(familial amyloid polyneuropathy)	家族性アミロイドポリニューロパチー
FAP(fluorouracil, adriamycin, cisplatin)	フルオロウラシル、アドリアマイシン、シスプラチン併用療法
FAS(fetal alcohol syndrome)	胎児性アルコール症候群
fasting hypoglycemia	空腹時低血糖
fatigue	疲労
fatigue fracture	疲労骨折
fatty cast	脂肪円柱
FBG(fasting blood glucose)	空腹時(朝食前)血糖=FBS
FBM(fetal breathing movement)	胎児呼吸様運動
FBS(fasting blood sugar)	空腹時(朝食前)血糖=FBG
FBS(flexible fiber bronchoscopy)	ファイバー気管支鏡検査
FC(febrile convulsion)	熱性痙攣
FCHL(familial combined hyperlipidemia)	家族性複合型高脂血症
FCL(fibular collateral ligament)	外側側副靱帯
FCMD(Fukuyama type congenital muscular dystrophy)	福山型先天性筋ジストロフィー
FCR(flexor carpi radialis)	橈側手根屈筋腱
FCR(flexor carpi radialis〔muscle〕)	橈側手根屈筋
FCS(fiberoptic colonoscopy)	大腸内視鏡検査
FCU(flexor carpi ulnaris)	尺側手根屈筋腱
FCU(flexor carpi ulnaris〔muscle〕)	尺側手根屈筋
FD(fetal distress)	胎児仮死
FD(forced diuresis)	強制利尿
FD(frontal dementia)	前頭葉型痴呆=FLD
FDIU(fetal death in uterus)	子宮内胎児死亡=IUFD
FDL(musculus flexor digitorum longus)	長指屈筋

FDM(musculus flexor digitorum minimi brevis)	短小指屈筋
FDP (fibrin(/fibrinogen)degradation products)	フィブリン(／フィブリノーゲン)分解産物
FDP(flexor digitorum profundus〔muscle〕)	深指屈筋
FDS(fiber-duodenoscope)	十二指腸ファイバースコープ
FDS(flexor digitorum superficialis〔muscle〕)	浅指屈筋
Fds(fundus)	眼底
Fe(ferrum)	鉄
FE(fetal echo)	胎児エコー
FE(focal emphysema)	巣状肺気腫
febrile convulsion	熱性痙攣＝FC
FEC(forced expiratory capacity)	努力性呼気肺活量＝FEV
FECG(fetal electrocardiogram)	胎児心電図
feeling	感情
FEFmax(maximal forced expiratory flow)	最大努力性呼気流量
FEFx(forced expiratory flow)	努力性呼気流量
FEM (fluorouracil, epirubicin, mitomycin-C)	フルオロウラシル、エピルビシン、マイトマイシンC併用療法
FENa(fractional excretion of filtered sodium)	尿中ナトリウム排泄率
fenestration operation	開窓術穿孔設置
fertility drug	排卵誘発剤
fertilized egg	受精卵
FES(fat embolism syndrome)	脂肪塞栓症候群
fetal malnutrition	胎児栄養失調
fetishism	フェティシズム
fetopathy	胎児病
fetus	胎児
FEV(forced expiratory volume)	努力性呼気肺活量＝FEC
FEV$_{1.0}$ (forced expiratory volume in 1second)	1秒量
fever	発熱
FF(filtration fraction)	濾過率
FFA(fluorescein fundus angiography)	蛍光眼底血管造影

FF

FFA(free fatty acid)	遊離脂肪酸
F-F bypass(femoro-femoral bypass)	大腿―大腿動脈バイパス
FFL(fetal femur length)	胎児大腿骨長
FFP(fresh frozen plasma)	新鮮凍結血漿
FGS(fibergastroscope)	胃ファイバースコープ
FGS(focal glomerular sclerosis)	巣状糸球体硬化症
FH(family history)	家族歴
FH(fulminant hepatitis)	劇症肝炎
FHB(fetal heart beat)	胎児心拍
FHF(fulminant hepatic failure)	劇症肝不全
FHL(familial hemophagocytic lymphohistiocytosis)	家族性血球貪食性組織球症
FHM(fetal heart movement)	胎児心拍動
FHR(fetal heart rate)	胎児心拍数
FHS(fetal heart sound)	胎児心音
FHT(fetal heart tone)	胎児心音
fibrinogen	フィブリノーゲン
fibromuscular dysplasia	線維筋性異形成症
fibrous ankylosis	線維性強直
fibrous cartilage	線維軟骨
fibrous dysplasia	線維性骨異形成症
FIFx(forced inspiratory flow)	努力性吸気流量
filtration	濾過
fine motor development	協調運動発達
finger tremor	手指振戦
FIO$_2$(fractional concentration of oxygen in inspired gas)	吸入気酸素濃度
Fishberg concentration test	フィッシュバーグ尿濃縮試験
FIV(forced inspiratory volume)	努力性吸気肺気量
FIVC(forced inspiratory vital capacity)	努力性吸気肺活量
fixation	固定
FL(fatty liver)	脂肪肝
FL(femoral length)	大腿骨長

fl(flexion)	屈曲
	対 伸展：ext
FL(frontal lobe)	前頭葉
flat foot	扁平足
FLD(fibrosing lung disease)	線維化性肺疾患
FLD(frontal lobe dementia)	前頭葉型痴呆＝FD
flexion contracture	屈曲拘縮
	対 伸展拘縮：extension contracture
flight of ideas	観念奔逸
FLKS(fatty liver and kidney syndrome)	脂肪肝・腎症候群
floppy infant	ぐにゃぐにゃ乳児
flow velocity	血流速度
FM(fetal movement)	胎動
FM(functional murmur)	機能性心雑音
FMD(fibromuscular dysplasia)	線維筋形成不全
FNF(femoral neck fracture)	大腿骨頚部骨折
FO(foramen ovale)	卵円孔
FO(fundus oculi)	眼底
focal segmental glomerulosclerosis	巣状分節性糸球体硬化症
forequarter amputation	肩甲帯離断術
Forestier's subset	フォレスター分類
FP(facial palsy)	顔面神経麻痺
FP(fluorouracil, cisplatin)	フルオロウラシル、シスプラチン併用療法
FP(food poisoning)	食中毒
FP(fresh plasma)	新鮮液状血漿
FPB(flexor pollicis brevis〔muscle〕)	短母指屈筋
FPCG(fetal phonocardiogram)	胎児心音図
FPD(feto-placental disproportion)	胎児胎盤不均衡
FPL(flexor pollicis longus〔muscle〕)	長母指屈筋
FPLN(focal proliferative lupus nephritis)	巣状増殖性ループス腎炎
fragile X syndrome	脆弱X症候群
FRC(functional residual capacity)	機能的残気量

free floating anxiety	浮動性不安
frem(fremitus vocalis)	音声振盪
Freudian psychoanalysis	フロイト精神分析
FRH(follicle stimulating hormone releasing hormone)	卵胞刺激ホルモン放出ホルモン
FRJM(full range of joint movement)	関節運動の最大域
frontal lobe syndrome	前頭葉症候群
frostbite	凍傷
frozen shoulder	五十肩
FRP(functional refractory period)	機能的不応期
Fru(fructose)	果糖(フルクトース)
FS(face scale)	フェイススケール
FS(fractional shortening)	円周短縮率
FSH(follicle stimulating hormone)	卵胞刺激ホルモン
FSHRH(follicle stimulating hormone releasing hormone)	卵胞刺激ホルモン放出ホルモン
FTA(femorotibial angle)	大腿脛骨角、膝外側角
FTA(fetal trunk area)	胎児躯幹面積
FTD(feto-thoracic diameter)	胎児胸郭横径
FTG(full thickness skin graft)	全層植皮術=FTSG
FTND(full term normal delivery)	満期正常分娩、満期産
FTNSD (full term normal and spontaneous delivery)	満期正常自然分娩
FTNVD(full term normal vaginal delivery)	満期正常経腟分娩
F to N(finger to nose test)	指鼻試験
FTRC(frozen thawed red blood cells)	解凍濃厚赤血球液
FTSG(full-thickness skin graft)	全層植皮術=FTG
FTT(fat tolerance test)	脂肪負荷試験
full-term infant	正期産児
functional position	良肢位
fundus uteri	子宮底
funnel chest	漏斗胸
FUO(fever of unknown origin)	原因不明熱

FV(femoral vein)	大腿静脈
	〈対〉大腿動脈:FA
FVC(forced vital capacity)	努力性肺活量
FWB(full weight-bearing)	全荷重
Fx(fracture)	骨折

G

G (Gaffky scale)	ガフキー度表
G (gastric juice)	胃液
G (germinoma)	胚細胞腫
G (gravida)	経妊回数
GA (gastric analysis)	胃液検査
GA (general anesthesia)	全身麻酔
	参照 局所麻酔：LA
GA (gestational age)	妊娠週数
GAD (generalized anxiety disorder)	全般性不安障害
Gal (galactose)	ガラクトース
galactosemia	ガラクトース血症
ganglion	結節腫、ガングリオン
GANS (granulomatous angiitis of the nervous system)	神経系肉芽腫性血管炎
Ganser's syndrome	ガンザー症候群
GAS (global assessment scale)	グローバル診断法
GAS (group A streptococcus)	A群溶血性連鎖球菌
gastrectomy	胃切除術
gastric dilatation	胃拡張
gastric lavage	胃洗浄
gastroptosis	胃下垂
gastrospasm	胃痙攣
GB (gallbladder)	胆嚢
GB exam (gallbladder examination)	胆嚢造影検査
GBK (Gallenblasen Karzinom)	胆嚢癌
GBM (glomerular basement membrane)	糸球体基底膜
GBMF (glioblastoma multiforme)	多形神経膠芽腫
GBS (gallbladder stone)	胆嚢胆石
GBS (gastric bypass surgery)	胃バイパス手術
GBS (group B streptococcal infection)	B群溶連菌感染症
GBS (group B streptococcus)	B群溶血性連鎖球菌
GBS (Guillain-Barre syndrome)	ギラン・バレー症候群

GC(Gastric Cancer)	胃癌
GC(glucocorticoid)	糖質コルチコイド
GCa(gastric carcinoma)	胃癌＝MK
GCS(Glasgow Coma Scale)	グラスゴー・コーマ・スケール
GCS(glucocorticosteroid)	副腎皮質ステロイド
G-CSF(granulocyte colony-stimulating factor)	顆粒球コロニー刺激因子
GCT(giant cell tumor)	巨大細胞腫
GCT(granular cell tumor)	顆粒細胞腫
GCU(growing care unit)	正常新生児室
GDA(gastroduodenal artery)	胃十二指腸動脈
GDM(gestational diabetes mellitus)	妊娠糖尿病
GDS(geriatric depression scale)	老年うつ病スケール
GDS(group D streptococcus)	D群溶血性連鎖球菌
GDU(gastroduodenal ulcer)	胃十二指腸潰瘍
GE(generalized epilepsy)	全般てんかん
GE(glycerin enema)	グリセリン浣腸
GEJ(gastroesophageal junction)	胃食道接合部
gene analysis	遺伝子解析
gene map	遺伝子地図
general fatigue	全身倦怠感
gene therapy	遺伝子治療
genu recurvatum	反張膝
genu valgum	外反膝、X脚＝knock knee
genu varum	内反膝、O脚＝bowleg
geographic tongue	地図状舌
GEP (gastro-entero-pancreatic endocrine system)	胃－腸－膵内分泌系
GEP(gastroenteropancreatic)	消化管ホルモン＝GIH
GER(gastroesophageal reflux)	胃食道逆流
GERD(gastroesophageal reflux disorder)	胃食道逆流性疾患
germinoma	胚細胞腫
Gerstmann's syndrome	ゲルストマン症候群
gestalt therapy	ゲシュタルト療法
GEU(gestation extra uterine)	子宮外妊娠＝EP, EUP

GF

GF(gastrofiberscope)	胃内視鏡、胃ファイバースコープ＝GFS
GF(griseofulvin)	グリセオフルビン
GFR(glomerular filtration rate)	糸球体濾過値(率)
GFS(gastrofiberscope)	胃ファイバイスコープ＝GF
GH(growth hormone)	成長ホルモン
GH-IH(growth hormone inhibiting hormone)	成長ホルモン分泌抑制ホルモン
GI(gastro-intestinal)	胃腸の
GI(glucose-insulin therapy)	グルコース・インスリン療法
GI(upper gastrointestinal radiography)	上部消化管撮影
giant negative T wave	巨大陰性T波
GID(gender identity disorder)	性同一性障害
giddiness	めまい
GIF(gastro intestinal fiberscopy)	胃腸ファイバースコープ検査
GIFT(gamete intra-fallopian transfer)	卵管内胚細胞移植
GIK(glucose insulin kalium)	グルコース・インスリン・カリウム療法
GIP(gastric inhibitory peptide)	胃酸分泌抑制ペプチド
GIP(gastric inhibitory polypeptide)	胃酸分泌抑制ポリペプチド
GIP(giant cell interstitial pneumonia)	巨細胞性間質性肺炎
Gips(gypsum)	ギプス
girdle pain	帯状痛
GIST(gastrointestinal stromal tumor)	消化管間質腫瘍
GIT(gastrointestinal tract)	消化管
GITT(glucose insulin tolerance test)	ブドウ糖インスリン負荷試験
giving way	膝くずれ
GJ stomy(gastrojejunostomy)	胃空腸吻合術
GL, Gla(glaucoma)	緑内障 ◀関連▶白内障：Cat
glenohumeral joint	肩甲上腕関節、肩関節
glioma	神経膠腫
glomerulosclerosis	糸球体硬化症
glossopharyngeal N	舌咽神経

Gr

Glu(glucose)	ブドウ糖＝glu
glucagon	グルカゴン
glycogen	グリコーゲン
glycosuria	糖尿
GM(grand mal)	大発作　関連 小発作：PM
GMS(grand mal seizures)	てんかん大発作
GN(glomerulonephritis)	糸球体腎炎
GNB(gram negative bacillus)	グラム陰性桿菌
GNC(gram negative coccus)	グラム陰性球菌
GnRH(gonadotropin releasing hormone)	ゴナドトロピン放出ホルモン
GnRHa (gonadotropin releasing hormone agonist)	ゴナドトロピン放出ホルモン作用薬
GO(gas oxygen anesthesia)	笑気麻酔
goiter	甲状腺腫
gonad	性腺
gonadotropic hormone	性腺刺激ホルモン
gonarthrosis	変形性膝関節症
GOT(glutamic-oxaloacetic transaminase)	グルタミン酸オキサロ酢酸トランスアミナーゼ＝AST
GOTS(great occipito-trigeminal syndrome)	大後頭三叉神経症候群
gout kidney	痛風腎
gouty arthritis	痛風性関節炎
GP(general paralysis)	進行性麻痺
GP(Goldmann perimeter)	ゴールドマン視野計
GP(grasping power)	握力
GPB(gram positive bacillus)	グラム陽性桿菌
GPC(gastric parietal cell)	胃壁細胞
GPC(gram positive coccus)	グラム陽性球菌
GPI(general paralysis of the insane)	精神病性進行性麻痺
GPT(glutamic-pyruvic transaminase)	グルタミン酸ピルビン酸トランスアミナーゼ＝ALT
graft schizophrenia	接枝統合失調症
graftable	バイパス術可能
Grawitz's tumor	グラビッツ腫瘍(腎細胞癌)

gr

greenstick fracture	若木骨折
GRF(gonadotropin releasing factor)	ゴナドトロピン放出因子
GRF(growth hormone releasing factor)	成長ホルモン放出因子
GRH(growth hormone releasing hormone)	成長ホルモン放出ホルモン
gross hematuria	肉眼的血尿
gross motor development	粗大運動発達
group psychotherapy	集団精神療法
growing fracture	成長性骨折
growing pain	成長痛
growth failure	成長障害
growth hormone deficiency	成長ホルモン分泌不全
growth retardation	発育遅延
GS(gallstone)	胆石症
GS(gastritis)	胃炎
GS(gestational sac)	胎嚢
GSD(glycogen storage disease)	糖原病
GSI(genuine stress incontinence)	真性腹圧性尿失禁
GT(gastric tube)	胃チューブ
GTC(generalized tonic-clonic convulsion)	全般性強直性間代性痙攣
GTCS(generalized tonic-clonic seizure)	全身性強直性間代性発作
GTT(glucose tolerance test)	ブドウ糖負荷試験
GU(gastric ulcer)	胃潰瘍
GU(genitourinary)	尿生殖器の
gul(gurgling)音	腸蠕動音、グル音
Guyon canal	尺骨管
GVH(graft-versus-host)	移植片対宿主
GVHD(graft versus host disease)	移植片対宿主病
GVHR(graft versus host reaction)	移植片対宿主反応
GXT(graded exercise test)	多段階運動試験
GYN(gynecology)	婦人科(ギネ)

H

H(hepar)	肝臓
H(horizontal plane)	水平面
H0〜3(hepatic metastasis)	肉眼的肝転移の程度の分類
H0. s.1-4	原発性肝癌の存在範囲を示す記号
HA(habitual abortion)	習慣性流産
HA(headache)	頭痛
HA(hemolytic anemia)	溶血性貧血
HA(hepatic artery)	肝動脈　対 肝静脈：HV
HA(hepatitis A)	A型肝炎
HA(hyaluronic acid)	ヒアルロン酸
HAA(hepatitis associated antigen)	肝炎関連抗原
HA-Ag(hepatitis A antigen)	A型肝炎抗原
HAART (highly active antiretroviral therapy)	高活性抗レトロウイルス療法（抗HIV薬併用療法）
habitual dislocation	習慣性脱臼
HACE(high-altitude cerebral edema)	高所性脳浮腫
HAD(high density area)	高濃度範囲
HAF(hepatic arterial flow)	肝動脈血流量＝HABF
HAIR-An syndrome	ヘア・アン症候群
hallucination	幻覚
hallux valgus	外反母趾
halo-pelvic traction	頭蓋輪骨盤牽引
halo traction	頭蓋輪牽引
HAM(HTLV-1-associated myelopathy)	HTLV-1(ヒトT細胞白血病ウイルス1)関連脊髄症
HAM-D(Hamilton depression rating scale)	ハミルトンうつ病評価尺度＝HDS
hammer toe	槌状趾
HAM syndrome(hypoparathyroidism-Addison-Monilia syndrome)	副甲状腺機能低下アジソン・モニリア症候群
hand-foot-and-mouth disease	手足口病

HA

HANE(hereditary angioneurotic edema)	遺伝性血管運動神経性浮腫
HAPE(high-altitude pulmonary edema)	高所性肺浮腫
HAR(hemagglutination reaction)	赤血球凝集反応
harelip	兎唇
Hasegawa dementia rating scale	長谷川式簡易知的機能診査スケール
HAV(hepatitis A virus)	A型肝炎ウイルス
Hb(hemoglobin)	ヘモグロビン(血色素)
HB(hepatitis B)	B型肝炎
HbA1c(hemoglobin A1c)	ヘモグロビンA1c
HBc-Ag(hepatitis B core antigen)	B型肝炎コア抗原
HBE(His bundle electrocardiogram)	ヒス束心電図
Hbe-Ag(hepatitis B e antigen)	B型肝炎e抗原
HBF(hepatic blood flow)	肝血流量
HB nephropathy	HB腎症
HBO therapy(hyperbaric oxygen therapy)	高圧酸素療法
HBP(high blood pressure)	高血圧　対 低血圧：LBP
HBs-Ag(hepatitis B surface antigen)	B型肝炎表面抗原
HBV(hepatitis B virus)	B型肝炎ウイルス
HC(head circumference)	頭囲
HC(hemorrhage cerebral)	脳出血
HC(Huntington chorea)	ハンチントン舞踏病
HCC(hepatocellular carcinoma)	肝細胞癌
HCG, hCG (human chorionic gonadotropin)	ヒト絨毛性ゴナドトロピン
HCL(hairy cell leukemia)	毛状細胞性白血病
HCM(hypertrophic cardiomyopathy)	肥大型心筋症
hCS (human chorionic somatomammotropin)	ヒト絨毛性乳腺刺激ホルモン
HCU(high care unit)	高度治療室
HCV(hepatitis C virus)	C型肝炎ウイルス
HCVD(hypertensive cardiovascular disease)	高血圧性心血管疾患
HD(hemodialysis)	血液透析
HD(hip disarticulation)	股関節離断

HD (Hodgkin's disease)	ホジキン病
HD (house dust)	ハウスダスト
HDF (hemodiafiltration)	血液透析濾過
HDL (high density lipoprotein)	高比重リポ蛋白
HDL-C (HDL-cholesterol)	HDLコレステロール
HDN (hemolytic disease of the fetus and the newborn)	新生児溶血性疾患
HDN (hemorrhagic disease of newborn)	新生児出血性疾患
HDS (Hamilton depression scale)	ハミルトンうつ病評価尺度＝HAM-D
HDS (herniated disk syndrome)	椎間板ヘルニア症候群
HDT (high-dose chemoradiotherapy)	大量化学療法
HE (hereditary elliptocytosis)	遺伝性楕円赤血球症
HE (hyperbaric enema)	高圧浣腸
headache	頭痛
head control	頚定
heart	心臓
heat rash	汗疹
heartburn	胸やけ
heat intolerance	暑がり 対 寒がり ：cold intolerance
heatstroke	熱射病
heavy metal nephropathy	重金属腎症
hebephrenic type	破瓜型（統合失調症）
HEEH (home elemental enteral hyperalimentation)	在宅成分栄養経管栄養法
hematemesis	吐血
hematochezia	鮮血便
hematuria	血尿
hemiarthroplasty	半関節形成術
hemicrania	片頭痛
hemiplegia	片麻痺
	参照 両麻痺：diplegia 対麻痺：paraplegia

He

Hemo(hemorrhoids)	痔核
hemophilia	血友病
hemophilic arthritis	血友病性関節炎
hemoptysis	喀血
hemorrhagic cystitis	出血性膀胱炎
hemostasis	止血
hemothorax	血胸
HEN(home enteral nutrition)	在宅経管経腸栄養法
HEP(hepatic metastasis)	肝転移
hepatic coma	肝性昏睡
hepatomegaly	肝腫
hepatorenal syndrome	肝腎症候群
hereditary fructose intolerance	遺伝性果糖不耐症
hereditary nephritis	遺伝性腎炎
hermaphroditism	半陰陽
HES(hypereosinophilic syndrome)	好酸球増多症候群
HF(heart failure)	心不全 参照 急性心不全：AHF 慢性心不全：CHF
HF(hemofiltration)	血液濾過
HFJV(high frequency jet ventilation)	高頻度ジェット換気
HFMD(hand-foot and mouth disease)	手足口病
HFO, HFOV (high frequency oscillatory ventilation)	高頻度振動換気
HFS(hemifacial spasm)	半側顔面痙攣
HFV(high frequency ventilation)	高頻度人工換気
HG(herpes gestationis)	妊娠性疱疹、妊娠性ヘルペス
HH(homonymous hemianopia)	同名半盲
HHD(hypertensive heart disease)	高血圧性心疾患
HHE(hemiconvulsion-hemiplegia-epilepsia syndrome)	片側痙攣片麻痺てんかん症候群
HHM (humoral hypercalcemia of malignancy)	腫瘍随伴体液性高カルシウム血症

HHNC(hyperglycemic hyperosmolar nonketotic coma)	高血糖性高浸透圧性非ケトン性昏睡
HI(head injury)	頭部外傷
hibernating myocardium	冬眠心筋
hiccup	吃逆（しゃっくり）
HID(headache, insomnia, depression)	頭痛、不眠、うつ
HID(herniated intervertebral disc)	椎間板ヘルニア＝PID
HIE(hypoxic ischemic encephalopathy)	低酸素性虚血性脳症
high-arched palate	高口蓋
high-pitched cry	甲高い泣き声
high risk pregnancy	ハイリスク妊娠
hilar shadow	肺門陰影
hilus	肺門
hip joint	股関節
hip spica cast	股関節ギプス包帯
HIP(pregnancy-induced hypertension)	妊娠高血圧症＝PIH
histrionic personality disorder	演技的人格障害
HIT(hysteroscopic insemination into tube)	子宮鏡下卵管内受精法
HIV (human immunodeficiency virus)	ヒト免疫不全性ウイルス、エイズ
hive	蕁麻疹
H-J(Hugh-Jones)	ヒュー・ジョーンズ分類
HL(hearing loss)	聴力損失、難聴
HL(hyperlipidemia)	高脂血症（脂質異常症）
HLA(human leukocyte antigen)	ヒト白血球抗原
HLHS(hypoplastic left heart syndrome)	左心形成不全症候群
HLR(heart lung ratio)	心肺係数
HLTx(heart-lung transplantation)	心肺移植
HM(hand motion)	手動弁
hMG (human menopausal gonadotropin)	ヒト閉経期尿性ゴナドトロピン
HMV(home mechanical ventilation)	在宅人工呼吸療法
HNCM(hypertrophic nonobstructive cardiomyopathy)	肥大型非閉塞性心筋症

HN

HNKC(hyperosmolar nonketotic coma)	高浸透圧性非ケトン性昏睡
HNP(herniated nucleus pulposus)	髄核ヘルニア
hoarseness	嗄声
HOCM(hypertrophic obstructive cardiomyopathy)	肥大型閉塞性心筋症
HOH(hard of hearing)	難聴
holoprosencephaly	全前脳胞遺残症
homocystinuria	ホモシスチン尿症
homosexuality	同性愛
HONK(hyperosmolar non-keton)	高浸透圧性非ケトン性(糖尿病)
HONK(hyperosmolar non-ketotic hyperglycemic coma)	高浸透圧性非ケトン性高血糖昏睡
hordeolum	ものもらい＝stye
HOT(home oxygen therapy)	在宅酸素療法
hot pack	ホットパック
Hp(haptoglobin)	ハプトグロビン
HP(Helicobacter pylori)	ヘリコバクターピロリ
HP(hemoperfusion)	血液灌流
HP(history of present illness)	現病歴＝PI **関連** 既往歴：PH
HPA axis(hypothalamic-pituitary-adrenal)	視床下部－下垂体－副腎系
HPD(hepato-pancreatoduodenectomy)	肝膵頭十二指腸切除
hPL(human placental lactogen)	ヒト胎盤性ラクトゲン
HPLC(high-performance liquid chromatography)	高性能液体クロマトグラフィー
HPLH(hypoplastic left heart)	左心形成不全
HPMV(high-pressure mechanical ventilation)	高圧機械呼吸
HPN(home parenteral nutrition)	在宅(中心)静脈栄養法
HPRH(hypoplastic right heart)	右心形成不全
HPS(hypertrophic pyloric stenosis)	肥厚性幽門狭窄症
HPT(hyperparathyroidism)	上皮小体機能亢進症
HPV(hepatic portal vein)	肝門脈

HPV(human papilloma virus)	ヒト乳頭腫ウイルス
Hr(harn)	尿
HR(heart rate)	心拍数
HREH(high-renin essential hypertension)	高レニン本態性高血圧症
HRT(hormone replacement therapy)	ホルモン補充療法
HS(heart sound)	心音
HS(hereditary spherocytosis)	遺伝性球状赤血球症
HS(herpes simplex)	単純疱疹
HSCT (hematopoietic stem cell transplantation)	造血幹細胞移植
HSE(herpes simplex encephalitis)	単純ヘルペス性脳炎
HSG(herpes simplex genitalis)	外陰部単純ヘルペス
HSG(hysterosalpingography)	子宮卵管造影
HSL(herpes simplex labialis)	口唇単純ヘルペス
HSP(Henoch- Schönlein purpura)	シェーンライン・ヘノッホ紫斑病
HSP(hereditary spastic paraplegia)	遺伝性痙性対麻痺
HSPN (Henoch-Schönlein purpura nephritis)	シェーンライン・ヘノッホ紫斑病性腎炎
HSV(herpes simplex virus)	単純疱疹(ヘルペス)ウイルス
Ht(height)	身長
Ht(hematocrit)	ヘマトクリット値
HT(high temperature)	高温、高体温
HT(hypertension)	高血圧(症)
HT(hypertropia)	上斜視
HTC(hepatoma cell)	肝癌細胞
HTLV(human T-cell leukemia virus)	ヒトT細胞白血病ウイルス
HTLV-1 (human T-cell lymphotropic virus type 1)	ヒトT細胞リンパ行性ウイルス1型
HTO(high tibial osteotomy)	高位脛骨骨切術
HTP(house-tree-person technique)	家・樹木・人物画法
HTX(heart transplantation)	心移植
Hu(Humphry field analyzer irrigation)	ハンフリー自動視野計灌流吸引チップ
Hubbard tank	ハバードタンク

Hu

Hunter syndrome	ハンター症候群
Hurler syndrome	ハーラー症候群
HUS(hemolytic uremic syndrome)	溶血性尿毒症症候群
HV(hallux valgus)	外反母趾
HV(hepatic vein)	肝静脈
	対 肝動脈：HA
HV(hyperventilation)	換気亢進、呼吸亢進(過呼吸)
HVA(homovanillic acid)	ホモバニリン酸
HVGR(host versus graft reaction)	宿主対移植片反応
HV interval(His-ventricular interval)	ヒス―心室時間
HVS(hyperventilation syndrome)	過換気症候群
HVS(hyperviscosity syndrome)	過粘稠度症候群
Hy(hysteria)	ヒステリー
hyaline cartilage	硝子軟骨
hydrocephaly	水頭症
hydronephrosis	水腎症
hydrops	水腫
hydroureter	水尿管
hypalgesia	痛覚鈍麻
hyperacidity	胃酸過多
hyperactivity	多動機能亢進
hyperbilirubinemia	高ビリルビン血症
hypercalcinuria	高カルシウム尿症
hypercapnia	高炭酸ガス血症
hypercholesterolemia	高コレステロール血症
hyperesthesia	知覚過敏
hyperglycemia	高血糖
	対 低血糖：hypoglycemia
hyperhidrosis	発汗過多
hyperkalemia	高カリウム血症
hyperkinesia	運動亢進症、多動
hyperlipidemia	高脂血症
hyperlipoproteinemia	高リポ蛋白血症
hypermenorrhea	月経過多

hy

hyperopia	遠視
	◀関連▶乱視：AS
	近視：My
hyperparathyroidism	副甲状腺機能亢進症
hyperpnea	過呼吸
hyperprolactinemia	高プロラクチン血症
hypertelorism	両眼隔離症
hypertension	高血圧
hyperthyroidism	甲状腺機能亢進症
hypertonic saline infusion	高張食塩水負荷
hypertriglyceridemia	高トリグリセリド血症
hyperventilation syndrome	過呼吸症候群
hypesthesia	知覚鈍麻
hypnotherapy	催眠療法
hypnotics	催眠薬
Hypo(hypodermic injection)	皮下注射
	参照 静脈内注射：IV, iv
	筋肉内注射：I.m.
	皮内注射：SC, sc
hypoalbuminemia	低アルブミン血症
hypochondriacal delusion	心気妄想
hypochondriasis	心気症
hypocomplementemic glomerulonephritis	低補体性糸球体腎炎
hypoglossal N(nerve)	舌下神経（第12脳神経）
hypoglycemia	低血糖
	◀対▶高血糖：hyperglycemia
hypoparathyroidism	副甲状腺機能低下症
hypopituitarism	下垂体機能低下症
hypoplastic kidney	低形成腎
hypothalamus	視床下部
hypothyroidism	甲状腺機能低下症
hypotonic bladder	低緊張性膀胱
hypovolemia	循環血液量減少

hy

hypoxia	低酸素血症
hysterical neurosis	ヒステリー神経症
hystero(hysterosalpingography)	子宮卵管造影
HZ(herpes zoster)	帯状疱疹
Hz(Hertz)	ヘルツ
HZ(Herz)	心臓
HZV(herpes zoster virus)	帯状疱疹ウイルス

I

I (ileum)	回腸
IA (induced abortion)	人工妊娠中絶
IA (infantile autism)	乳児自閉症
IA (intraarterial)	動脈内
	対 静脈内(の)：IV
IA (intraarticular)	関節内
IAA (ileo-anal anastomosis)	回腸肛門吻合術
IAA (interruption of aortic arch)	大動脈弓遮断
IABP (intra aortic balloon pumping)	大動脈内バルーンパンピング
IADL (instrumental activities of daily life)	器具による日常生活動作
IAJ (isthmo-ampullary junction)	峡部膨大部境界
IAM (internal auditory meatus)	内耳道
IAR (interferon beta, nimustine and radiation)	インターフェロンβ、ニムスチンと放射線照射の併用療法
IARF (ischemic acute renal failure)	虚血性急性腎不全
IAS (interatrial septum)	心房中隔
IBD (inflammatory bowel disease)	炎症性腸疾患
IBL (immunoblastic lymphadenopathy)	免疫芽球性リンパ腺症
IBS (immunoblastic sarcoma)	免疫芽球性肉腫
IBS (irritable bowel syndrome)	過敏性腸管症候群
IC (informed consent)	インフォームド・コンセント
IC (inspiratory capacity)	最大吸気量
IC (intercostal)	肋間の
IC (intermittent claudication)	間欠性跛行
IC (internal carotid artery)	内頚動脈＝ICA
IC (invasive carcinoma)	浸潤癌
IC (ischemic colitis)	虚血性大腸炎
ICA (ileocolic artery)	回腸結腸動脈
ICA (internal carotid artery)	内頚動脈
	対 外頚動脈：ECA
ICA (islet cell antibody)	抗膵島細胞抗体
ICCE (intracapsular cataract extraction)	水晶体嚢内摘出術

IC

ICD(implantable cardiac defibrillator)	植込型除細動器
ICD(International Classification of Diseases)	国際疾病分類
ICF(intracellular fluid)	細胞内液(量)
ICG test(indocyanine green test)	インドシアニングリーン試験
ICH(intracranial hematoma)	頭蓋内血腫
ICH(intracranial hemorrhage)	脳内出血
ICH(intracranial hypertension)	頭蓋内圧亢進=IICP
ICL(intraocular contact lens)	眼内コンタクトレンズ
ICM(idiopathic cardiomegaly)	特発性心拡大
ICP(intracranial pressure)	頭蓋内圧
ICPC(internal carotid posterior communicating aneurysm)	内頚動脈後交通動脈分岐部動脈瘤
IC-PC(internal carotid - posterior communicating artery)	内頚動脈後交通動脈
ICR(ileocecal resection)	回盲部切除術
ICS(intercostal space)	肋間腔
ICS(irritable colon syndrome)	過敏性結腸症候群
ICSI(intracytoplasmic sperm injection)	卵実質内精子注入法、顕微受精
ICT(induction chemotherapy)	術前化学療法
ICT(intracoronary thrombolysis)	冠動脈内血栓溶解療法
ICT(intracranial tumor)	頭蓋内腫瘍
ICU(intensive care unit)	集中治療室
ID(identification)	IDカード
I&D(incision and drainage)	切開排膿
IDA(iron deficiency anemia)	鉄欠乏性貧血
IDDM(insulin-dependent diabetes mellitus)	インスリン依存性糖尿病
	参照 インスリン非依存性糖尿病：NIDDM
idea of reference	関連妄想
identity	アイデンティティ
IDK(internal derangement of knee)	膝内障
IDM(idiopathic disease of the myocardium)	特発性心筋疾患
IDM(infant of diabetic mother)	糖尿病母体児

IDS(immunity deficiency syndrome)	免疫不全症候群
IDUS(intraductal ultrasonography)	胆管腔内超音波検査法
IDV(intermittent demand ventilation)	間欠的強制呼吸
IE(infective endocarditis)	感染性心内膜炎
I/E(inspiratory time/expiratory time)	吸気時間／呼気時間
IFN(interferon)	インターフェロン
Ig(immunoglobulin)	免疫グロブリン
IgA(immunoglobulin A)	免疫グロブリンA
IgA nephropathy	IgA腎症
IGE(idiopathic generalized epilepsy)	特発性全般てんかん
IGF(insulin-like growth factor)	インスリン様成長因子
IgG(immunoglobulin G)	免疫グロブリンG
IgM(immunoglobulin M)	免疫グロブリンM
IGT(impaired glucose tolerance)	耐糖能異常
IGTT(intravenous glucose tolerance test)	静脈性糖負荷試験
IH(infectious hepatitis)	流行性肝炎
IHA(infusion hepatic angiography)	持続注入肝動脈血管造影
IHB(infantile hyperbilirubinemia)	新生児高ビリルビン血症
IHC(intrahepatic cholestasis)	肝内胆汁うっ滞
IHD(intrahepatic bile duct)	肝内胆管
IHD(ischemic heart disease)	虚血性心疾患
IHF(immune hydrops fetalis)	免疫性胎児水腫
IHPH(intrahepatic portal hypertension)	肝内門脈圧亢進
IHSS(idiopathic hypertrophic subaortic stenosis)	特発性肥大型大動脈弁下狭窄症
IIA(internal iliac artery)	内腸骨動脈
	対 外腸骨動脈：EIA
IICP(increased intracranial pressure)	頭蓋内圧亢進＝ICH
IIP(idiopathic interstitial pneumonia)	特発性間質性肺炎
IL(interleukin)	インターロイキン
ILBBB(incomplete left bundle branch block)	不完全左脚ブロック
ILD(interstitial lung disease)	間質性肺疾患
ILV(independent lung ventilation)	片側肺換気
IM(infectious mononucleosis)	伝染性単核球症

Im

I.m.(intramuscular injection)	筋肉内注射
	参照 皮下注射：Hypo
	静脈内注射：IV, iv
	皮内注射：SC, sc
Im(middle intrathoracic esophagus)	胸部中部食道
IM, im(intramuscle〔injection〕)	筋肉（筋肉内注射）
IMA(inferior mesenteric artery)	下腸間膜動脈
IMD(ischemic myocardial damage)	虚血性心筋障害
IMF(intermaxillary fixation)	顎間固定
immune complex glomerulonephritis	免疫複合体腎炎
immunochemotherapy	免疫化学療法
impacted fracture	くいこみ骨折
implantatio tubae	卵管移植術
impulse control disorder	衝動抑制障害
IMR(interferon-beta, ranimustine and radiation)	インターフェロンβ、ラニムスチンと放射線照射の併用療法
IMV(inferior mesenteric vein)	下腸間膜静脈
IMV(intermittent mandatory ventilation)	間欠的強制換気法
IN(icterus neonatorum)	新生児黄疸
inc(increasing)	増加
incarceration of hernia	嵌頓ヘルニア
incest	近親相姦
incoherence	散乱
incontinence of urine	尿失禁
increased muscle tonus	筋トーヌス亢進
incubator	保育器
index finger	人差し指
indigestion	消化不良
INE (infantile nectrotizing encephalomyelopathy)	乳児壊死性脳脊髄障害
INF(infiltration)	浸潤、癌浸潤度
Inf(inflammatory changes)	炎症
infancy	乳児期

infantile sexuality	小児性欲
infection	感染
infectious arthritis	感染性関節炎
inferiority complex	劣等感
INFH(idiopathic necrosis of the femoral head)	特発性大腿骨頭壊死
inflammation	炎症
influence of thought	思考干渉
inguinal hernia	鼠径ヘルニア
inhalation	吸入
	対 吸引：suction/asporation
inj(injection)	注射　関連 点滴：DI
inoculation	予防接種
INPB (intermittent negative pressure breathing)	間欠的陰圧呼吸
INPV (intermittent negative pressure ventilation)	間欠的陰圧換気
INS(idiopathic nephrotic syndrome)	特発性ネフローゼ症候群
insanity	精神錯乱
insight	病識
insight therapy	洞察療法
Insp(inspiration)	吸気
	対 呼気：expiration/exhalation
instinct	本能
insulin	インスリン
insulinoma	インスリノーマ
intelligence	知能
intercostal artery	肋間動脈
intercostal neuralgia	肋間神経痛
intermittent explosive disorder	間欠性爆発性障害
interpersonal relations	対人関係
interstitial nephritis	間質性腎炎
interview	面接

in

intracranial hypertension increased	頭蓋内圧亢進
intractable diarrhea in infancy	乳児性難治性下痢症
intrinsic muscle	内在筋
in-utero diagnosis	羊水診断
INVAGI(invagination)	腸重積症
invagination	腸重積症＝INVAGI
IO(inferior oblique muscle)	下斜筋
IO(intestinal obstruction)	腸閉塞
IOH(idiopathic orthostatic hypotension)	特発性起立性低血圧症
IOL(intraocular lens)	眼内レンズ
ION(idiopathic osteonecrosis of femoral head)	特発性大腿骨頭壊死
IOP(intraocular pressure)	眼圧
IP(ifosfamide, cisplatin)	イホスファミド、シスプラチン併用療法
IP(interphalangeal)	指節間関節＝IPJ
IP(interstitial pneumonia)	間質性肺炎
IP(intraperitoneal)	腹腔内の
IP(intravenous pyelography)	静脈性腎盂造影
IP(irinotecan, cisplatin)	イリノテカン、シスプラチン併用療法
IPD(intermittent peritoneal dialysis)	間欠的腹膜透析
IPF(idiopathic pulmonary fibrosis)	特発性肺線維症
IPH(idiopathic portal hypertension)	特発性門脈圧亢進症
IPH(idiopathic pulmonary hemosiderosis)	特発性肺ヘモジデリン沈着症
IPJ(interphalangeal joint)	指節間関節＝IP
IPL (idiopathic plasmacytic lymphadenopathy)	特発性プラズマ細胞性リンパ腺症
IPNPB(intermittent positive negative pressure breathing)	間欠的陽陰圧呼吸
IPNPV(intermittent positive negative pressure ventilation)	間欠的陽陰圧換気
IPP(intrahepatic portal pressure)	肝内門脈圧

IPPB (intermittent positive pressure breathing)	間欠的陽圧呼吸
IPPF (immediate postsurgical prosthetic fitting)	術直後義肢装着法＝IPSF
IPPV (intermittent positive pressure ventilation)	間欠的陽圧換気法
IPSF(immediate postsurgical fitting)	術直後義肢装着法＝IPPF
IPSP(inhibitory postsynaptic potentials)	抑制性シナプス後電位
IQ(intelligence quotient)	知能指数
IR(internal rotation)	内旋　対 外旋：ER
IRA(ileo-rectal anastomosis)	回腸直腸吻合術
IRA(inferior rectal artery)	下直腸動脈
IRBBB (incomplete right bundle branch block)	不完全右脚ブロック
IRD(idiopathic respiratory distress)	特発性呼吸窮迫
IRDNI(idiopathic respiratory distress of the newborn infant)	特発性新生児呼吸障害
IRDS (idiopathic respiratory distress syndrome)	特発性呼吸窮迫症候群
IRDS(infantile respiratory distress syndrome)	新生児呼吸窮迫症候群
IRI(immuno reactive insulin)	免疫反応性インスリン
iritis	虹彩炎
iron deficiency anemia	鉄欠乏性貧血
irritability	被刺激性
IRSA (idiopathic refractory sideroblastic anemia)	特発性不応性鉄芽球性貧血
IRV(inspiratory reserve volume)	予備吸気量
ischemic contracture	阻血性拘縮
ischemic kidney	虚血腎
ischial spine	坐骨棘
ischioneuralgia	坐骨神経痛＝sciatica
ischuria	尿閉
ISD(immunosuppressive drug)	免疫抑制薬
ISD(interventricular septal defect)	心室中隔欠損

IS

ISO(international organization for standardization)	国際標準化機構
ISS(injury severity score)	外傷重症度スコア
I-S stomy(ileo-sigmoidostomy)	回腸S状結腸吻合術
IT(inhalation therapy)	吸入療法
ITP(idiopathic thrombocytopenic purpura)	特発性血小板減少性紫斑病
ITP(intrathoracic pressure)	胸腔内圧
ITT(insulin tolerance test)	インスリン負荷試験
IU(international unit)	国際単位
Iu(upper intrathoracic esophagus)	胸部上部食道
IUCD(intrauterine contraceptive device)	子宮内避妊器具
IUD(intrauterine device)	子宮内避妊器具
IUFD(intrauterine fetal death)	子宮内胎児死亡＝FDIU
IUGR(intrauterine growth retardation)	子宮内胎児発育不全(遅延)
IUP(intrauterine pressure)	子宮内圧
IV(intravenous)	静脈内(の) 対 動脈内：IA
IV, iv(intravenous)	静脈
I.v.(intravenous injection)	静脈内注射 参照 筋肉内注射：I.m. 皮下注射：Hypo 皮内注射：SC, sc
IVC(inferior vena cava)	下大静脈
IVC(inspiratory vital capacity)	吸気肺活量
IVC(intravenous cholecystography)	経静脈的胆嚢造影
IVCY(intermittent pulse intravenous cyclophosphamide therapy)	シクロホスファミド大量静注療法
IVF(in vitro fertilization)	体外受精
IVF-ET (in-vitro fertilization and embryo transfer)	体外受精胚移植
IVH(intravenous hyperalimentation)	中心静脈栄養 対 末梢静脈栄養：PVN
IVH(intraventricular hemorrhage)	脳出血

IVM(involuntary movement)	不随意運動
	対 随意運動：autokinesia
IVP(intravenous pyelography)	静脈性腎盂造影
IVS(interventricular septum)	心室中隔
IVSD(interventricular septum defect)	心室中隔欠損
IVU(intravenous urography)	静脈性尿路造影

JB(Jetzing Brille)	現在のメガネ
JCAHO(joint commission on accreditation of healthcare organization)	米国病院医療評価機構
JCML(juvenile type chronic myelocytic leukemia)	若年性慢性骨髄性白血病
JCS(Japan Coma Scale)	日本昏睡(ジャパン・コーマ)スケール
JDM(juvenile diabetes mellitus)	若年性糖尿病
JE(Japanese encephalitis)	日本脳炎
jeopardized collateral	危機に瀕した側副血行路
JGA(juxtaglomerular apparatus)	傍糸球体装置
JJ(jaw jerk)	下顎反射
JMDP(Japanese marrow donation program)	日本骨髄バンク
JOD(juvenile onset diabetes)	若年性糖尿病
joint capsule	関節包
JPD(jejunal pouch double tract)	空腸再建術
JRA(juvenile rheumatoid arthritis)	若年性関節リウマチ
Judkins's method	ジャドキンス法
Jug.(jugular venous pulse wave)	頸静脈波
juvenile cataract	若年性白内障
juvenile diabetes	若年性糖尿病
JVD(jugular venous distention)	頸静脈怒張

K(kalium)	カリウム
K(keratosis)	角化上皮
KAFO(knee-ankle-foot orthosis)	長下肢装具＝LLB, SKA orthosis
KAS(Katz adjustment scales)	カッツ法
KBN(Kondylonbettung Münster)	ミュンスター式果部荷重下腿義足
K cell(killer cell)	キラー細胞
KCP(knee chest posture)	膝胸位
KCT(kaolin clotting time)	カオリン凝固時間
Kent bundle	ケント束
keratoplasty	角膜移植
Kernicterus	核黄疸
ketogenic hypoglycemia	ケトン血性低血糖症
ketone body	ケトン体
ketonuria	ケトン体尿
ketosis	ケトーシス
ketotic hypoglycemia	ケトン性低血糖症
KICU(kidney intensive care unit)	腎疾患集中治療室
kidney	腎臓
kidney calculi	腎結石
kidney transplantation	腎移植
Killip's classification	キリップ分類
kinesitherapy	運動療法
KIP(Klinische Intelligenz Prüfung)	慶応式臨床知能検査
KJ(knee jerk)	膝蓋腱反射＝PTR
KK(Kollumkarzinom)	子宮体部癌
KKK(Kehlkopfkrebs)	喉頭癌
kleptomania	窃盗癖
Kluver-Bucy syndrome	クリューバー・ビューシー症候群
KM(Kuhmilch)	牛乳
knee cap	膝蓋骨＝patella

•kn•

knee jerk	膝蓋腱反射＝KJ, PTR
knee joint	膝関節
knock-knee	X脚　◀関連▶ O脚：bowleg
Korsakoff's psychosis	コルサコフ精神病
Korsakoff's syndrome	コルサコフ症候群
kot	便（コートと読む）
KP(keratic precipitates)	角膜後面沈着物
KPE(Kelman's phacoemulsification)	超音波水晶体乳化吸引術
KS(Kaposi sarcoma)	カポジ肉腫
KSD(keratitis superficialis diffusa)	びまん性表層角結膜炎
KSS(Kearns-Sayre syndrome)	カーンズ・セイヤー症候群
KUB(kidney, ureter and bladder)	腎、尿管、膀胱（撮影）
Kussmaul breathing	クスマウル呼吸
KVO(keep vein open)	静脈確保
KW(Keith-Wagener classification)	キース・ワグナーの分類
Kymo(kymography)	動態撮影
kyphosis	脊柱後弯症、後弯（症）

L

L(lateral segment)	左葉外側区域（肝）
L(left)	左　対 右：R
L(lues)	梅毒
L(lumbar)	腰椎の、腰髄の
L(lumbar spine)	腰椎
L1, L2, L3,…L5(lumbar vertebrae first, second, third,…fifth)	第1（2、3、5）腰椎
L1(primary lung cancer)	原発性肺癌
L2(metastatic lung cancer)	転移性肺癌
LA(left atrium)	左心房　対 右心房：RA
LA(left renal artery)	左腎動脈
LA(local anesthesia)	局所麻酔
	参照 全身麻酔：GA
LA(lumbar artery)	腰動脈
LABC(lymphadenosis benigna cutis)	皮膚良性リンパ腺腫症
labor	陣痛
labyrinthitis	内耳炎
LAC(laparoscopic assisted colectomy)	腹腔鏡補助下大腸切除術
laceration	裂傷、破裂傷
lactate	乳酸
LAD(left anterior descending coronary artery)	左冠動脈前下行枝
LAD(left axis deviation)	左軸偏位
LAD(leukocyte adhesion deficiency)	白血球接着不全症
LAFR(laminar air flow room)	無菌室
LAH(left anterior hemiblock)	左脚前枝ブロック
LAH(left atrial hypertrophy)	左房肥大
laminar air flow unit	無菌室＝LAFR
laminectomy	椎弓切除術
laminotomy	椎弓切開術（椎弓形成）
language disorder	言語障害
languor	倦怠
lanugo	産毛

la

lap(laparotomy)	開腹(術)
LAP(left atrial pressure)	左(心)房圧
Lapa(ro)(laparoscopy)	腹腔鏡検査
laparoscopic surgery	腹腔鏡下手術
LAR(late allergic response)	遅延型アレルギー反応
LAR(late asthmatic response)	遅発型喘息反応
LAR(low anterior resection)	低位前方切除術
laryngeal cancer	喉頭癌=KKK
laryngomalacia	喉頭軟化症
LASER(light amplification by stimulated emission of radiation)	レーザー
LASIK, Lasik(laser in situ keratomileusis)	レーザー生体内角膜切開(術)
lassitude	(精神的、肉体的な)だるさ
late deceleration	遅発性一過性徐脈
latent infection	潜伏感染
lateral recumbent position	側臥位 ◀関連▶仰臥位：dorsal position 腹臥位：proneness
LATS(long-acting thyroid stimulator)	持続性甲状腺刺激物質
LAV(lymphadenopathy-associated virus)	リンパ節症関連ウイルス
LAVH (laparoscopic-assisted vaginal hysterectomy)	腹腔鏡補助下子宮摘出術
laxative	下剤、緩下薬
LB(low back)	背下部
LBBB(left bundle branch block)	左脚ブロック ◀関連▶右脚ブロック：RBBB
LBC(lymphadenosis benigna cutis)	皮膚良性リンパ腺腫症
LBP(low back pain)	腰痛
LBP(low blood pressure)	低血圧 ◀対▶高血圧：HBT, HT
LBW, LBWI(low birth weight〔infant〕)	低出生体重児
LC(laparoscopic cholecystectomy)	腹腔鏡下胆嚢摘出術
LC(laryngitis chronica)	慢性喉頭炎

LD

LC(liver cirrhosis)	肝硬変
LC(loss of consciousness)	意識障害
LC(lung cancer)	肺癌
LCA(left colic artery)	左結腸動脈
LCA(left common carotid artery)	左総頚動脈
LCA(left coronary artery)	左冠状動脈
	◀関連▶ 右冠状動脈：RCA
	左回旋枝：LCX
Lcc(liver cell carcinoma)	肝細胞癌＝HCC
LCC(luxatio coxae congenita)	先天性股関節脱臼
LCCA(late cerebellar cortical atrophy)	晩発性小脳皮質萎縮症
LCCS(low cervical cesarean section)	低子宮頚部帝王切開（術）
LCL(laparoscopic choledocholithotomy)	腹腔鏡下総胆管切石術
LCL(lateral collateral ligament)	外側側副靭帯
LCM(lymphocytic choriomeningitis)	リンパ球性脈絡髄膜炎
LCOS(low cardiac output syndrome)	低心拍出量症候群
LCV(leukocytoclastic vasculitis)	白血球破壊性血管炎
LCX(left circumflex)	左回旋枝
	◀関連▶ 右冠状動脈：RCA
	左冠状動脈：LCA
LCX(left circumflex artery)	左冠動脈回旋枝
LD(learning disability)	学習障害
LD(lethal dose)	致死量
LDA(left dorsoanterior〔position〕)	左背前位（胎位）
LDA(low density area)	低吸収濃度域
LDGL(lymphoproliferative disease of granular lymphocytes)	顆粒リンパ球増多症
LDH(lactase dehydrogenase)	乳酸脱水素酵素
LDH(lumber disk herniation)	腰椎椎間板ヘルニア
LDL(low density lipoprotein)	低比重リポ蛋白
L-DLE(localized disseminated lupus erythematosus)	限局性播種性エリテマトーデス
LDMC(latissimus dorsi myocutaneous flap)	広背筋皮弁
LDP(left dorsoposterior〔position〕)	左背後位（胎位）

LE

LE(left eye)	左眼　対　右眼：RE
LE(lupus erythematosus)	紅斑性狼瘡、ループスエリテマトーデス
lead nephrotoxicity	鉛腎毒性
learning theory	学習説
LECV(late extra cephalic version)	妊娠末期骨盤位外回転術
LED(lupus erythematosus disseminatus)	播種性紅斑性狼瘡
Leigh subacute necrotizing encephalopathy	リー亜急性壊死性脳症
LEL(lymphoepithelial lesion)	リンパ上皮性病変
LEP(lupus erythematosus profundus)	深在性エリテマトーデス
leprosy	癩、ハンセン病
LES(lower esophageal sphincter)	下部食道括約筋
LET(leukocyte esterase test)	白血球エステラーゼテスト
lethargy	嗜眠
leukemia	白血病
leukorrhea	帯下
Levin tube	経鼻胃管
Levine 1／6, 2／6, 3／6, 4／6, 5／6, 6／6	レバイン心雑音強度分類1〜6度
LFA(left frontoanterior〔position〕)	左前頭前位(胎位)
LFD(large for dates infant)	不当重量児
LFD(least fatal dose)	最小致死量
LFD infant(large for dates infant)	日数不当重量児
LFP(left frontoposterior〔position〕)	左前頭後位(胎位)
LFT(left frontotransverse〔position〕)	左前頭横位(胎位)
LFT(liver function test)	肝機能検査
LFT(lung function test)	肺機能検査
LG(limb-girdle〔muscular dystrophy〕)	肢帯型筋ジストロフィー
LGA(left gastric artery)	左胃動脈
LGEA(left gastroepiploic artery)	左胃大網動脈
LGL(large granular lymphocyte leukemia)	大型顆粒リンパ球性白血病
LGL(Lown-Ganong-Levine syndrome)	ローン・ギャノング・レバイン症候群

LGV(lymphogranuloma venereum)	性病性リンパ肉芽腫
LH(luteinizing hormone)	黄体形成ホルモン
LH-RH (luteinizing hormone releasing hormone)	黄体形成ホルモン放出ホルモン
LHA(lateral hypothalamic area)	外側視床下部
LHA(left hepatic artery)	左肝動脈 ◀対▶ 右肝動脈：RHA
LHB(left heart bypass)	左心バイパス
LHC(left heart catheterization)	左心カテーテル法
LHD(luetic heart disease)	梅毒性心疾患
LHF(left side heart failure)	左心不全 ◀関連▶ 右心不全：RHF
LHV(left hepatic vein)	左肝静脈 ◀対▶ 右肝静脈：RHV
LI(lamellar ichthyosis)	葉状魚鱗癬
libido	リビドー、性欲
lichen	苔癬
life prolonging measure	延命処置
ligament injury	靭帯損傷
light reflex absent	対光反射なし
LIH(left inguinal hernia)	左鼠径ヘルニア
LIMA(left internal mammarial artery)	左内胸動脈
limited operation	縮小手術
Lin(liniment)	塗布剤
linac(linear accelerator)	直線加速器
LIP(lymphocytic interstitial pneumonia)	リンパ球性間質性肺炎
lipoid nephrosis	リポイドネフローゼ
Liq(liquor cerebrospinalis)	リコール（髄液）
Lisfranc joint	足根中足関節
lissencephaly	脳回欠損
LITA(left internal thoracic artery)	左内胸動脈
liver transplantation	肝移植
LK(locus Kiesselbach)	キーゼルバッハ部位
LK(lungenkrebs)	肺癌

LL

LL(lower lid)	下眼瞼
LL(lower lobe)	下肺葉
LL(lymphocytic leukemia)	リンパ球性白血病
LLB(long leg brace)	長下肢装具
LLC(laparoscopic laser cholecystectomy)	腹腔鏡下レーザー胆嚢摘出術
LLC(long leg cast)	長下肢ギプス包帯
LLN(lower limits of normal)	正常下限
LLQ(left lower quadrant)	左下腹部
LLSB(left limits of sternal border)	胸骨下部左縁
LLV(lymphatic leukemia virus)	リンパ性白血病ウイルス
LM(lateral meniscus)	外側半月
	対 内側半月：MM
LMA(left mentoanterior〔position〕)	左頤部前位(体位)
LMD(local medical doctor)	近医、開業医
LMDF(lupus miliaris disseminatus faciei)	顔面播種状粟粒性狼瘡
LMM(lentigo maligna melanoma)	悪性黒子黒色腫
LMP(last menstrual period)	最終月経＝LPM, LR
LMP(left mentoposterior〔position〕)	左頤部後位(胎位)
LMRP(local medical review policy)	地球医療再検討方策
LMT(left main coronary trunk)	冠動脈主幹部
LMT(left mentotransverse〔position〕)	左頤部横位(胎位)
LMWP(low molecular weight protein)	低分子蛋白
LN(lipoid nephrosis)	微小変化群＝MC
LN(lupus nephritis)	ループス腎炎
LN(lymph node)	リンパ節
L/N(lymph node)	リンパ節
LOA(left occipitoanterior〔position〕)	第1頭位第1分類(胎位)
lobe	葉、裂片
LOC(loss of consciousness)	意識消失
lochia	悪露
Logo therapy	ロゴ療法
LOM(limitation of motion)	運動制限
loop diuretic	ループ利尿薬
loosening	ゆるみ

LS

LOP(left occipito-posterior〔position〕)	第1頭位第2分類(胎位)
lordosis	脊柱前弯症、前弯(症)
LOS(low output syndrome)	低心拍出量症候群
loss of consciousness	意識消失、意識喪失＝LOC
LOT(left occipito-transverse〔position〕)	第1頭位(胎位)
low set ear lobe	耳介低位
Lowe syndrome	ロー症候群
lower extremity	下肢
	対 上肢：upper extremity
lowest part	先進部
LP(late ventricular potential)	心室遅延電位
Lp(lipoprotein)	リポ蛋白
LP(lumbar puncture)	腰椎穿刺(ルンバール)
LPD(lymphoproliferative disease)	リンパ増殖性疾患
LPDS(lyophilized porcine dermal skin)	凍結乾燥豚真皮
LPH(low perfusion hyperemia)	低灌流充血
LPL(lipoprotein lipase)	リポ蛋白リパーゼ
LPM(last period of menstruation)	最終月経＝LMP, LR
LPM(low potential malignancy)	低悪性度腫瘍
LPRC(leukocyte poor red cells)	白血球除去赤血球
L-P shunt(lumbo-peritoneal shunt)	腰椎クモ膜下腔－腹腔短絡術
LpX(lipoprotein X)	リポ蛋白X
LR(letzte Regel)	最終月経(期)＝LMP, LPM
LR(light reflex)	対光反射
L-R shunt(left to right shunt)	左右短絡
LS(lymphosarcoma)	リンパ肉腫
L-S(lumbo-sacral)	腰仙部、腰仙椎、腰仙髄
LSA(left sacrum anterior)	第1骨盤位第1分類(胎位)
LSA(lichen sclerosus et atrophicus)	硬化性萎縮性苔癬
LSA(liver specific antigen)	肝特異抗原
LSB(left sternal border)	胸骨左縁
LSC, LSCT(laparoscopic cholecystectomy)	腹腔鏡下胆嚢摘出術(ラパコレ)

LS

LScP(left scapula posterior〔position〕)	左肩甲骨後位
LSCS(lumber spinal canal stenosis)	腰部脊柱管狭窄症
LSO(left salpingo-oophorectomy)	左側付器摘出(術)
LSP(left sacroposterior〔position〕)	第1骨盤位第2分類(胎位)
LSS(life support system)	生命維持装置
LST(lateral spreading tumor)	側方伸展型(大腸)腫瘍
LST(left sacrotransverse〔position〕)	第1骨盤位(胎位)
LST(lymphocyte stimulation test)	リンパ球刺激テスト
LSVC(left superior vena cave)	左上大静脈
Lt(lower thoracic esophagus)	胸部下部食道
LTA(laryngotracheal anesthesia)	喉頭気管麻酔
LTG(low-tension glaucoma)	低眼圧緑内障
LTH(luteotrop(h)ic hormone)	黄体刺激ホルモン
LTM(long-term memory)	長期記憶
	◀関連▶ 短期記憶：STM
LTOT(long term oxygen therapy)	長期酸素療法
LTP(laser trabeculoplasty)	レーザー線維柱帯形成術
LTV(long term variability)	緩やかな胎児心拍数基線細変動
LTX(lung transplantation)	肺移植
LUF(luteinized unruptured follicle)	黄体形成未破裂卵胞
LUL(left upper lobe)	左(肺)上葉
LUL(left upper lobectomy)	左肺上葉切除
lumbago	腰痛
lumbar disc herniation	椎間板ヘルニア
lumbosacral strain	ぎっくり腰
lung base	肺底部
lupus	狼瘡、皮膚結核
lupus nephritis	ループス腎炎
LUQ(left upper quadrant)	左上腹部
Luschka joint	椎鉤(ルシュカ)関節
LV(left ventricle)	左心室　◀対▶右心室：RV
LV(left vision, left visus)	左眼視力
	◀関連▶右眼視力：RV

LV(live vaccine)	生ワクチン
LVAD(left ventricular assist device)	左室補助装置＝LVAS
LVAS(left ventricular assist system)	左室補助装置＝LVAD
LVD(left ventricular diameter dimension)	左室径
LVD(left ventricular dysfunction)	左室機能不全
LVEDD (left ventricular end-diastolic dimension)	左室拡張末期径
LVESD (left ventricular end-systolic dimension)	左室収縮末期径
LVET(left ventricular ejection time)	左心室駆出時間
LVF(left ventricular failure)	左室不全 ◀関連▶右心不全：RVF
LVG(left ventriculography)	左室造影
LVH(left ventricular hypertrophy)	左室肥大 ◀関連▶右室肥大：RVH
LV mass(left ventricular mass)	左室体積
LV out(left ventricular outflow tract)	左室流出路
LVPW(left ventricular posterior wall)	左室後壁
LVSW(left ventricular stroke work)	左室1回仕事量
LVSWI(left ventricular stroke work index)	左室1回仕事係数
LVV(left ventricular volume)	左室容量
LW(Lendenwirbel)	腰椎
LX(luxation)	脱臼、転位
LYM(lymph node metastasis)	リンパ節転移
Lym(lymphocyte)	リンパ球 ◀関連▶単球：MO/monocyte 顆粒球：granulocyte
lymphoma	リンパ腫 ◀関連▶悪性リンパ腫：malignant lymphoma

M

M(malignant)	悪性の
M(medial segment)	左葉内側区域(肝)
M(meningioma)	髄膜腫
M(metastasis)	遠隔転移(TNM分類)
M(mosaic)	モザイク
m癌(mucosa)	粘膜層の癌(壁深達度)
M領域	胃角部領域(胃中部1/3)
MA(megaloblastic anemia)	巨赤芽球貧血
MA(microaneurysm)	毛細血管瘤
MA(mitral atresia)	僧帽弁閉鎖症
MAAS (massive amnion aspiration syndrome)	羊水過量吸引症候群
MABP(mean arterial blood pressure)	平均血圧＝MBP
MAC(maximal acid concentration)	最高酸濃度
macroadenoma	巨大腺腫
macroglobulinemia	マクログロブリン血症
macroglossia	巨大舌
MAD(major affective disorder)	大感情障害
MAD(maximum allowable dose)	最大許容線量
Mahaim fibers	マハイム束、線維
MAHC (malignancy associated hypercalcemia)	悪性腫瘍随伴性高カルシウム血症
maintain patient airway	気道確保
maintenance	継続投与
Maj(major curvature of stomach)	胃大弯 ◀関連▶ 胃小弯：Min
major tranquilizer	神経安定薬
maladjustment	適応障害
malaise	倦怠(感)
mal-alignment	歯列不正
malignant	悪性、悪性の ◀対▶ 良性の：benign

malignant GCT (malignant giant cell tumor)	悪性巨細胞腫
malignant nephrosclerosis	悪性腎硬化症
mallet finger	つち指
Mallory-Weiss syndrome	マロリー・ワイス症候群
malnutrition	栄養不良、栄養失調症
malocclusion	不正咬合
malposition	不良肢位
MALT (mucosa-associated lymphoid tissue)	粘膜関連リンパ組織
mal-union	変形癒合
mandibular respiration	下顎呼吸
manic depressive psychosis	躁うつ病
manic excitement	躁病興奮
manic type	躁状態
manifest anxiety test	顕在性不安検査
manipulation	徒手整復
mannerism	衒奇（わざとらしさ）
MAO (maximal acid output)	最高酸分泌量
MAO (mesenteric arterial occlusion)	腸間膜動脈閉塞症
MAO (monoamine oxidase)	モノアミン酸化酵素
MAP (mannitol-adenine-phosphate solution)	ヒト赤血球濃厚液（マンニトール、アデニン、リン酸液）
MAP (mitral annuloplasty)	僧帽弁（弁輪）形成術
MAPCA (major aorto-pulmonary collateral artery)	主要体肺側副動脈
MAR (bone marrow metastasis)	骨髄転移
march hemoglobinuria	行軍血色素尿症
marital therapy	夫婦療法
mark	傷、しみ、あざ
MAS (malabsorption syndrome)	吸収不良症候群
MAS (Manifest Anxiety Scale〔Taylor〕)	テイラー不安検査（顕在性不安尺度）
MAS (massive aspiration syndrome)	過量吸引症候群

・MA・

MAS (massive aspiration syndrome of newborn)	新生児過量吸引症候群
MAS(meconium aspiration syndrome)	胎便吸引症候群
masked depression	仮面うつ病
masochism	被虐嗜愛
mass transfer coefficient	質量転移係数
MAS syndrome(malabsorption syndrome)	吸収不良症候群
mastication	咀嚼
MAT(multifocal atrial tachycardia)	多源性心房性頻脈
maternal transport	母体搬送＝MT
MAVR(mitral and aortic valve replacement)	僧帽弁大動脈弁置換
maximal pressure	最高血圧
MB(medulloblastoma)	髄芽腫
MBC(maximum bladder capacity)	最大膀胱許容量
MBC(maximum breathing capacity)	最大換気量、分時最大呼吸量
MBD(minimal brain damage〔syndrome〕)	微小脳損傷(症候群)
MBD(minimal brain dysfunction)	微小脳障害
MBL(menstrual blood loss)	月経量
MBP(mean blood pressure)	平均血圧＝MABP
MC(mineralocorticoid)	鉱質コルチコイド
MC(minimal change)	微小変化群
MC(molluscum contagiosum)	伝染性軟属腫
MCA(middle cerebral artery)	中大脳動脈
MCA(middle colic artery)	中結腸動脈
MCA(multiple congenital anomaly)	多発性先天異常
McB(McBurney's point)	マックバーニー圧痛点
MCC(median cervical cyst)	正中頚嚢胞
MCD(medullary cystic disease)	腎髄質嚢胞性疾患
M-C flap(muscle cutaneous flap)	筋肉皮弁
MCG(mechanocardiography)	心機図
MCG(micturition cystography)	排尿時膀胱造影法
MCGN(mesangiocapillary glomerulonephritis)	脈管膜毛細管性糸球体腎炎

MCH(mean corpuscular hemoglobin)	平均赤血球ヘモグロビン(血色素)量
MCH(muscle contraction headache)	筋緊張性頭痛＝TTH
MCHC (mean corpuscular hemoglobin concentration)	平均赤血球ヘモグロビン(血色素)濃度
MCL(medial collateral ligament)	内側側副靱帯
MCL(midclavicular line)	鎖骨中線
MCLS (mucocutaneous lymph node syndrome)	川崎病、急性熱性皮膚粘膜リンパ節症候群
MCNS (minimal change nephrotic syndrome)	微小変化型ネフローゼ症候群
MCOS(mucocutaneous ocular syndrome)	粘膜皮膚眼症候群
MCP, MCPJ(metacarpophalangeal joint)	中手指節間関節
M-CSF (macrophage-colony stimulating factor)	マクロファージコロニー刺激因子
MCT(medium chain triglyceride)	中鎖トリグリセリド
MCT(microwave coagulation therapy)	マイクロ波凝固療法
MCTD(mixed connective tissue disease)	混合性結合組織病
MCT milk(medium chain triglyceride milk)	中鎖脂肪酸ミルク
MCV(mean corpuscular volume)	平均赤血球容積
MCV, MNCV (motor nerve conduction velocity)	運動神経伝導速度
MD(major depression)	大うつ病
MD(manic depressive)	躁うつ病＝MDI
MD(medical doctor)	医師、医学博士
MD(Meniere's disease)	メニエール病
MD(mental deficiency)	精神発達遅滞
MD(muscular dystrophy)	筋ジストロフィー
MD(myotonic dystrophy)	筋緊張性ジストロフィー
MDI(manic-depressive illness)	躁うつ病
MDI(metered-dose inhaler)	定量噴霧吸入器
MDL(magendurchleuchtung)	胃透視
MDR(minimum daily requirement)	1日最低必要量
MDS(myelodysplastic syndrome)	骨髄異形成症候群

MD

MDSO(mentally disordered sex offender)	異常性格性攻撃者
ME(benign myalgic encephalomyelitis)	良性筋痛性脳脊髄炎
ME(medical electronics)	医用電子工学
ME(medical engineering)	医用工学
ME(myoclonus epilepsy)	ミオクローヌスてんかん
MEA, MEN (multiple endocrine adenomatosis)	多発性内分泌腺腫症
measles	麻疹(はしか)
meconium	胎便
Med(mediastinum)	縦隔
MED(minimum erythema dose)	最小紅斑量
MED(multiple epiphyseal dysplasia)	多発性骨端骨異形成症
median nerve	正中神経 ◀関連▶橈骨神経： radial nerve 尺骨神経： ulnar nerve
median sternotomy	胸骨縦切開
mediastinal tumor	縦隔腫瘍
mediastinoscopy	縦隔鏡
meditation	瞑想
medulla oblongata	延髄
medullary carcinoma	髄様癌
medullary cystic kidney	髄質嚢胞腎
medullary nailing	骨髄釘固定術
medulloblastoma	髄芽腫
MEF(maximal expiratory flow)	最大呼気流量
megalocystis	巨大膀胱
megaloureter	巨大尿管
megrim	片頭痛
MEL(micro-explosion lithotripsy)	微小発破砕石術
MELAS(mitochondrial encephalo myopathy; lactic acidosis and stroke-like attack)	メラス型ミトコンドリア脳筋症
melena	下血

melena neonatorum	新生児メレナ
memory	記憶
	参照 短期記憶：STM
	長期記憶：LTM
menarche	初潮, 月経
Meniere disease	メニエール病
meningeal irritation	髄膜刺激症侯
meninges	髄膜
meniscectomy	半月板切除術
meniscus	関節半月
menopausal disease	更年期障害
menopause	閉経
menorrhagia	月経過多
menstrual cramps pain	生理痛
menstruation	月経
MEP (maximal expiratory pressure)	最大呼気圧
mercy killing	安楽死
mesangial proliferative glomerulonephritis	メサンギウム増殖性糸球体腎炎
mesothelioma	胸膜中皮腫
MET (metabolic equivalents)	代謝当量（代謝率）
meta (metastasis)	癌の転移
metabolic bone disease	代謝性骨疾患
metaphysis	骨幹端
metastasis	（腫瘍の）転移
metastatic lung tumor	転移性肺腫瘍
methylmalonic acidemia	メチルマロン酸血症
METS (metabolic equivalents)	メッツ（安静時の酸素摂取量＝1 MET）
metyrapone test	メチラポン試験
MF (mycosis fungoides)	菌状息肉症
MF (myelofibrosis)	骨髄線維症
MF (myocardial fibrosis)	心筋線維症
MFD (minimum fatal dose)	最小致死量

・MF・

MFH(malignant fibrous histiocytoma)	悪性線維性組織球腫
m flac(membrana flaccida)	弛緩膜
MG(Magen geschwür)	胃潰瘍
Mg(magnesium)	マグネシウム
MG(Meulengracht)	黄疸指数
MG(myasthenia gravis)	重症筋無力症
Mgk(megakaryocyte)	巨核球
MGN(membranous glomerulonephritis)	膜性糸球体腎炎
MH(malignant histiocytosis)	悪性組織球症
MH(malignant hyperthermia)	悪性高体温症、悪性高熱症
MH(menstrual history)	月経歴
MHA(microangiopathic hemolytic anemia)	微小血管障害性溶血性貧血
MHC(major histocompatibility complex)	主要組織適合複合体
MHC(mental health center)	精神保健センター
MHE(malignant hemangioendothelioma)	悪性血管内皮腫
MHN(morbus hemolyticus neonatorum)	新生児溶血性黄疸
MHV(middle hepatic vein)	中肝静脈
MI(maturation index)	成熟度指数
MI(mitral insufficiency)	僧帽弁閉鎖不全
MI(motility index)	運動指数
MI(myocardial infarction)	心筋梗塞
MIC(microinvasive carcinoma)	微小浸潤癌
MIC(minimum inhibitory concentration)	最小発育阻止濃度
microadenoma	微小腺腫
microcephaly	小頭症
microscopic hematuria	顕微鏡的血尿
microsurgery	顕微鏡下手術
miction pain	排尿痛
MID(multiple infarct dementia)	多発梗塞性痴呆
midbrain	中脳
	◀関連▶ 大脳：cerebrum
	小脳：cerebellum
	間脳：diencephalon
middle finger	中指

midtarsal joint	横足根関節
MIH (melanotropin release-inhibiting hormone)	メラノトロピン放出抑制ホルモン
milk vomit	吐乳
MIM(Mendelian inheritance in man)	ヒトにおけるメンデル遺伝
Min(minor curvature of stomach)	胃小弯
	◀関連▶胃大弯：Maj
mind reading	思考察知
minimal pressure	最低血圧
	◀関連▶最高血圧：maximal pressure
minor tranquilizer	穏和精神安定薬
miosis, myosis	縮瞳
	対 散瞳：mydriasis
MIP(maximum inspiratory pressure)	最大吸気圧
miscarriage	流産
misdiagnosis	誤診
MIT(minimum invasive therapy)	最小侵襲手術
mite	ダニ
mixed infection	混合感染
Miyake retention test	三宅式記銘力検査
MK(Magenkrebs)	胃癌
ML(malignant lymphoma)	悪性リンパ腫
ML(middle lobe of lung)	肺中葉
MLD(mmanual lymph drainage)	リンパ管内マッサージによる間質液吸収促進
MLD(myelogenous leukemia)	骨髄性白血病
MLG(myelography)	脊髄造影
MLN(membranous lupus nephritis)	膜性ループス腎炎
MLNS(minimal lesion nephrotic syndrome)	微小変化型ネフローゼ症候群
MM(malignant melanoma)	悪性黒色腫
MM(medial meniscus)	内側半月
	対 外側半月：LM
MM(Menschenmilch)	母乳

mm

mm (motus manus)	手動弁
MM (multiple myeloma)	多発性骨髄腫
mm (muscularis mucosae)	粘膜筋板
MM (Muttermund)	子宮口
MMC (meningomyelocele)	脊髄髄膜瘤
MMD (myotonic muscular dystrophy)	筋緊張性筋ジストロフィー
MMF (maximal midexpiratory flow)	最大中間呼気流量
MMG (mammography)	乳房撮影法、マンモグラフィー
MMK (Mammakrebs)	乳癌（マンマ）
MMM (myelosclerosis with myeloid metaplasia)	骨髄化生を伴う骨髄硬化症
MMPI (Minnesota multiphasic personality inventory)	ミネソタ多面的人格検査
MMR (measles-mumps-rubella vaccine)	麻疹・流行性耳下腺炎・風疹混合ワクチン
MMT (manual muscle test)	徒手筋力テスト
MMT (mixed mesodermal tumor)	混合性中胚葉腫瘍
MMV (mandatory minute volume)	強制分時換気量
MN (membranous nephropathy)	膜性腎症
MND (motor neuron disease)	運動ニューロン疾患
MNMS (myonephropathic metabolic syndrome)	筋腎代謝性症候群
Mo (monocyte)	単球
	▶関連 リンパ球：Lym
	顆粒球：granulocyte
Mo (mother)	母親
mobilization operation	授動術
MOD (maturity onset diabetes mellitus)	成人型糖尿病
MODS (multiple organ dysfunction syndrome)	多臓器不全症候群
MODY (maturity onset diabetes in youth)	若年性成人型糖尿病
MOF (multiple organ failure)	多臓器不全
moist rale	湿性ラ音
	▶対 乾性ラ音：dry rale
MoL (monocytic leukemia)	単球性白血病
mole	ほくろ、黒あざ、胞状奇胎

Mole (Blasenmole)	胞状奇胎
mood	気分
moon face	満月様顔貌
Morita therapy	森田療法
morning sickness	悪阻、つわり
Moro reflex	モロー反射
morphinism	モルヒネ中毒
MOSF (multiorgan system failure)	多臓器機能不全
motor aphasia	運動性失語 参照 感覚性失語：sensory aphasia
motor weakness	運動麻痺
moyamoya disease	もやもや病
MP, MPJ, MP joint (metacarpophalangeal joint)	中手指節関節
MP (multipara)	経産　参照 初産：PP
mp癌 (muscularis propria)	固有筋層までの癌（壁深達度）
mPAP (mean pulmonary arterial pressure)	平均肺動脈圧
MPD (minimal phototoxic dose)	最小光毒量
MPD (multiple personality)	多重人格障害
MPD (myeloproliferative disorder)	骨髄増殖性疾患
MPGN (membranoproliferative glomerulonephritis)	膜性増殖性糸球体腎炎
MPGN, MPN (mesangial proliferating glomerulonephritis)	メサンギウム性増殖性糸球体腎炎
MPI (Mausley personality inventory)	モズリー性格検査
MPNST (malignant peripheral nerve sheath tumor)	悪性末梢性神経鞘腫瘍
MPP (mycoplasma pneumonia)	マイコプラズマ肺炎
MPPV (malignant persistent positional vertigo)	悪性持続性頭位眩暈症
MPS (mucopolysaccharidosis)	ムコ多糖体沈着症
MR (Magenresektion)	胃切除術
MR (magnetic resonance)	磁気共鳴

MR

MR(measles-rubella vaccine)	麻疹、風疹ワクチン
MR(medical representative)	製薬企業の医療品情報担当者
MR(mental retardation)	精神(発達)遅滞
MR(mitral regurgitation)	僧帽弁逆流症、僧帽弁閉鎖不全
MRA(magnetic resonance angiography)	磁気共鳴血管造影法
MRA(malignant rheumatoid arthritis)	悪性関節リウマチ
MRA(middle rectal artery)	中直腸動脈
MRAO(modified right anterior oblique)	修正右前斜位
MRBF(mean renal blood flow)	平均腎血流量
MRC(medullary respiratory chemoreceptor)	延髄呼吸化学受容体
MRC(metastatic renal cell carcinoma)	転移性腎細胞癌
MRCP(magnetic resonance cholangiopancreatography)	磁気共鳴膵胆管造影
MR-CT(magnetic resonance computerized tomography)	磁気共鳴コンピュータ画像診断法
MRD(minimal residual disease)	微小残存病変(腫瘍)
MRDM(malnutrition related diabetes mellitus)	栄養障害関連糖尿病
MRI(magnetic resonance imaging)	磁気共鳴画像診断装置 参照 コンピュータ断層撮影：CT
MRSA (methicillin resistant *staphylococcus aureus*)	メチシリン耐性黄色ブドウ球菌 参照 院内感染：nosocomial infection
MRTK (malignant rhabdoid tumor of the kidney)	腎横紋筋肉腫瘍様腫瘍
MS(maxillary sinus)	上顎洞
MS(Meniere's syndrome)	メニエール症候群
MS(mitral stenosis)	僧帽弁狭窄症
MS(morning stiffness)	朝のこわばり
MS(multiple sclerosis)	多発性硬化症
MS, MSA(multiple system atrophy)	多系統萎縮症
MSBP(Munchausen Syndrome by Proxy)	代理ミュンヒハウゼン症候群

MSH(melanocyte-stimulating hormone)	メラニン細胞刺激ホルモン
MSK(medullary sponge kidney)	髄質海綿腎
MSL(midsternal line)	胸骨中線
MSOF(multiple systemic organ failure)	系統的多臓器不全
MSR, MSI(mitral stenosis & regurgitation)	僧帽弁狭窄兼閉鎖不全
MSUD(maple syrup urine disease)	メープルシロップ尿症
MSW(medical social worker)	医療ソーシャルワーカー
MT(Magen tube)	胃チューブ
MT(maternal transport)	母体搬送
MT(mediastinal tumor)	縦隔腫瘍
MT(membrana tympani)	鼓膜
Mt(middle thoracic esophagus)	胸部中部食道
MTPJ(metatarsophalangeal joint)	中趾節関節
MTP joint(metatarsophalangeal joint)	中趾節関節
MTT(mean transit time)	平均循環時間
MTX(methotrexate)	メトトレキサート(メソトレキセート)
MUC(mucosal ulcerative colitis)	粘膜性潰瘍性大腸炎
mucous	粘性の炎症、カタル
multiple	多発性
multiple personality	多重人格
multiple sclerosis	多発性硬化症
mumps	おたふく風邪、流行性耳下腺炎
MUO(myocardiopathy of unknown origin)	原因不明の心筋症
MUGA(multiple-gated acquisition scan)	多関門集積スキャン
muscle strain	肉離れ
music therapy	音楽療法
mutism	無言症
MV(mechanical ventilation)	機械的人工換気
MV(minute ventilation)	分時換気量
MV(mitral valve)	僧帽弁
	◀関連▶ 三尖弁：TV
MVD(micro-vascular decompression)	微小神経血管減圧術
MVO(midventricular obstruction)	心室中部閉塞症

MV

MVO₂(myocardial oxygen consumption)	心筋酸素消費量
MVP(mitral valve plasty)	僧帽弁形成術
MVP(mitral valve prolapse syndrome)	僧帽弁逸脱症候群
MVR(massive vitreous retraction)	増殖硝子体網膜症
MVR(mitral valve replacement)	僧帽弁置換術
MVV(maximal voluntary ventilation)	最大換気量
M-W syndrome (Mallory Weiss syndrome)	マロリー・ワイス症候群
My(myopia)	近視
	◀関連▶ 遠視：hyperopia
	乱視：AS
myalgia	筋肉痛
MyD(myotonic muscular dystrophy)	筋緊張性ジストロフィー
mydriasis	散瞳
	◀対▶ 縮瞳：miosis, myosis
Myelo(myelography)	脊髄造影法(ミエロ)
myeloma	骨髄腫
myeloma kidney	骨髄腫腎
myelosuppression	骨髄抑制
myocarditis	心筋炎
myogenic torticollis	筋性斜頚
myoglobinuria	ミオグロビン尿症
myoma(myoma uteri)	子宮筋腫
mysophobia	不潔恐怖
myxedema	粘液水腫
MZ(monozygotic twins)	一卵性双生児＝EZ
	参照 二卵性双生児：DZ

N

N(nerve)	神経
N(Neurosis)	神経症
N(neutrophilic leukocyte)	好中球
	◀関連▶ 好酸球：Eo, Eos 好塩基球：Bas
N(regional lymph nodes)	所属リンパ節転移の程度（TNM分類）
Na(natrium)	ナトリウム
NA(necrotizing angiitis)	壊死性血管炎
NA(neurologic age)	神経学的年齢
NA(noradrenaline)	ノルアドレナリン
NAA(no apparent abnormalities)	はっきりした異常なし
NAC(neo adjuvant chemotherapy)	新導入化学療法
NAD(nicotinamide-adenine dinucleotide)	ニコチン酸アデニンジヌクレオチド
NAD(no appreciable disease)	特記すべき疾患なし
NAD(nothing abnormal detected)	検査結果に異常認めず
Na-K pump	ナトリウム−カリウムポンプ
NANB, NANBH(nonA-nonB hepatitis)	非A非B肝炎
NAP(nerve action potential)	神経活動電位
NAP(neutrophil alkaline phosphatase)	好中球アルカリホスファターゼ
narcissism	自己陶酔、自己愛
narcissistic personality disorder	自己愛性人格障害
NARES(non-allergic rhinitis with eosinophilia syndrome)	非アレルギー性好酸球増多性鼻炎症候群
narrowing of consciousness	意識野の狭窄
natural position	中間（立）位、基本肢位
nausea	悪心、吐き気、嘔気
nausea and vomiting of pregnancy	つわり
NB(Nasenbepinseln)	点鼻
NB(neuroblastoma)	神経芽細胞腫
NB(neurogenic bladder)	神経因性膀胱

NB

NB(new born)	新生児
NB(Nichts Besonders)	異常なし
N-B(noso-biliary)	鼻-胆嚢チューブ
NBAS(newborn behavioral assessment scale)	新生児行動評価
NBD(neurogenic bladder dystion)	神経性膀胱機能障害
NBD(no brain damage)	脳障害なし
NBL(normoblast)	正常赤血球
NBM(nothing by mouth)	経口摂取不可、禁食
NBN(newborn nursery)	新生児室
NBP(nonbacterial pharyngitis)	非細菌性咽頭炎
NBTE(non-bacterial thrombotic endocarditis)	非細菌性血栓性心内膜炎
NC(no change)	不変、特記事項なし
nc(non corrigent)	視力矯正不能
n.c.(non corrigibile)	視力矯正不能
NC(nurse call)	ナースコール
NCA(neuro circulatory asthenia)	神経循環無力症
NCC(nucleated cell count)	有核細胞数
NCCHD (non-cyanotic congenital heart disease)	非チアノーゼ性先天性心疾患
NCCP(noncardiac chest pain)	非心原性胸痛
NCE(noncardiac edema)	非心原性浮腫
NCE(nonconvulsive epilepsy)	非痙攣性てんかん
NCE(normal chromatic erythrocyte)	正常色素性赤血球
NCF(normal colposcopic findings)	正常所見
NCLM(nodular cutaneous lupus mucinosis)	結節性皮膚ループスムチン症
NCN(nevus cell nevus)	母斑細胞母斑
NCPF(noncirrhotic portal fibrosis)	非硬変症性門脈線維症
NCV(nerve conduction velocity)	神経伝導速度
ND(nerve deafness)	神経難聴
ND(neurotic depression)	神経性うつ病
ND(not detectable)	検出できない
nd(numerus digitorum)	指数弁
ndE(nach dem essen)	毎食後　参照　毎食前:vdE　食間に:zwdE

Ne

NDI(nephrogenic diabetes insipidus)	腎性尿崩症
NE(norepinephrine)	ノルエピネフリン
NEAA(non-essential amino acid)	非必須アミノ酸
	◀関連▶必須アミノ酸：EAA
nearmiss SIDS(nearmiss sudden infant death syndrome)	未然型乳児突然死症候群
NEC(necrotizing enterocolitis)	壊死性腸炎
NEC(neonatal necrotizing enterocolitis)	新生児壊死性腸炎
neck	首、頚部
necrophilia	死体嗜愛
necrosis	壊死
needle biopsy	針生検
NeF(nephritic factor)	腎炎因子
Neg(negative)	陰性
negativism	拒絶症
NEL(no-effect level)	無影響量
neonatal death	新生児死亡
neonatal hepatitis syndrome	新生児肝炎症候群
neonatal period	新生児期
nephritic syndrome	腎炎症候群
nephroblastoma	腎芽細胞腫（ウィルムス腫瘍）
nephrocalcinosis	腎石灰化症
nephrogenic diabetes insipidus	腎性尿崩症
nephrolithiasis	腎結石
nephron	ネフロン
nephroptosis	腎下垂
nephrosis	ネフローゼ
nephrotic syndrome	ネフローゼ症候群
nephrotoxicity	腎毒性
nerve injury	神経損傷
nesidioblastosis	膵島細胞症
NET(nerve excitability test)	神経興奮性検査
nettle rash	蕁麻疹
Neuro(neurology, neurologic)	神経内科、神経学、神経学の

ne

neuroblastoma	神経芽細胞腫
neuroectodermal tumor	神経外胚葉性腫瘍
neuro-endoscopic surgery	神経内視鏡手術
neurogenic bladder	神経因性膀胱
neurological deficit	神経脱落症候
neurolysis	末梢神経剥離術
neurotic	神経症の
Neutro(neutrophilic leukocyte)	好中球
newborn	新生児
NF(neurofibromatosis)	神経線維腫症
NF(neutral fat)	中性脂肪
NFTT(nonorganic failure-thrive syndrome)	非器質性発育不良症候群
NG(nephrography)	腎造影
NG(new growth)	新生物
NG(nitroglycerin)	ニトログリセリン
NG tube(nasogastric tube)	経鼻胃管
NHC(non-ketotic hyperosmolar coma)	非ケトン性高浸透圧性昏睡
NHL(non-Hodgkin's lymphoma)	非ホジキンリンパ腫
NHS(neonatal hepatitis syndrome)	新生児肝炎症候群
NICU(neonatal intensive care unit)	新生児集中治療部
NIDDM (non-insulin dependent diabetes mellitus)	インスリン非依存性糖尿病 参照 インスリン依存性糖尿病：IDDM
night sweat	寝汗、盗汗
night terrors	夜驚症
NIHF(non-immunologic hydrops fetalis)	非免疫性胎児水腫
nihilistic delusion	虚無妄想
nitrogen metabolism	窒素代謝
niveau	鏡面像、ニボー像
NK cell(natural killer cell)	ナチュラルキラー細胞
NL(normal limits)	正常範囲
NLA(neurolept-anesthesia)	ニューロレプト麻酔
NLE(neonatal lupus erythematosus)	新生児エリテマトーデス
NLP(no light perception)	光覚なし

NM(nodular melanoma)	結節性黒色腫
NMA(neurogenic muscular atrophy)	神経原性筋萎縮
NME(necrolytic migratory erythema)	壊死性遊走性紅斑
NMJ(neuromuscular junction)	神経筋接合部
NMR(nuclear magnetic resonance)	核磁気共鳴
NMU(neuromuscular unit)	神経筋単位
NN(neurinoma)	神経鞘腫
NNJ(neonatal jaundice)	新生児黄疸＝IN
NNT(number needed to treat)	治療必要数
NO(nasal obstruction)	鼻閉
NO(nitric oxide)	一酸化窒素
NO(nitrous oxide)	笑気、亜酸化窒素
NOAEL(no observed adverse effect level)	無毒性量
nocturia	夜尿
nocturnal dyspnea	夜間呼吸困難
nocturnal hemoglobinuria	夜間血色素尿症
nodule	結節
NOEL(no observed effect level)	無影響量
non-directive psychotherapy	非指示的療法
non-Freudian psychoanalysis	非フロイト精神分析
non-union	偽関節
no pl(no perception of light)	光覚なし＝NLP
NOS(not otherwise specified)	詳細不明
nosocomial infection	院内感染
	参照 メシチリン耐性黄色ブドウ球菌：MRSA
nosogenesis	発病
NOx(nitrogen oxides)	窒素酸化物
NP(nasal polyp)	鼻ポリープ
NP(neuropsychiatry)	精神神経医学
NP(no particular)	異常なし＝OB
n.p.(nothing particular)	異常なし
NPC(nasopharyngeal carcinoma)	鼻咽頭癌
NPD(narcissistic personality disorder)	自己愛性人格障害

NP

NPD(nephrophthisis dextra)	右腎結核
NPH(neutral-protamine-hagedorn insulin)	中間型インスリン
NPH(normal pressure hydrocephalus)	正常圧水頭症
NPH(nucleus pulposus herniation)	椎間板ヘルニア髄核脱出
NPMA(neural progressive muscle atrophy)	神経性、進行性筋萎縮症
NPN(non protein nitrogen)	非蛋白性窒素
NPO(non per os)	禁飲食
NPS(nephrophthisis sinistra)	左腎結核症
NPT(nocturnal penile tumescence)	夜間陰茎勃起(現象)
NR(normal range)	正常範囲
NRBC(normal red blood cell)	正常赤血球
NREM, NREM sleep (non rapid eye movement〔sleep〕)	ノンレム睡眠、徐波睡眠
NS(Nasenspulumg)	鼻洗
NS(nephrose syndrome)	ネフローゼ症候群
NS(nervous system)	神経系 参照 中枢神経系：CNS, ZNS 自律神経系：ANS 末梢神経系：PNS
NS(normal saline solution)	生理食塩水
NS(normal serum)	正常血清
NSAID (non-steroidal anti-inflammatory drug)	非ステロイド系抗炎症薬
NSD(normal spontaneous delivery)	経腟自然分娩
NSFTD (normal spontaneous fullterm delivery)	正常自然満期産
NSR(normal sinus rhythm)	正常洞調律
NSRH(nonspecific reactive hepatitis)	非特異性反応性肝炎
NST(non stress test)	ノンストレステスト
NTB(necrotizing tracheobronchitis)	壊死性気道粘膜炎
NTD(neural tube defect)	中枢神経管欠損
NTG(nitroglycerin)	ニトログリセリン
NTG(normal-tension glaucoma)	正常眼圧緑内障

NUD(non-ulcer dyspepsia)	非潰瘍性消化不良
NUG(necrotizing ulcerative gingivitis)	壊死性潰瘍性歯肉炎
Nv(naked vision)	裸眼視力
NV(Nasenverstopfung)	鼻閉
N&V(nausea and vomiting)	悪心・嘔吐
NV(neurovascular)	神経血管性
NVC(neurovascular compression syndrome)	神経血管圧迫症候群
NVD(neovascularization on the disc)	乳頭状新生血管
NWB(non-weight bearing)	免荷
Ny(nystagmus)	眼振
nyctalopia	夜盲症
nycturia	夜間頻尿
NYHA (New York Heart Association classification)	ニューヨーク心臓協会心機能分類
nystagmus	眼振＝Ny

O (objective data)	客観的情報
	対 主観的情報：S
O (occipital)	後頭部の
	対 前頭部の：F
O (occiput)	後頂
O (oral)	経口的
O (oxygen)	酸素
OA (occiput anterior)	後頭骨前方
OA (orthostatic albuminuria)	起立性蛋白尿
OA (osteoarthritis)	変形性関節症
OAC (open aortic commissurotomy)	直視下大動脈弁交連切断術
OAD (obstructive airway disease)	閉塞性気道障害
OAP (ophthalmic artery pressure)	眼動脈圧
OAP (osteoarthropathy)	骨関節症
OA-PICA (occipital artery -posterior inferior cerebellar artery 〔anastomosis〕)	後頭動脈・後下小脳動脈
Ob (oblique)	斜位
OB (obstetrics)	産科(学)
OB (occult blood 〔bleeding〕)	潜血
OB (ohne Befunde, ohne Besondere, ohne Beschwerde)	所見なし、異常なし、苦痛(訴え)なし＝NP
OBD (organic brain disease)	器質性脳疾患
OBLA (onset of blood lactate accumulation)	乳酸蓄積閾値
obese	肥満した
obesity	肥満(症)
	対 痩せ：emaciation
OB-GYN (obstetrics and gynecology)	産婦人科
object	対象
object relations	対象関係
object symptom	他覚症状
	参照 自覚症状：subject symptom

OD

OBS(organic brain syndrome)	脳器質症候群
obsessive compulsive disorder	強迫性障害＝OCD
obsessive idea	強迫思考
obsessive-compulsive neurosis	強迫神経症
obsessive thinking	強迫観念
obstetric palsy	分娩麻痺
obstruction	障害(物)閉塞
obstructive enterocolitis	閉塞性腸炎
obstructive nephropathy	閉塞性腎症
OC(obstetrical conjugate)	産科的結合線
OC(oral condition)	口腔内所見
OC(oral contraceptive)	経口避妊薬
OC(oxygen consumption)	酸素消費量
occipital lobe syndrome	後頭葉症候群
OCC th(occupational therapy)	作業療法
occult blood	潜血＝OB
OCD(obsessive-compulsive disorder)	強迫性障害
OCD(occupational cervicobrachial disorders)	職業性頚肩腕障害
OC-DIC(oc-drip infusion cholangiography)	経口経静脈胆嚢胆管造影
OCG(oral cholecystography)	経口胆嚢造影(法)
OCH(oral contraceptive hormone)	経口避妊ホルモン
OCPD (obsessive compulsive personality disorder)	強迫性人格障害
OCT(oxytocin challenge test)	オキシトシン負荷テスト
oculomotor N	Ⅲ動眼神経
OCV(opacitas corporis vitrei)	硝子体混濁
Od(oculus dexter)	右眼　対 左眼：Os
OD(open drip)	開放点滴
OD(orthostatic dysregulation)	起立性調節障害
OD(outside diameter)	外径
OD(over dose)	過剰投与
ODA(occipitodextra anterior〔position〕)	右前方後頭位(胎位)
ODC(oxygen dissociation)	酸素解離曲線
ODM(ophthalmodynamometry)	眼底血圧測定

OD

ODN(ophthalmodynamometer)	眼底血圧計
ODT(occlusive dressing technique)	閉鎖密封療法
OD test(orthostatic disturbance test)	自律神経失調症テスト
OE(otitis externa)	外耳炎
	◀関連▶中耳炎：OM
Oedipus complex	エディプスコンプレックス
OF(occipitofrontal〔diameter〕)	前後径、後前頭径
OGI(osteogenesis imperfecta)	骨形成不全症＝OI
OGTT(oral glucose tolerance test)	経口ブドウ糖負荷試験
OH(occupational history)	職歴
OH(orthostatic hypotension)	起立性低血圧症
OHA(oral hypoglycemic agent)	経口血糖降下薬
OHD(organic heart disease)	器質性心疾患
OHP(oxygen under high pressure)	高圧酸素療法
OHS(obesity-hypoventilation syndrome)	肥満性低換気症候群
OHS(open heart surgery)	開心術、直視下心臓手術
OHSS(ovarian hyperstimulation syndrome)	卵巣過剰刺激症候群
OI(opportunistic infection)	日和見感染
OI(orgasmic impairment)	オルガスムス障害
OI(orientation inventory)	見当識調査票
OI(osteogenesis imperfecta)	骨形成不全症＝OGI
OI(oxytocin induction)	オキシトシン分娩誘導
OICU(obstetric intensive care unit)	産科集中治療室
OIH(ovulation inducing hormone)	排卵誘発ホルモン
OJ(obstructive jaundice)	閉塞性黄疸
OK(oesophaguskrebs)	食道癌
OKAN(optokinetic after nystagmus)	視運動性眼振＝OKN
OKK(Oberkieferkrebs)	上顎癌
OKN(optokinetic nystagmus)	視運動性眼振＝OKAN
OLA(occipitolevoanterior〔position〕)	左後頭前方位（胎位）
OLF(ossification of ligamentum flavum)	黄色靱帯骨化症＝OYL
olfactory N	Ⅰ嗅神経
OLG(oligodendroglioma)	乏突起膠腫
oliguria	乏尿

OLP(occipitolevoposterior〔position〕)	左後頭後方位(胎位)
OLT(occipitolevotransverse〔position〕)	左後頭横位(胎位)
OM(obtuse marginal branch)	鈍縁枝
OM(osteomalacia)	骨軟化症
OM(otitis media)	中耳炎
OMC(open mitral commissurotomy)	直視下僧帽弁交連切開術
OMD(organic mental disorder)	器質性精神疾患
OME(otitis media with effusion)	滲出性中耳炎
OMI(old myocardial infarction)	陳旧性心筋梗塞
omn quad hor(omni quadrante hora)	4時間ごとに 参照 毎時：quaque hora 隔日に：quaque die
OMPC(otitis media purulenta chronica)	慢性化膿性中耳炎
ON(optic nerve)	視神経
ON(osteonecrosis)	骨壊死
oncotic pressure	膠質浸透圧
OP(occiput posterior)	後頭骨後方
OP(operation)	手術
OP(outpatient)	外来患者
OPCA(olivo-ponto-cerebellar atrophy)	オリーブ橋小脳萎縮症
OPCD (olivo-pontine cerebellar degeneration)	オリーブ橋小脳皮質変性
OPD(ocular psychosomatic disease)	眼精神身体症
OPD(out patient department)	外来診療部門
OPD(out patient dispensary)	外来用薬局
open fracture	開放骨折
operant conditioning approach	オペラント的方法
Oph(ophthalmoscope)	検眼鏡
Ophth(ophthalmology)	眼科学
ophthalmalgia	眼痛
ophthalmopathy	眼症状
opistho-tonus	後弓反張
OPLL(ossification of posterior longitudinal ligament)	後縦靭帯骨化症

op

opportunistic infection	日和見感染＝OI
OPSI	脾摘痕重症感染症
(overwhelming post-splenectomy infection)	
optic N	Ⅱ視神経
OPV(oral polio vaccine)	経口ポリオワクチン
OR(operating room)	手術室
oral	口の、経口の
oral contraceptive	経口避妊薬＝OC
organ	器官、臓器
organic affective syndrome	器質性感情症候群
organic brain syndrome	器質性精神症候群
organic delusional syndrome	器質性妄想症候群
organic mental disorder	器質性精神障害
organic personality syndrome	器質性人格症候群
organic psychosis	器質性精神病
orientation	見当識
ORL(oto-rhino-laryngology)	耳鼻咽喉科学
ORS(oral surgeon)	口腔外科医
ORT(operating room technician)	手術室技師
ORT(oral rehydration therapy)	経口輸液療法
ORT(orthoptist)	視能訓練士
Ortho(orthopaedics)	整形外科、整形外科医
orthopnea	起座呼吸
orthostatic dizziness	立ちくらみ
orthostatic proteinuria	起立性蛋白尿
OS(occipitosacral〔position〕)	後頭仙骨位(胎位)
Os(oculus sinister)	左眼　対　右眼：Od
OS(opening snap)	オープニングスナップ、僧帽弁開放音
OS(orthopedic surgeon)	整形外科医
OS(osteosarcoma)	骨肉腫
OSAS(obstructive sleep apnea syndrome)	閉塞性睡眠時無呼吸症候群
osmotic diuresis	浸透圧利尿
osmotic pressure	浸透圧

OSS(bone metastasis)	骨転移
osteo(osteomyelitis)	骨髄炎
osteoarthritis of the hip joint	変形性股関節症
osteoarthritis of the knee joint	変形性膝関節症
osteomalacia	骨軟化症
osteomyelitis	骨髄炎
osteopenia	骨減少
osteophyte	骨棘
osteoporosis	骨粗鬆症
ostium of vagina	腟口
OT(occiput transverse〔position〕)	後頭横位(胎位)
OT(occiput transverse presentation)	低在横定位
OT(occupational therapist)	作業療法士
	◀関連▶ 理学療法士:PT
OT(occupational therapy)	作業療法
OT(ocular tension)	眼圧
OT(old tuberculin)	陳旧性結核
OT(orientation test)	見当識検査
OT(orotracheal)	口腔気管の
OT(oxytocin)	オキシトシン
otalgia	耳痛
OTC(ornithine transcarbamylase)	オルニチントランスカルバミラーゼ
OTC(over the counter)	市販薬(カウンターごしに買える薬剤という意味)
OTH(metastasis to other organs)	他臓器転移
otitis media	中耳炎
	◀関連▶ 外耳炎:otitis externa
otitis media with effusion	滲出性中耳炎
Oto(otology)	耳科学
OU(oculi unitas)	両眼
	参照 右眼:Od、左眼:Os
OVA(old vascular accident)	陳旧性脳血管障害
Ova Ca(ovarian carcinoma)	卵巣癌

OV

ovary	卵巣
OVC(obarian cancer)	卵巣癌
overhead traction	頭上方向牽引
ovulation	排卵
OW(oral wedge)	肉眼的癌口側断端
OW(oval window)	卵円窓
OX, OXY(oxytocin)	オキシトシン
oxygen inhalation	酸素吸入
oxytocics	子宮収縮薬
OYL(ossification of yellow ligament)	黄色靭帯骨化症＝OLF
OYL(progesterone)	プロゲステロン

P

P(para)	経産回数
	◀関連▶ 経産：MP
P(parietal)	頭頂部の
P(part)	部分
P(peritoneum)	腹膜
P(phosphorus)	リン
P(plan)	計画
P(plasma)	血漿
P(posterior)	後の
P(posterior segment)	右葉後区域(肝)
P(pressure)	圧
P(proctos)	肛門管
P(psychiatrist)	精神(科)医
P(psychiatry)	精神医学
P(psychosis)	精神病
P(pulse)	脈拍
P(punctation)	赤点斑
PA(atrial pressure)	心房圧
PA(panarteritis)	汎動脈炎
PA(paralysis agitans)	振戦麻痺
Pa(paranoia)	パラノイア
PA(periarteritis)	動脈周囲炎
PA(pernicious anemia)	悪性貧血
PA(pituitary adenoma)	下垂体腺腫
PA(plasma absorption)	血漿吸着
PA(polyarteritis)	多発性動脈炎
PA(posterior-anterior)	後前方向
PA(pression arterielle)	動脈圧＝ABP
	◀対▶ 静脈圧：VP
PA(psoriatic arthritis)	乾癬性関節炎
PA(pulmonary artery)	肺動脈
	◀対▶ 肺静脈：PV

PA

PA(pulmonary atresia)	肺動脈閉鎖症
PAB(premature atrial beat)	心房性期外収縮＝PAC
PAB(pulmonary artery banding)	肺動脈絞扼術
PAC(papillary adenocarcinoma)	乳頭腺癌
PAC(papular acrodermatitis of childhood)	小児丘疹性末端皮膚炎、ジャノッティ皮膚炎
PAC(premature atrial contraction)	心房性期外収縮＝PAB
PACG(primary angle-closure glaucoma)	原発性閉塞隅角緑内障
pachygyria	厚脳回
pacing failure	ペースメーカー不全
$PaCO_2$(arterial carbon dioxide tension)	動脈血炭酸ガス分圧
PACS (picture archive and communication system)	画像収集通信解析システム
PACU(post anesthesia care unit)	麻酔後回復室
PAD(primary affective disorder)	原発性感情疾患
PAD(primary afferent depolarization)	一次性求心性線維脱分極
PAD(psycho-affective disorder)	精神情動疾患
PADP(pulmonary arterial diastolic pressure)	肺動脈拡張期圧
PAE(post antibiotic effect)	抗生物質持続効力
PAEDP (pulmonary artery end-diastolic pressure)	肺動脈拡張終(末)期圧
PAF(paroxysmal atrial fibrillation)	発作性心房細動
PAF(platelet activating factor)	血小板活性化因子
PAF(progressive autonomic failure)	進行性自律神経機能不全症
PAG(pelvic angiography)	骨盤内血管造影
PAG(pelvic arteriography)	骨盤動脈造影
PAG(pulmonary angiography)	肺血管造影
PAH(para-aminohippuric acid)	パラアミノ馬尿酸
PAH(pregnancy associated hypertension)	妊娠高血圧症
PAH(pulmonary arterial hypertension)	肺高血圧
PAI(inferior pulmonary artery)	下肺動脈
pain	疼痛
painless myocardial infarction	無痛性心筋梗塞
pal(palpitation)	動悸

palliation	（病気、痛みなどの）軽減、一時的な抑え
palliative operation	姑息(的)手術、保存的手術
palpation	触診
palpitation	動悸、心悸亢進＝pal
palsy	運動麻痺
PAM(primary amebic meningoencephalitis)	原発性アメーバ性髄膜脳炎
PAN (periarteritis nodosa, polyarteritis nodosa)	結節性動脈周囲炎、(結節性)多発性動脈炎
PAN(periodic alternating nystagmus)	周期性方向交代性眼振
panaritium	ひょう疽
pancreas	膵臓
pancreatic	膵臓に関する
panic attack	パニック発作
panic disorder	恐慌症、恐慌性障害
pantalar arthrodesis	汎距骨固定術
PAO(peak acid output)	最大刺激時酸分泌量
PaO$_2$(arterial O$_2$ pressure)	動脈血酸素分圧
PAP(Papanicolaou staining)	パパニコロー染色法
Pap(papilloma)	乳頭腫、パピローマ
PAP(platelet agglutinating protein)	血小板凝集因子
PAP(primary atypical pneumonia)	原発性非定型肺炎
PAP(prostatic acid phosphatase)	前立腺性酸性ホスファターゼ
PAP(prostatic cancer associated antigen)	前立腺癌関連抗原
PAP(pulmonary arterial pressure)	肺動脈圧
papillary muscle dysfunction	乳頭筋機能不全
papillary necrosis	腎乳頭壊死
papilledema	うっ血乳頭、乳頭浮腫
Pap smear(Papanicolaou's smear)	パパニコロー標本
Pap test(Papanicolaou's test)	パパニコロー試験
papula	丘疹
PAPVC(partial anomalous pulmonary venous connection)	部分的肺静脈還流異常

•PA•

PAPVD(partial anomalous pulmonary venous drainage)	部分肺静脈還流異常
PAPVR(partial anomalous pulmonary venous return)	部分的肺静脈還流異常
PAR(postanesthetic recovery)	麻酔後の回復
Para(paraplegia)	対麻痺
paracen(paracentesis)	鼓膜切開術
paradoxical motion	奇異性運動
paralysis	麻痺
paramnesia	記憶錯誤
paranoid personality disorder	妄想性人格障害
paranoid type	妄想型(統合失調症)
paraphilia	性倒錯
paraplegia	対麻痺 ◀関連▶ 四肢麻痺：tetraplegia
parathyroid gland	副甲状腺 ◀関連▶ 甲状腺：thyroid gland
parent(parenteral)	非経口的、腸管外の
parenteral nutrition	非経口栄養
paresis	運動麻痺
paresthesia	異常感覚
parietal lobe syndrome	頭頂葉症候群
Parkinson disease	パーキンソン病＝PD
Parkinsonian syndrome	パーキンソン症候群
Parkinsonism	パーキンソン症
parox(paroxysmal)	発作の、痙攣の
paroxysmal dyspnea	発作性呼吸困難
parrot fever	オウム熱
partial amnesia	部分健忘 ◀参照▶ 完全健忘：total amnesia
PARU(postanesthetic recovery unit)	麻酔後回復室
PAS(peripheral anterior synechia)	周辺虹彩前癒着

PAS(pituitary adrenal system)	下垂体副腎皮質系
PASA(primary acquired sideroblastic anemia)	原発性後天性鉄芽球性貧血
PASI(psoriasis area and severity index)	乾癬病巣範囲重症度指数
passive aggressive personality disorder	受動性攻撃性人格障害
Past(pasta)	パスタ(泥膏)〔剤〕(油脂と粉剤とを練和して泥状とした膏剤)
PAT(paroxysmal atrial tachycardia)	発作性心房性頻拍
pathologic dislocation	病的脱臼
pathologic fracture	病的骨折
pathological drunkenness	病的酩酊
pathological reflex present	病的反射出現
pathophobia	疾病恐怖
Paw(airway pressure)	気道内圧
PAWP(pulmonary artery wedge pressure)	肺動脈楔入圧
PB(barometric pressure)	大気圧
PB(parotid basic type)	PB型(耳下腺唾液)
PB(phenobarbital)	フェノバルビタール
PB(premature beat)	期外収縮
PBC(primary biliary cirrhosis)	原発性胆汁性肝硬変=PBI
PBF(pulmonary blood flow)	肺血流量
PBI(primary bilary cirrhosis)	原発性胆汁性肝硬変=PBC
PBI(protein-bound iodine)	蛋白結合ヨウ素
PBL(peripheral blood lymphocyte)	末梢血リンパ球
P-BLR(ponto-bulbar locomotor region)	橋-延髄歩行誘発野
PBP(penicillin-binding protein)	ペニシリン結合蛋白
PBP(progressive bulbar palsy)	進行性球麻痺
PBP(pseudobulbar palsy)	仮性球麻痺
PBSCT(peripheral blood stem cell transplantation)	末梢血幹細胞移植
PBV(pulmonary blood volume)	肺血流量
PC(penicillin)	ペニシリン

•PC•

PC(pericarditis constrictiva)	収縮性心膜炎
PC(pharyngitis chronica)	慢性咽頭炎
PC(pheochromocytoma)	褐色細胞腫
PC(photocoagulation)	光凝固
PC(platelet concentrate)	血小板濃厚液
PC(pneumotaxic center)	呼吸調節中枢
pc(post cibum)	食後　参照 食前：a.c.
PC(posterior communicating artery)	後交通動脈
PC(position change)	体位変換
PC(pseudotumor cerebri)	偽脳腫瘍
PC(pulmonary capillary)	肺毛細血管
PC, PCa(prostatic carcinoma)	前立腺癌
PCA(portacaval anastomosis)	門脈大静脈吻合
PCA(posterior cerebral artery)	後大脳動脈
	対 前大脳動脈：ACA
PCAG(primary closed angle glaucoma)	原発性閉塞隅角緑内障
PCD(plasma cell dyscrasia)	形質細胞異常症
PCD(polycystic ovary)	多嚢胞性卵巣＝PCO
PCE(polyarthritis chronique évolutive)	慢性進行性多発性関節炎
PCF(pharyngoconjunctival fever)	咽頭結膜熱
PCG(penicillin-G)	ペニシリンG
PCG(phonocardiogram)	心音図
PCG(plan craniography)	単純頭蓋撮影法
PCH(paroxysmal cold hemoglobinuria)	発作性寒冷ヘモグロビン(血色素)尿症
PCH(primary chronic hepatitis)	原発性慢性肝炎
PCKD(polycystic kidney disease)	多発性嚢胞腎＝PKD
PCL(posterior chamber lens)	後房内レンズ
PCL(posterior contact lens)	後房コンタクトレンズ
PCL(posterior cruciate ligament)	後十字靭帯
PCM(protein calorie malnutrition)	蛋白栄養代謝障害
PCN(percutaneous nephrostomy)	経皮的腎瘻造設術
PCN, PCNL(percutaneous nephrolithotomy)	経皮的腎切石術

PCNA(proliferating cell nunclear antigen)	増殖細胞核（蛋白）抗原
PCO(poly cystic ovary)	多嚢胞性卵巣＝PCD
PCO2(partial pressure of blood CO2)	炭酸ガス分圧
P com(posterior communicating artery)	後交通動脈 対 前交通動脈：Acom
Pcom(A)(posterior communicating〔artery〕)	後交通動脈
PCOS(polycystic ovary syndrome)	多嚢胞性卵巣症候群
PCP(pneumocystis pneumonia)	ニューモシスチス肺炎
PCPS(partial cardiopulmonary support)	部分的心肺補助装置
PCPS(percutaneous cardio-pulmonary support)	経皮的心肺補助装置
PCR(polymerase chain reaction)	ポリメラーゼ連鎖反応
PCS(peroral cholangioscopy)	経口胆管鏡検査
PCS(portacaval shunt)	門脈下大静脈吻合（術）
PCT(porphyria cutanea tarda)	晩発性皮膚ポルフィリン症
PCT(postcoital test)	性交後試験
PCT(proximal convoluted tubule)	近位曲尿細管
PCU(palliative care unit)	緩和ケア病棟
PCV(packed cell volume)	赤血球容積
PCV(penicillin-V〔phenoxymethylpenicillin〕)	ペニシリンV（フェノキシメチルペニシリン）
PCWP(pulmonary capillary wedge pressure)	肺動脈楔入圧
PD(pancreaticoduodenectomy)	膵頭十二指腸切除術
PD(panic disorder)	パニック障害、恐怖症候群
PD(paralyzing dose)	麻痺量
PD(parasite density)	寄生虫密度
PD(Parkinson's disease)	パーキンソン病
PD(Parkinsonian dementia)	パーキンソン認知症
PD(peritoneal dialysis)	腹膜透析
PD(personality disorder)	人格障害
PD(Pick disease)	ピック病
PD(posterior descending coronary artery)	冠状動脈下行枝
PD(postural drainage)	体位ドレナージ

PD

PD(progression of the disease)	（病気の）進行
PD(prostatodynia)	前立腺痛
PD(provisional diagnosis)	仮診断、暫定診断
PD(psychotic depression)	精神的うつ病
PD(pulmonary disease)	肺疾患
PD(pupillary distance)	瞳孔間距離
PDA(patent ductus arteriosus)	動脈管開存症
PDA-division (patent ductus arteriosus division)	動脈管開存（ボタロー管）切断術
PDC(parkinsonism dementia complex)	パーキンソン認知症症候群
PDD(pervasive developmental disorder)	広汎性発達障害
PDD(primary degenerative dementia)	一次性変性痴呆
PDE(paroxysmal dyspnea on exertion)	運動時発作的呼吸困難
PDGF(platelet-derived growth factor)	血小板由来増殖因子
PDHC(pyruvate dehydrogenase complex〔deficiency〕)	ピルビン酸脱水素酵素（欠損症）
PDLL(poorly differentiated lymphocytic lymphoma)	未分化型リンパ性リンパ腫
PDN(prednisolone)	プレドニゾロン
PDR(proliferative diabetic retinopathy)	増殖型糖尿病網膜症
PDS(placental dysfunction syndrome)	胎盤機能不全症候群
PDT(photo-dynamic therapy)	光線力学療法
PE(panlobular emphysema)	汎小葉型肺気腫
PE(partial epilepsy)	部分てんかん
PE(pericardial effusion)	心嚢貯留液
PE(physical examination)	理学的検査、身体検査
PE(plasma exchange)	血漿交換
PE(Portio-erosion)	腟部びらん
PE(pulmonary embolism)	肺塞栓症
PE(pulmonary emphysema)	肺気腫
PEA(phaco-emulsification & aspiration)	超音波水晶体乳化吸引術
pear-shaped	洋梨型の
pectus excavatum	漏斗胸
PED(pediatrics)	小児科

pedophilia	小児嗜愛
PEEP(positive end-expiratory pressure)	呼気終末陽圧
PEF(peak expiratory flow)	最大呼気流量
PEFR(peak expiratory flow rate)	最大呼気速度
PEG(percutaneous endoscopic gastrostomy)	経皮内視鏡的胃瘻造設術
PEG(pneumo-encephalography)	気脳撮影
PEI(phosphorus excretion index)	リン酸排泄係数
PEIT (percutaneous ethanol injection therapy)	経皮的エタノール注入療法
pelvic examination	内診
pelvis	腎盂
PEM(protein energy malnutrition)	蛋白エネルギー栄養失調症
pemphigus	天疱瘡
PEO(progressive external ophthalmoplegia)	進行性外眼筋麻痺
PEP(pigmentation, edema, polyneuropathy〔syndrome〕)	色素沈着、浮腫、多発神経障害症候群
PEP(pre-ejection period)	前駆出期
PEP/(V)ET(pre-ejection period/ventricular ejection time)	心室前駆出期・駆出時間比
PER(peak ejection rate)	最大駆出率
PER(peritoneum metastasis)	腹膜転移
percussion	打診法
perforation	穿孔
perfusion	血流
perfusion defect	灌流欠損
pericardium	心膜
perinatal	周産期の
perinatal period	周産期
periodic depression	周期性うつ病
periodical mania	周期性躁病
peripheral vertigo	末梢性眩暈
perirenal abscess	腎周囲膿瘍
peritoneal catheter	腹膜カテーテル
peritonitis	腹膜炎

pe

peroneal nerve	腓骨神経
perseveration	保続
persistent infection	持続感染
personality	人格
personality disorder	人格障害
perspiration	発汗
pertussis	百日咳
perverseness	ひねくれ
Pes(esophageal pressure)	食道内圧
PET(peritoneal equilibration test)	腹膜機能検査
PET (positron emission computed tomography)	ポジトロン断層シンチグラフィー
PET(psychiatry emergency team)	精神科救急チーム
petechiae	点状出血
petit mal	小発作 ◀関連▶ 大発作：gland mal
PF(pars flaccid)	弛緩部
PF(patellofemoral)	膝蓋大腿部
PF(peak flow)	ピークフロー、最大流量
PF(personality factor)	人格因子
PF(pulmonary function)	肺機能
PFA(perifimbrial adhesion)	卵管采周囲癒着
PFC(persistent fetal circulation)	胎児循環遺残
PFD(pancreatic function diagnosis)	膵機能診断テスト
PFFD(proximal femoral focal deficiency)	先天性大腿骨欠損
PFI(physical fitness index)	体力指数
PFJ(patellofemoral joint)	膝蓋大腿関節＝PF joint
PF joint(patellofemoral joint)	膝蓋大腿関節＝PFJ
PFO(patent foramen ovale)	卵円孔開存
PFR(peak filling rate)	最大充満速度
PFR(peak flow rate)	最大流速
PFS(pressure flow study)	圧力尿流試験
PFT(pancreatic function test)	膵機能テスト
PFT(picture frustration test)	絵画・欲求不満テスト

PFT(pulmonary function test)	肺機能検査
PG(prognosis)	予後
PG(prostaglandin)	プロスタグランジン
PG(pyoderma gangraenosum)	壊疽性膿皮症
PGA(polyglandular autoimmune 〔syndrome〕)	多腺性自己免疫(症候群)
PGE(primary generalized epilepsy)	原発性全般てんかん
PGE₁(prostaglandin E₁)	プロスタグランジンE_1
PGL(persistent generalized lymphadenopathy)	持続性全身性リンパ節腫脹
PGN(proliferative glomerulonephritis)	増殖性糸球体腎炎
PGR(psychogalvanic reflex)	精神皮膚電流反射
PGTT(prednisolone glucose tolerance test)	プレドニゾロンブドウ糖負荷試験
PGU(postgonococcal urethritis)	淋疾後尿道炎
PH(past history)	既往歴　関連　現症歴：PI
PH(personal history)	個人歴
Ph(hypopharynx)	下咽頭
PH(plasmapheresis)	血漿交換
PH(portal hepatitis)	門脈肝炎
PH(pulmonary hypertension)	肺高血圧症
phantom feeling	幻想
phantom pain	幻想痛
pharmacologic convulsive therapy	薬剤痙攣療法
PHC(photocoagulation)	光凝固
PHC(primary health care)	プライマリヘルスケア
PHC(primary hepatic carcinoma)	原発性肝癌＝PLC
phenothiazine derivative	フェノチアジン誘導体
pheochromocytoma	褐色細胞腫
PHIN (progressive hypertrophic interstitial neuritis)	進行性肥厚性間質性神経炎
PHN(postherpetic neuralgia)	帯状疱疹後神経痛
PHN(public health nurse)	保健師
phobic disorder	恐怖症
PHP(primary hyperparathyroidism)	原発性副甲状腺機能亢進症

PH

PHP(pseudohypoparathyroidism)	偽性副甲状腺機能低下症
PHPT(primary hyperparathyroidism)	原発性副甲状腺機能亢進症
PHT(phenytoin)	フェニトイン
PHT(portal hypertension)	門脈圧亢進症
PHT(pulmonary hypertension)	肺高血圧症
Physiol(physiology)	生理学
Ph⁺(Philadelphia〔chromosome〕)	フィラデルフィア染色体＝Ph1
Ph1(Philadelphia chromosome)	フィラデルフィア染色体＝Ph⁺
PI(peripheral iridectomy)	周辺虹彩切除
PI(plasma iron)	血漿鉄
PI(premature infant)	未熟児
PI(present illness)	現病歴　◀関連▶ 既往歴：PH
PI(pulmonary insufficiency)	肺動脈弁閉鎖不全（症）
pia mater	軟膜
PIB(partial ileal bypass)	部分的回腸バイパス術
PIC(personality inventory for children)	小児用人格調査表
PIC(picibanil)	ピシバニール
PICA(posterior inferior cerebellar artery)	後下小脳動脈
	◀対▶ 前下小脳動脈：AICA
PICC(peripherally inserted central catheter)	末梢挿入中心静脈カテーテル
PICU(pediatric intensive care unit)	小児集中治療室
PICU(perinatal intensive care unit)	周産期集中治療室
PICU(psychiatric intensive care unit)	精神科集中管理室
PID(pelvic inflammatory disease)	骨盤内炎症性疾患
PID(Protrusion of the Intervertebral Disk)	椎間板ヘルニア
PIDR(plasma iron disappearance rate)	血漿鉄消失率
PIE(pulmonary infiltration with eosinophilia)	好酸球増加を伴う肺浸潤
PIE(pulmonary interstitial emphysema)	間質性肺気腫
PIF(prolactin inhibiting factor)	プロラクチン抑制因子
PIF(prolactin release-inhibiting factor)	プロラクチン放出抑制因子
Pig deg(pigmentary degeneration)	網膜色素変性症
pigeon chest	鳩胸
pigmentation	色素沈着
pigmented spot	色素斑

PIGN(postinfectious glomerulonephritis)	感染後糸球体腎炎
PIH(pregnancy induced hypertension)	妊娠高血圧症候群
PIH(primary intracerebral hemorrhage)	原発性脳内出血
PIH(prolactin-release inhibiting hormone)	プロラクチン放出抑制ホルモン
piles	痔核
pimple	面皰(にきび)
PION(posterior ischemic optic neuropathy)	虚血性後部視神経ニューロパチー
PIP(peak inspiratory pressure)	最大吸気圧
PIP, PIPJ(proximal interphalangeal joint)	近位指節間関節
PIP joint(proximal interphalangeal joint)	近位指節間関節
PIT(R)(plasma iron turnover)	血漿鉄交代(率)
pitressin test	ピトレシンテスト
pituitary adenoma	下垂体腺腫
pituitary dwarfism	下垂体性小人症
pituitary gigantism	下垂体性巨人症
pituitary gland	下垂体
pityriasis	枇糠疹
PIVKA(protein induced by vitamin K absence)	ビタミンK非存在下誘導蛋白
P-J catheter(pancreatojejunostomy catheter)	膵空腸吻合カテーテル
PK(Pankreaskrebs)	膵臓癌
PK(Prostatakrebs)	前立腺癌
PKC(phlyctenular keratoconjunctivitis)	フリクテン性角膜結膜炎
PKD(polycystic kidney disease)	多発性嚢胞腎=PCKD
PKK(Pankreaskopfkrebs)	膵頭部癌
PKN(parkinsonism)	パーキンソン症候群
PKU(phenylketonuria)	フェニルケトン尿症
PL(palmaris longus muscle)	長掌筋
PL(perception of light)	光覚
PL(phospholipid)	リン脂質

PL

PL(placental alkaline phosphatase)	胎盤アルカリホスファターゼ
pl(pleura)	胸膜, 肋膜
PL(posterolateral artery branch)	後側壁枝
PL(prolactin)	プロラクチン
placental transfusion syndrome	胎盤輸血症候群
plasma exchange	血漿交換法
plaster	ギプス
plaster cast	ギプス包帯
plastic operation	形成手術
play therapy	遊戯療法
PLC(perivascular lymphocytic cuffing)	血管周囲リンパ球浸潤
PLC(primary liver cancer)	原発性肝癌
PLE(pleura metastasis)	胸膜転移
PLE(polymorphous light eruption)	多形日光疹
pleura	胸膜
pleural cavity	胸膜腔
pleural effusion	胸水
pleural friction rub	胸膜摩擦音
pleural indentation	胸膜陥凹
pleural thickening	胸膜肥厚
pleurisy	胸膜炎
PLL(posterior longitudinal ligament)	後縦靱帯
PLL(prolymphocytic leukemia)	前リンパ球性白血病
PLS(prolonged life support)	長期間救命処置
PLSVC(persistent left superior vena cava)	左上大静脈遺残症
PLT(platelet)	血小板
plus celer	速脈
plus tardus	遅脈
PM(pacemaker)	ペースメーカー
PM(papillary muscle)	乳頭筋
PM(petit mal)	小発作　関連 大発作：GM
PM(pneumomediastinum)	気縦隔(症)
PM(polymyositis)	多発性筋炎
pm(post meridiem / afternoon)	午後　参照 午前：am

PM(powder milk)	調整粉乳
pm(proper muscle layer)	固有筋層
PMA(progressive muscular atrophy)	進行性筋萎縮症
PMB(post menopausal bleeding)	閉経後出血
PMCT(percutaneous microwave coagulation therapy)	経皮的マイクロ波凝固療法
PMD(primary myocardial disease)	原発性心筋疾患
PMD(progressive muscular dystrophy)	進行性筋ジストロフィー
PMF(progressive massive fibrosis)	進行性塊状線維症
PMH(pure motor hemiplegia)	純粋運動性片麻痺
PMI(pacemaker implantation)	ペースメーカー植え込み術
PMI(perioperative myocardial infarction)	術中心筋梗塞
PMI(point of maximal impulse)	最大拍動点
PMI(posterior myocardial infarction)	後壁心筋梗塞
PMI (post-myocardial infarction〔syndrome〕)	心筋梗塞後症候群
PMI(pulmonary gas-mixing index)	肺内ガス混合指数
PML(posterior mitral leaflet)	僧帽弁後尖
PML (progressive multifocal leukoencephalopathy)	進行性多巣性白質脳症
PMM-C flap (pectoralis major muscle cutaneous flap)	大胸筋皮弁
PMN(polymorphonuclear〔neutrophilic〕leukocyte)	多形核(好中性)白血病
PMP(patient management problem)	患者管理問題
PMPO(postmenopausal palpable ovary)	閉経後卵巣腫大
PMR(peak metabolic rate)	最高代謝率(寒冷時)
PMR(polymyalgia rheumatica)	リウマチ性多発筋痛
PMR(postural miosis reaction)	体位性縮瞳反応
PMS(postmenopausal syndrome)	閉経後症候群
PMS(premenopausal syndrome)	月経前症候群
PN(parenteral nutrition)	非経口的栄養補給、静脈栄養
PN(periarteritis nodosa)	結節性動脈周囲炎

PN

PN(peripheral nerve)	末梢神経
Pn(pneumonia)	肺炎
PN(polyarteritis nodosa)	結節性多発性動脈炎
PN(progress notes)	経過記録
PN(psychoneurologic)	精神神経学
PN(psychoneurotic)	精神神経症の
PN(pyelonephritis)	腎盂腎炎
PNC(periarteritis nodosa cutaneous)	皮膚結節性動脈周囲炎
PND(paroxysmal nocturnal dyspnea)	発作性夜間呼吸困難
PND(postnasal drip)	後鼻漏、鼻後方滴注(法)
PNET(primitive neuroectodermal tumor)	未分化神経外胚葉(性)腫瘍
pneumococcus	肺炎球菌
pneumomediastinum	気縦隔＝PM
pneumonectomy	肺摘除術
pneumothorax	気胸＝Pnx
PNF (proprioceptive neuromuscular facilitation)	固有受容器神経筋促進法
PNH(paroxysmal nocturnal hemoglobinuria)	発作性夜間ヘモグロビン(血色素)尿症
PNI(perineural invasion)	癌神経周囲浸潤
PNI(prognostic nutritional index)	予後判定栄養指標
PNL(perceived noise level)	騒音レベル
PNL(percutaneous nephrolithotomy)	経皮的腎砕石術
PNMA(progressive neural muscular atrophy)	進行性神経性筋萎縮症
PNO(progressive nuclear ophthalmoplegia)	進行性核性眼筋麻痺
PNP(peripheral neuropathy)	末梢神経障害
PNPB(positive negative pressure breathing)	陽陰圧呼吸法
PNPV(positive negative pressure ventilator)	(自動)陽陰圧呼吸装置
PNS(parasympathetic nervous system)	副交感神経系 ◀関連▶ 交感神経系：SNS
PNS(percutaneous nephrostomy)	経皮的腎瘻(術)
PNS(peripheral nervous system)	末梢神経系 対 中枢神経系：CNS, ZNS
Pnx(pneumothorax)	気胸

PO (per os)	経口的(口から摂取する)
PO (phone order)	音階
Po (polyp)	ポリープ
PO (post operative)	術後
PO (pump-oxygenator)	人工心肺装置
PO_2 (partial pressure of blood O_2)	酸素分圧
POA (primary optic atrophy)	原発性視神経萎縮
POAG (primary open angle glaucoma)	原発性開放隅角緑内障
POD (post operative day)	術後日
POF (premature ovarian failure)	早発卵巣不全
polio (poliomyelitis anterior acuta)	急性灰白髄炎(ポリオ)
pollakiuria	頻尿(症)
pollinosis	花粉症
polydactyly	多指症
polydipsia	多飲
polymicrogyria	多小脳回
polyostotic fibrous dysplasia	多骨性線維性骨形成異常症
polyphagia	過食
polypnea	多呼吸、頻呼吸
polyuria	多尿
POM (pain on motion)	運動痛
POMC (postoperative maxillary cyst)	術後性上顎嚢胞
pompholyx	汗疱
POMR (problem oriented medical record)	問題志向型診療録
pons	橋
POPS (peroral pancreatoscopy)	経口的膵管鏡検査
POS (problem-oriented system)	問題思考型システム
Posm (plasma osmolality)	血漿浸透圧
post (posterior wall stomach)	胃後壁
posterior fontanel	小泉門
	◀関連▶ 大泉門：anterior fontanel
posterior pituitary	下垂体後葉
postoperative atelectasis	術後性無気肺

po

postoperative complications	術後合併症
postoperative delirium	術後せん妄
postprandial	食後の
postrenal acute renal failure	腎後性急性腎不全
post-term infant	過期産児
postural drainage	体位ドレナージ
posture	姿勢
POW (prisoner of war syndrome)	戦争捕虜症候群
POWZ (postoperative Wangenzyste)	術後性頬部嚢胞
P0〜3 (peritoneal dissemination)	肉眼的腹膜播種性転移の程度の分類
PP (periodic paralysis)	周期性四肢麻痺
PP (phthisis pulmonum)	肺結核
PP (plasmapheresis)	血漿交換
PP (presenting part)	胎児先進部
PP (primipara)	初産　参照 経産：MP
PP (progressive paralysis)	進行麻痺
PP (proximal phalanx)	基節骨
PP (pulse pressure)	脈圧
PP (pyloroplasty)	幽門形成術
PPB (positive pressure breathing)	陽圧呼吸
PPC (pneumopericardium)	心膜気腫、気心膜症
PPC (progressive patient care)	段階別患者ケア
PPD (purified protein derivative of tuberculin)	精製ツベルクリン
PPDP (persistent pulmonary dysfunction in premature infant)	未熟児の持続性呼吸障害
PPF (plasma protein fraction)	血漿蛋白分解
PPG (pylorus-preserving gastrectomy)	幽門輪保存胃切除術
PPH (post partum hemorrhage)	分娩後出血
PPH (posterior pituitary hormone)	下垂体後葉ホルモン
PPH (primary pulmonary hypertension)	原発性肺高血圧症
PPHN (persistent pulmonary hypertension of newborn)	新生児遷延性肺高血圧症

PPHP(pseudopseudohypoparathyroidism)	偽性偽性副甲状腺機能低下症
PPI(proton pump inhibitor)	プロトンポンプ阻害薬
ppm(parts per million)	百万分量単位中の絶対数
PPP(palatopharyngoplasty)	口蓋咽頭形成(術)
PPP(pigmented pretibial patches)	前脛骨部色素斑
PPP(pruritic papules of pregnancy)	妊娠性掻痒性丘疹
PPP(pseudoprecocious puberty)	仮性早熟
PPP(pustulosis palmaris et plantaris)	掌蹠膿疱症
PPPD(porokeratosis plantaris, palmaris et disseminata)	播種状掌蹠孔角化症
PPPD, PpPD(pylorus-preserving pancreato duodenectomy)	幽門輪温存膵頭十二指腸切除術
PPPPPP(pain, pallor, paresthesia, pulselessness, paralysis, prostration)	急性動脈閉塞症時にみられる症候の6つのP
PPRF(paramedian pontine reticular formation)	傍正中橋網様体
PPS(algesic substance)	発痛物質
PPS(postpolio syndrome)	ポリオ後症候群
PPS(prospective payment system)	診断群別包括払い
PPS(pure pulmonary stenosis)	純型肺動脈弁狭窄症
PPSM(plantar-palmar-subungual melanoma)	掌蹠爪下黒色腫
PPT(plasma prothrombin time)	血漿プロトロンビン時間
Ppt(precipitate)	沈殿物
PPV(phacomatosis pigmento vascularis)	色素血管母斑症
PPV(positive pressure ventilation)	陽圧換気
PQ(atrio-ventricular conduction〔time〕)	房室伝導時間
PR(partial remission)	部分寛解
	◀関連▶ 完全寛解:CR
Pr(presbyopia)	老視
PR(pulmonary regurgitation)	肺動脈弁逆流(症)
PR(pulmonic regurgitation)	肺動脈弁閉鎖不全
PR(pulse rate)	脈拍数
PRA(plasma renin activity)	血漿レニン活性

PR

PRC (plasma renin concentration)	血漿レニン濃度
PRCA (pure red cell anaemia)	純赤血球性貧血
PRCA (pure red cell aplasia)	赤芽球癆
PRE (progressive resistive exercise)	漸増抵抗運動
precocious puberty	思春期早発症
preconscious	前意識
precordial pain	前胸部痛
predilection place	好発部位
preg (pregnancy)	妊娠
premature delivery	早産
pre-medi (preanesthetic medication)	前投薬
premedication	前投薬
premenstrual syndrome	月経前症候群
prenatal period	出生前期
preoperative management	術前管理
prerenal acute renal failure	腎前性急性腎不全
presbycusis	老人性難聴
preschool period	幼児期
presenting part	先進部
preserved blood	保存血
pressure symptom	圧迫症状
pre-term infant	早期産児
prevention	予防
PRF (prolactin-releasing factor)	プロラクチン放出因子
prickly heat	汗疹(あせも)
primal therapy	プライマル(原初)療法
primary	原発
primary syndrome	初発症状
primary teeth	乳歯
	◀関連▶永久歯：secondary teeth
principal effect	主作用
	参照 副作用：side effect

PRIND(prolonged reversible ischemic neurological deficits)	遷延性可逆性虚血性神経脱落
PRK(photorefractive keratectomy)	レーザー屈折矯正角膜切除術
PRL(prolactin)	プロラクチン
PRN(polyradiculoneuritis)	多発神経炎
prn(pro re nata)	患者の状況によって／必要に応じて
productive cough	痰咳(湿性咳)
progeria	早老症
progesterone	プロゲステロン
prognosis	予後
progressive	進行性の
prohibition	禁止
projection	投影
projective testing	投影法
PROM(premature rupture of membranes)	前期破水
PROMM(proximal myotonic myopathy)	近位筋緊張性筋障害
prominent eyes	眼球突出
prone	腹臥位の、うつぶせになる
proneness	腹臥位
	◀関連▶仰臥位：dorsal position 側臥位：lateral recumbent position
PROST(pronuclear stage tubal transfer)	体外受精卵卵管内移植＝ZIFT
prostatic cancer	前立腺癌
prostatitis	前立腺炎
protective inoculation	予防接種
protein-losing enteropathy	蛋白漏出性腸症
proteinuria	蛋白尿
protruding tongue	舌突出
PRP(panretinal photocoagulation)	汎網膜光凝固

PR

PRP(platelet rich plasma)	多血小板血漿
PRP(pressure rate product)	ダブルプロダクト(心拍数×収縮期血圧)
PRP(progressive rubella panencephalitis)	進行性風疹性全脳炎
PRRF(postrenal renal failure)	腎後性腎不全
PRS(personality rating scale)	人格評点スケール
PRT(pendular rotation test)	振子様回転検査
prurigo	結節性痒疹、痒疹
pruritus	痒症
PS test(pancreozymin-secretin test)	パンクレオザイミン・セクレチン試験
PS(paradoxical sleep)	逆説睡眠
PS(patient serum)	患者血清
PS(photic stimulation)	光刺激
PS(pressure systolic)	収縮気圧
PS(psychiatric)	精神医学の
PS(pulmonary stenosis)	肺動脈(弁)狭窄症
PS(pyloric stenosis)	幽門狭窄症
PSA(prostate specific antigen)	前立腺特異抗原
PSAGN(poststreptococcal acute glomerulonephritis)	急性溶連球菌感染後糸球体腎炎
PSC(posterior subcapsular cataract)	後嚢下白内障
PSC(primary sclerosing cholangitis)	原発性硬化性胆管炎
PSD(psychosomatic diseases)	心身症
PSE(partial splenic embolization)	部分的脾動脈塞栓術
PSE(present state examination)	現在症検査
PSE(progressive symmetric erythrokeratodermia)	進行性対称性紅斑角皮症
pseudoarthrosis	偽関節
pseudocroup	仮性クループ
pseudocyesis	想像妊娠
PSG(polysomnogram)	睡眠脳波検査
PSH(periarthritis scapulohumerals)	肩関節周囲炎、五十肩
PSH(post spinal headache)	脊髄麻酔後頭痛

PSL(prednisolone)	プレドニゾロン
PSM(presystolic murmur)	前収縮期雑音
PSMA(progressive spinal muscular atrophy)	進行性脊髄性筋萎縮症
PSNS(parasympathetic nervous system)	副交感神経系
	◀関連▶交感神経系：SNS
PSO(psoriasis vulgaris)	尋常性乾癬
psoriasis	乾癬
psoriatic arthritis	乾癬性関節炎
PSP(progressive supranuclear palsy)	進行性核上性麻痺
PSp(pseudopregnancy)	偽妊娠
PSP(test)(phenolsulfonphthalein〔test〕)	フェノールスルホンフタレイン（PSP排泄）試験
PSR(patellar sehnen-reflex)	膝蓋腱反射
PSR(positive supporting reflex)	陽性支持反射
PSR(pulmonary stenosis and regurgitation)	肺動脈弁狭窄兼閉鎖不全症
PSS(physiological saline solution)	生理食塩水
PSS(progressive systemic sclerosis)	進行性全身性強皮症
PST(paroxysmal supraventricular tachycardia)	発作性上室性頻拍
PSTT(placental site trophoblastic tumor)	胎盤着床部絨毛性腫瘍
PSV(pressure support ventilation)	圧維持換気法
PSVT(paroxysmal supraventricular tachycardia)	発作性上室性頻拍
PSW(psychiatric social worker)	精神科ソーシャルワーカー
Psy(psychiatry)	精神医学、精神科
psycho pharmaco therapy	向精神薬療法
psychoanalysis	精神分析
psychoanalytical psychotherapy	精神分析療法
psychodrama	心理劇
psychological testing of personality	性格テスト
psychomotor excitement	精神運動興奮
psychomotor retardation	精神運動抑制
psychomotor stimulant	精神運動刺激薬

ps

psychopathy	精神病質
psychosexual disorder	精神性的障害
psychosomatic disorder	精神身体障害
psychotherapy	精神療法
psychotropic drug	向精神薬
PT(paroxysmal tachycardia)	発作性頻脈
PT(pars tensa)	緊張部
PT(percussion tone)	打診音
PT(physical therapist)	理学療法士
	◀関連▶作業療法士：OT
PT(physical therapy)	理学療法
PT(prothrombin time)	プロトロンビン時間
PT(pyramidal tract)	錐体路
Pt, pt(patient)	患者　参照 外来患者：OP
PTA(percutaneous transluminal angio-dilatation)	経皮的血管拡張(術)
PTA(percutaneous transluminal angioplasty)	経皮的血管形成(術)
PTA(peritonsillar abscess)	扁桃周囲膿瘍
PTA(peritubal adhesion)	卵管周囲癒着
PTA(persistent truncus arteriosus)	総動脈幹遺残
PTA(posttraumatic amnesia)	外傷後健忘
PTA(pure tone audiometry)	純音聴力検査
PTAD(percutaneous transhepatic abscess drainage)	経皮経肝肝膿瘍ドレナージ
PTB(patellar tendon bearing)	膝蓋腱支持装具
PTB(posttraumatische Beschwerde)	頭部外傷後遺症
PTBD(percutaneous transhepatic biliary drainage)	経皮経肝胆道ドレナージ
PTC(percutaneous transhepatic cholangiography)	経皮経肝胆道造影
PTCA(percutaneous transluminal coronary angioplasty)	経皮経管冠動脈形成術
PTCD(percutaneous transhepatic cholangiodrainage)	経皮経肝胆管ドレナージ

PT

PTCR(percutaneous transluminal coronary recanalization)	経皮冠動脈血栓溶解療法
PTCS(percutaneous transhepatic cholangioscopy)	経皮経肝胆道鏡検査
PTD(persistent trophoblastic disease)	存続絨毛症
PTE(pulmonary thromboembolism)	肺動脈血栓塞栓(症)
PTG(parathyroid gland)	上皮小体
PTG(pneumatic tonography)	気体眼圧計
PTGBD(percutaneous transhepatic gallbladder drainage)	経皮経肝胆道ドレナージ
PTH(parathyroid hormone)	副甲状腺ホルモン ◀関連▶ 甲状腺ホルモン:TH
PTH(post-transfusion hepatitis)	輸血後肝炎
PTK(phototherapeutic keratectomy)	治療的レーザー角膜切除術
PTL(preterm labor)	切迫早産
PTMC(percutaneous transvenous mitral commissurotomy)	経皮経静脈僧帽弁交連切開術
PTN(pyramidal tract neuron)	錐体路ニューロン
PTO(percutaneous transhepatic obliteration of esophageal varices)	経皮経肝食道静脈瘤塞栓術
PTP(percutaneous transhepatic portography)	経皮経肝門脈造影
PTPA(posterior thalamoperforating artery)	後視床穿通動脈
PTPE(percutaneous transhepatic portal embolization)	経皮経肝門脈塞栓術
PTPE(percutaneous transhepatic portal vein embolization)	経皮経肝門脈枝塞栓術
PTR(patellar tendon reflex)	膝蓋腱反射
PTR(pulmonary valve replacement)	肺動脈弁置換術
PTSD(post traumatic stress disorder)	外傷性ストレス障害
PTT(partial thromboplastin time)	部分トロンボプラスチン時間
PTT(patellar tendon transfer)	膝蓋腱移行術
PTT(photo-toxic therapy)	光毒性治療法
PTX(parathyroidectomy)	副甲状腺全摘出術
PTX(pertussis toxin)	百日咳毒素

PT

PTX(pneumothorax)	気胸
PU(peptic ulcer)	消化性潰瘍
PUA(primary unknown adenocarcinoma)	原発不明癌
pubic arch	恥骨弓
PUE, FUE (pyrexia [fever] of unknown etiology)	原発不明熱＝PUO
PUJ(pelvic-ureteral junction)	腎盂尿細管移行部
PUL(percutaneous ultrasonic lithotripsy)	経皮的腎結石超音波砕石術
pulmonary	肺の
pulmonary abscess	肺膿瘍
pulmonary agenesis	肺無形成
pulmonary atelectasis	無気肺
pulmonary congestion	肺うっ血
pulmonary cystic disease	肺囊胞症
pulmonary edema	肺水腫
pulmonary fibrosis	肺線維症
pulmonary large cell carcinoma	肺大細胞癌
pulmonary markings	肺紋理
pulmonary periphery	肺野
pulmonary renal syndrome	肺腎症候群
pulmonary segmentectomy	肺区域切除
pulmonary sequestration	肺分画症
pulmonary small cell carcinoma	肺小細胞癌
pulmonary tuberculosis	肺結核
pulmonary valve	肺動脈弁
pulsatile secretion	脈状分泌
pulse Doppler	パルスドプラー法
pulse therapy	パルス療法
puncture	穿刺
PUO(pyrexia of unknown origin)	原発不明熱＝PUE
pupillary dilatation	瞳孔散大
pupillary reflex	瞳孔反射
PUPPP(pruritic urticarial papules and plaques of pregnancy)	妊娠性掻痒性蕁麻疹様丘疹兼局面症

purpura	紫斑
pursed lip breathing	口すぼめ呼吸
purulent	化膿性の、化膿した
pus	膿(うみ)
pustula	膿疱
PUVA(psoralen ultraviolet A therapy)	ソラレン紫外線療法
PV(pemphigus vulgaris)	尋常性天疱瘡
PV(plasma volume)	血漿量
PV(polycythemia vera)	真性多血症
PV(portal vein)	門脈静脈
PV(pulmonary valve)	肺動脈弁
PV(pulmonary vein)	肺静脈 　対　肺動脈：PA
PVC(premature ventricular contraction)	心室性期外収縮
PVC(pulmonary venous congestion)	肺静脈うっ血
PVD(peripheral vascular disease)	末梢血管疾患
PVD(posterior vitreous detachment)	後部硝子体剥離
PVE(prosthetic valve endocarditis)	人工弁心内膜炎
PVF(portal venous flow)	門脈血流量
PVFS(postviral fatigue syndrome)	ウイルス感染後疲労症候群
PVG(pneumo-ventriculography)	気脳室撮影
PVI(pressure-volume index)	圧・容積指標
PVL(periventricular leukomalacia)	脳室周囲白質軟化症
PVN(peripheral venous nutrition)	末梢静脈栄養 　対　中心静脈栄養：IVH
PVN(predictive value of negative test)	陰性反応的中度
PVO(pulmonary venous obstruction)	肺静脈閉塞
PVOD (pulmonary vascular obstructive disease)	肺血管閉塞性病変
PVOV(pulmonic valve opening velocity)	肺動脈弁開放速度
PVP(peripheral venous pressure)	末梢静脈圧 　対　中心静脈圧：CVP
PVP(predictive value of positive test)	陽性反応的中度
PVR(peripheral vascular resistance)	末梢血管抵抗
PVR(postvoid residual urine volume)	排尿後残尿量

PV

PVR(pressure-volume relationship)	圧・容積関係
PVR(pressure-volume response)	圧・容積反応
PVR(proliferative vitreoretinopathy)	増殖硝子体網膜症
PVR(pulmonary vascular resistance)	肺血管抵抗
PVS(persystent vegitative state)	遷延性植物状態
PVS(pigmented villonodular synovitis)	色素性絨毛結節性滑膜炎
P-V shunt(peritoneo-venous shunt)	腹腔—静脈短絡術
PVT(paroxysmal ventricular tachycardia)	発作性心室性頻拍
PVT(portal vein thrombosis)	門脈血栓症
PWB(partial weight-bearing)	部分荷重
PWBC(peripheral white blood cells)	末梢血白血球
Px(pneumothorax)	気胸
pyelonephritis	腎盂腎炎
pylon	仮義足
pyogenic arthritis	化膿性関節炎
pyothorax	膿胸
pyramidal system	錐体路系
pyramidal tract signs	錐体路症候
pyromania	放火癖
pyrosis	胸やけ
pyruvate	ピルビン酸
pyuria	膿尿

Q

QC(quality control)	（血清値の）精度管理
QCA(quantitative coronary arteriography)	定量的冠状動脈造影(法)
QCT(quantitative computed tomography)	定量的CT法
qdx(quantities duplex)	二倍量
qh(quaque hora)	毎時　参照 4時間ごとに：omn quad hor
q.i.d.(quater in die)	1日4回 参照 1日2回：b.d. 1日3回：t.i.d.
Qm(every morning / quaque mane)	毎朝
Qn(enery night / quaque nocte)	毎夜
QNS(quantity not sufficient)	量不足
QOD(quaque die)	隔日に
QOL(quality of life)	生命の質、生活の質
qp(quantum placet)	任意の量
QPA(pulmonary arterial flow)	肺動脈血流量
Qp/Qs(pulmonary/somatic arterial flow ratio)	肺／体血流比
QR(quantum rectum)	正量
Qs(quantum sufficiat)	十分量、適量
QS(shunt flow)	シャント血流量
QSE(quadriceps setting exercise)	大腿四頭筋セッティング運動
QS/QT(right to left shunt ratio)	肺シャント率
Qt(total blood flow)	心拍出量
Q-test(Queckenstedt test)	クエッケンシュテット検査
Q2h(every two hours)	2時間毎
quad id(quater in die)	1日4回
quadriplegia	四肢麻痺
quadruplet	四胎
querulous delusion	好訴妄想
Qw(every week)	毎週

R

R(resistance)	耐性、抵抗力
R(respiration)	呼吸、呼吸数
R(right)	右 対 左：L
Ra(rectum above the peritoneal reflection)	上部直腸
RA(refractory anemia)	不応性貧血
RA(rest angina)	安静時狭心症
RA(rheumatoid arthritis)	慢性関節リウマチ
RA(right atrium)	右心房 対 左心房：LA
RAA(renin-angiotensin-aldosterone)	レニン・アンギオテンシン・アルドステロン系
RAA(right atrial appendage)	右心耳
rabies	狂犬病
RAD(right axis deviation)	右軸偏位
Rad DX(radio-logical-diagnosis)	放射線学的診断
radial nerve	橈骨神経 参照 尺骨神経：ulner nerve 正中神経：median nerve
radiating pain	放散痛
radical operation	根治手術＝rad op
Radiol(radiology)	放射線医学
radiotherapy	放射線治療
rad op(radical operation)	根治手術
RAEB(refractory anemia with excess of blasts)	芽球増加性不応性貧血
RAfactor(rheumatoid factor)	リウマチ因子
RAG(renal arteriography)	腎動脈造影(法)
RAH(right anterior hemiblock)	右脚前枝ブロック
RAH(right atrial hypertrophy)	右心房肥大
RAHA(rheumatoid arthritis hemagglutination〔test〕)	慢性関節リウマチ赤血球凝集(試験)
RAI(radioactive iodine)	放射性ヨード
RAIU(radioactive iodine uptake test)	放射性ヨード摂取試験

rale	ラ音
RAO(right anterior oblique)	右斜位
RAP(renal artery pressure)	腎動脈圧
RAP(right atrial pressure)	右心房圧
rapid ACTH test	迅速ACTH試験
rapport	疎通性、信頼関係
RARS (refractory anemia with ring sideroblast)	環状鉄芽球を伴う不応性貧血
RAS(recurrent aphthous stomatitis)	再発性アフタ性口内炎
RAS(renal artery stenosis)	腎動脈狭窄
rash	発疹
RAST(radioallergosorbent test)	放射性アレルギー吸着試験
rational emotive psychotherapy	論理療法＝RET
Raw(airway resistance)	気道抵抗
Rb(rectum below the peritoneal reflection)	下部直腸
RB(renal biopsy)	腎生検
RB(reticular body)	網様体
RB(retinoblastoma)	網膜芽細胞腫
RB(Riemenbügel)	リーメンビューゲル（先天性股関節脱臼治療用装具）
RBBB(right bundle branch block)	右脚ブロック ◀関連▶ 左脚ブロック：LBBB
RBC(red blood cell〔count〕)	赤血球(数) ◀関連▶ 白血球：WBC
RBF(renal blood flow)	腎血流量
RC(respiration cease)	呼吸停止
RC(respiratory center)	呼吸中枢
RC(respiratory compensation)	呼吸性補正
R ca(rectal cancer)	直腸癌
RCA(right colic artery)	右結腸動脈
RCA(right coronary artery)	右冠動脈 ◀関連▶ 左冠動脈：LCA　左回旋枝：LCX
rCBF(regional cerebral blood flow)	局所脳血流

RC

RCC(renal cell carcinoma)	腎癌
RCC(renal cell carcinoma)	腎細胞癌
RCC(right coronary cusp)	右冠尖
RCI(respiratory control index)	呼吸調節率
RCIT(red cell iron turnover)	赤血球鉄代謝
RCM(restrictive cardiomyopathy)	拘束型心筋症
RCP(respiratory care practitioner)	呼吸ケア実施士
RCR(round the circadian rhythm)	生体リズムに基づく内服
RCS(reticulum cell sarcoma)	細網肉腫
RCS(right coronary sinus)	右冠状静脈洞
RC sign(red-color sign)	発赤所見
RCU(red cell iron utilization)	赤血球鉄利用率
RCU(respiratory care unit)	呼吸集中治療室
RCV(red cell volume)	赤血球容積
RD(Raynaud's disease)	レイノー病
RD(recessively inherited form of dystonia)	劣性遺伝性ジストニー
RD(retinal detachment)	網膜剥離
RD(rheumatic disease)	リウマチ性疾患
RdA(reading age)	読書年齢
RDA(recommended daily allowance)	1日量許容（1日に摂取すべき栄養素量）
RDC(rapidly destructive coxarthropathy)	急性破壊性股関節症
RDC(research diagnostic criteria)	研究のための診断基準
RDE(receptor destroying enzyme)	受容体失活酵素
RDEB (recessive dystrophic epidermolysis bullosa)	劣性栄養障害性表皮水疱症
RDPA(right descending pulmonary artery)	右下行肺動脈
RDS(respiratory distress syndrome)	呼吸窮迫症候群
RE(right eye)	右眼 対 左眼：LE
reaction formation	反応形成
reactive depression	反応性うつ病
reactive hypoglycemia	反応性低血糖
reality therapy	現実療法
receptor	受容器、感覚器官

recidivation	再発
recipient	臓器を提供される人
	対 提供者：donor
reconstruction	再建
rectal	直腸の
recurrence	再発、反復
recurrent dislocation	反復性脱臼
redistribution	再分布
redness	発赤
REE(resting energy expenditure)	安静時熱量消費量
reentry	興奮回帰性(リエントリー)
ref(reflex)	反射
referred pain	関連痛
reflux nephropathy	逆流性腎症
reg(regular)	規則的
regional	限局性
regression	退行
Rehabili(rehabilitation)	リハビリテーション
rejection	拒絶反応
reject transplant	移植拒絶
relapse	再発
relative curative operation	準治癒手術
relaxation therapy	リラクセーション療法
religious delusion	宗教妄想
REM, REM sleep	レム睡眠
(rapid eye movement〔sleep〕)	関連 ノンレム睡眠：NREM, NREM sleep
remission	寛解 参照 部分寛解：Pr 完全寛解：CR
remodeling	改構(再造形)、リモデリング
renal	腎臓の
renal abscess	腎膿瘍
renal anemia	腎性貧血
renal arterial embolism	腎動脈塞栓症

re

renal cell carcinoma	腎細胞癌＝RCC
renal cortex	腎皮質
renal diabetes insipidus	腎性尿崩症
renal failure	腎不全
renal glycosuria	腎性糖尿
renal hypertension	腎性高血圧症
renal infarction	腎梗塞
renal osteodystrophy	腎性骨異栄養症
renal parenchymal	腎実質性の
renal scintigraphy	腎シンチグラフィー
renal transplantation	腎移植
renin-angiotensin system	レニン-アンギオテンシン系
renovascular hypertension	腎血管性高血圧症
REP(retrograde pyelography)	逆行性腎盂造影法
REPE(re-expansion pulmonary edema)	再拡張性肺水腫
reperfusion arrhythmia	再灌流不整脈
reperfusion injury	再灌流障害
replantation	再接着術
repolarization	再分極
repression	抑圧
RES(reticuloendothelial system)	細網内皮系
residual type	残遺型（統合失調症）
resistance	抵抗
resonance	共鳴
resp(respiration)	呼吸
respiratory arrest	呼吸停止
REST(regressive electroshock treatment)	逆行性電気ショック療法
resuscitation	蘇生法
	参照 心肺蘇生法：CPR
	心肺脳蘇生法：CPCR
RET(rational emotive therapy)	論理療法
Ret(reticulocyte)	網状赤血球
RETDIAB(retinopathia diabetica)	糖尿病性網膜症
retinal detachment	網膜剥離＝RD

retrograde amnesia	逆行健忘
retroperitoneal fibrosis	後腹膜線維症
reverse redistribution	逆再分布
reversible ischemia	可逆的虚血
RF(rapid filling)	急速充満期
RF(relative function of the kidney)	相対的腎機能
RF(renal failure)	腎不全
RF(respiratory failure)	呼吸不全
RF(rheumatic fever)	リウマチ熱
RF(rheumatoid factor)	リウマチ因子
RFA(right frontoanterior〔position〕)	右後前頭位(胎位)
RFC(rosette-forming cell)	ロゼット形成細胞
RFP(rifampicin)	リファンピシン
RFT(right frontotransverse)	右横前頭位(胎位)
RGA(right gastric artery)	右胃動脈
RGE(right gastroepiploic artery)	右胃大網動脈
RGP(rigid gas permeable〔contact lens〕)	酸素透過性ハードコンタクトレンズ
RH(regional heparinization)	局所ヘパリン化
RH(releasing hormone)	放出ホルモン
Rh(rhesus factor)	Rh因子
rh(rhonchus)	ラ音
RHA(right hepatic artery)	右肝動脈
	◀対 左肝動脈：LHA
rhabdomyolysis	横紋筋融解症
rhagades	亀裂
RHC(right heart catheterization)	右心カテーテル(法)
RHD(rheumatoid heart disease)	リウマチ性心疾患
rheumatism	リウマチ
RHF(rightsided heart failure)	右心不全
	◀関連 左心不全：LHF
rhinitis	鼻炎
rhino-pollinosis	鼻花粉症
RHL(right hepatic lobe)	肝右葉

rH

rHL(right hepatic lobectomy)	肝右葉切除術
RHS(Ramsay Hunt syndrome)	ラムゼイ・ハント症候群
RHS(right heart strain)	右心負荷
RHV(right hepatic vein)	右肝静脈
	対 左肝静脈：LHV
RI(radioisotope)	ラジオアイソトープ（放射性同位元素）
RI(regular insulin)	レギュラーインスリン
RI(respiratory index)	呼吸指数
RIA(radioimmunoassay)	ラジオイムノアッセイ（放射免疫測定法）
RICE(rest, ice, compression, elevation)	安静、冷却、圧迫、挙上（応急処置）
RI(radioisotope)cisternography	ラジオアイソトープ脳槽造影
rickets	くる病
RICU(respiratory intensive care unit)	呼吸器疾患集中治療室
RIF(right iliac fossa)	右腸骨窩
RIH(right inguinal hernia)	右鼠径ヘルニア
RILD(radiation induced lung disease)	放射線誘発肺疾患
RILvD(radiation induced liver disease)	放射線誘発肝疾患
RIND (reversible ischemic neurological deficit)	可逆性虚血性神経脱落症状
ring finger	薬指
ringworm	たむし、水虫、白癬
RIP(radioimmunoprecipitation)	放射線免疫沈降法
RIST(radioimmunosorbent test)	放射性免疫吸着試験
RITA(right internal thoracic artery)	右内胸動脈
RK(Rectumkrebs)	直腸癌
RK(radial keratotomy)	放射状角膜切開術
R-L(rechts-links Storung)	左右障害
RLE(right lower extremity)	右下肢
RLF(retrolental fibroplasia)	後水晶体線維増殖（症）
RLH (reactive lymphoreticular hyperplasia)	反応性リンパ細網細胞増成（症）

RLL(right lower lobe of lung)	右肺下葉
RLN(recurrent laryngeal nerve)	反回神経
RLND (retroperitoneal lymph node dissection)	後腹膜リンパ節摘除(術)
RLQ(right lower quadrant)	右下腹部
RM(repetition maximum)	最大反復回復
RM(respiratory metabolism)	呼吸代謝
RM(respiratory movement)	呼吸運動
RM(resting metabolism)	安静代謝量
RMA(right mentoanterior〔position〕)	右頤前方位(胎位)
rMBF(regional myocardial blood flow)	局所心筋血流量
RME(resting metabolic expenditure)	安静時エネルギー消費量
RMI(recent myocardial infarction)	亜急性心筋梗塞
RML(right middle lobe of lung)	右中葉
RMP(right mentoposterior〔position〕)	右頤後方位(胎位)
RMR(relative metabolic rate)	エネルギー代謝率
RMS(rhabdomyosarcoma)	横紋筋肉腫
RMT(right mentotransverse〔position〕)	右頤横位(胎位)
RMTD (right main trunk coronary artery disease)	右冠動脈主幹部病変
RN(reflux nephropathy)	逆流性腎症
RNA(ribonucleic acid)	リボ核酸
RNCA(radionuclide cerebral angiography)	核医学的脳血管撮影
RND(radical neck dissection)	根本的頚部郭清術
RND(retroperitoneal node dissection)	後腹膜リンパ節郭清(術)
RNFL(retinal nerve fiber layer)	網膜神経線維束
RNP(ribonucleoprotein)	リボ核蛋白
RO(reality orientation)	(認知症老人への)リアリティ・オリエンテーション、現実見当識訓練
RO(reverse osmosis)	逆浸透
ROA(right occipitoanterior〔position〕)	右前方後頭位(胎位)
ROA(right occiput anterior)	第2頭位第1分類(胎位)
rocker-bottom foot	舟底足

RO

ROD(renal osteodystrophy)	腎性骨異栄養症
ROI(region of interest)	関心領域
ROM(range of motion)	関節可動域
ROM(rupture of membranes)	破水
ROME(range of motion exercise)	関節可動域訓練
ROMT(range of motion test)	関節可動域テスト
rooting reflex	口唇探索反射、哺乳反射
root sign	神経根症状
ROP(retinopathy of prematurity)	未熟児網膜症
ROP(right occipito-posterior〔position〕)	第2頭位第2分類(胎位)
Rorschach test	ロールシャッハ法
ROSC(return of spontaneous circulation)	心拍再開
roseola	バラ疹
ROT(right occipito-transverse〔position〕)	第2頭位(胎位)
rotation	関節の回旋
RP(rectal prolapse)	直腸脱
RP(retrograde pyelography)	逆行性腎盂造影法
Rp/Rs	肺／体血管抵抗比
Rp, Rx(recipe, prescription)	処方
RPC(radial peripapillary capillaries)	放射性乳頭周囲血管炎
RPCA(reversed passive cutaneous anaphylaxis)	逆受身皮膚アナフィラキシー
RPE(retinal pigment epithelium)	網膜色素上皮
RPF(relaxed pelvic floor)	弛緩骨盤底部
RPF(renal plasma flow)	腎血漿流量
RPGN(rapidly progressive glomerulonephritis)	急速進行性糸球体腎炎
RPLND(retroperitoneal lymph node dissection)	後腹膜リンパ節郭清(術)
RPO(right posterior oblique)	右後斜位
RPP(rate pressure product)	心筋酸素消費量(心拍数×収縮期血圧)
RPS(renal pressor substance)	腎昇圧物質
RQ(respiratory quotient)	呼吸商
RR(radiation response)	放射線効果

RT

RR(recovery room)	回復室
RR(relative risk)	相対危険度
RR(residual rate)	残尿率
RR(respiratory rate)	呼吸数
RR(response rate)	反応率
RRA(radioreceptor assay)	放射受容体測定
RRF(residual renal function)	残存腎機能
RRP(relative refractory period)	相対不応期
RRPM(rate responsive pacemaker)	心拍応答型ペースメーカー
RS(Raynaud syndrome)	レイノー症候群
Rs(rectosigmoid)	直腸S状部
RS(Reed-Sternberg〔cell〕)	リード・スタンバーグ細胞
RS(respiratory sound)	呼吸音
R-S(response-shock interval)	反応・ショック間隔
RS(Reye's syndrome)	ライ症候群
RSA(right sacroanterior〔position〕)	右仙骨前位(胎位)
RSA(right sacrum anterior)	第2骨盤位第1分類(胎位)
RSA(right subclavian artery)	右鎖骨下動脈
RSD(reflex sympathetic dystrophy)	反射性交感神経性ジストロフィー
RSI(repetitive strain injury)	反復性緊張障害
RSO(right salpingo-oophorectomy)	右付属器摘出術
RSP(right sacroposterior〔position〕)	第2骨盤位第2分類(胎位)
RST(right sacrotransverse〔position〕)	第2骨盤位(胎位)
RSV(respiratory syncytial virus)	呼吸器合胞体ウイルス
RT(radiation therapy)	放射線療法
RT(rectal tube)	直腸チューブ
RT(respiratory therapy)	呼吸療法
RTA(renal tubular acidosis)	腎尿細管性アシドーシス
RTA(renal tubular alkalosis)	腎尿細管性アルカローシス
RTC(round the clock〔therapy〕)	定時的服薬、24時間療法
RTC, rtc(return to clinic)	再診
RTH(radical total hysterectomy)	広汎性子宮全摘術
RTI(respiratory tract infection)	気道感染

·RT

RTI(reverse transcriptase inhibitor)	逆転写酵素阻害薬
RTP(radiation therapy planning)	放射線治療計画
RTX(renal transplantation)	腎移植
rubella	風疹
RUL(right upper limb)	右上肢
RUL(right upper lobe of lung)	右肺上葉
RUM(residual urine measurement)	残尿測定
running nose	鼻風邪、鼻感冒
ruptured suture	縫合不全
rupture of bag	破水
RUQ(right upper quadrant)	右上腹部
RV(renal vein)	腎静脈
RV(residual volume)	残気量
RV(right ventricle)	右心室
	対 左心室：LV
RV(right visus)	右眼視力
	関連 左眼視力：LV
RVD(respiratory viral disease)	ウイルス性呼吸器疾患
RVDP (right ventricular end diastolic pressure)	右室拡張期圧
RVE(right ventricular enlargement)	右心室拡大
RVF(right ventricular failure)	右室不全
	関連 左室不全：LVF
RVG(right ventriculography)	右室造影
RVH(right ventricular hypertrophy)	右室肥大
RVH, RVHT(renovascular hypertension)	腎血管(動脈)性高血圧症
RVI(residual volume index)	残気率
RVI(right ventricular infarction)	右室梗塞
RV infarction(right ventricular infarction)	右室梗塞
RVO(right ventricular outflow)	右心室流出量
RV out(right ventricular outflow tract)	右室流出路
RVP(renal venous pressure)	腎静脈圧
RVP(right ventricular pressure)	右室圧
RVR(renal vascular resistance)	腎血管抵抗

RVRR(renal vein renin ratio)	腎静脈血レニン比
RVSP(right ventricular systolic pressure)	右室収縮期圧
RVSTI (right ventricular systolic time interval)	右室収縮時間
RVSW(right ventricular stroke work)	右室一回仕事量
RVSWI(RV stroke work index)	右室一回仕事係数
RVT(renal vein thrombosis)	腎静脈血栓症
RWM(red wale marking)	みみず腫れ様所見
R-Y(Roux-en-Y anastomosis)	ルーY型腸吻合(術)
Rx(prescription)	処方, 処方箋＝ recipe, formula

S

S(original squamous epithelium)	扁平上皮
S(sacral)	仙骨の、仙髄の
S(sacrum)	仙骨
S(sagittal plane)	矢状面
S(schizophrenic disorder)	統合失調症
S(senile)	老年の、老人(性)の
S(serum)	血清
S(sigmoid colon)	S状結腸
	◀関連▶上行結腸：A
	横行結腸：T
	下行結腸：D
S(sinister)	左の　◀対▶右の：dextro
S(S-wave)	S波
SⅠ(first sound)	1音
SⅡ(second sound)	2音
SⅢ(third sound)	3音
SⅣ(fourth sound)	4音
s癌(serosa)	漿膜までの癌(壁深達度)
SA(sensory aphasia)	感覚性失語
SA(single atrium)	単心房
SA(splenic artery)	脾動脈　◀対▶脾静脈：SV
SA(spontaneous abortion)	流産
SA(stable angina)	安定性狭心症
	◀参照▶不安定性狭心症：UA
SA(suicide attempt)	自殺企図
SAA(serum amyloid A)	血清アミロイドA
SAA(severe aplastic anemia)	重度再生不良性貧血
SAB(selective alveolo-bronchography)	選択的肺胞気管支造影法
SAB(sinoatrial block)	洞房ブロック＝SA block
SA block(sinoatrial block)	洞房ブロック＝SAB
SACH(solid ankle cushion heel)	サッチ足
sacroiliac joint	仙腸関節

SACT(sinoatrial conduction time)	洞房伝導時間
SAD(seasonal affective disorder)	季節性感情障害
SAD(self-administered depression)	自己評価うつ病尺度
SAD(social anxiety disorder)	社会不安障害
sadism	加虐嗜愛
SADS(schedule for affective disorders and schizophrenia)	感情障害ならびに統合失調症面接基準
SAH(subarachnoid hemorrhage)	クモ膜下出血(ザー)
SAI(social adequacy index)	社会適合係数
SAM(systolic anterior movement)	僧帽弁前尖の収縮期前方運動
SAN(sinoatrial node)	洞結節
Sanfilippo syndrome	サンフィリッポ症候群
SANS(scale for the assessment of negative symptoms)	陰性症状評価尺度
SaO₂(arterial O₂ saturation)	動脈血酸素飽和度
SAP(sensory action potential velocity)	感覚神経伝導速度
SAP(systemic arterial pressure)	全身血圧
Sar(sarcoidosis)	サルコイドーシス
SARS(severe acute respiratory syndrome)	重症急性呼吸器症候群
SAS(self-rating anxiety scale)	自己評価不安尺度
SAS(shoulder arm syndrome)	肩腕症候群
SAS(sleep apnea syndrome)	睡眠時無呼吸症候群
SASP(salazosulfapyridine)	サラゾスルファピリジン(サラゾピリン)
SASS(supra aortic stenosis syndrome)	大動脈弁上狭窄症候群
SAT(sperm agglutination test)	精子凝集試験
SAT(structural atypism)	(悪性腫瘍の)構造模型
SAT(subacute thyroiditis)	亜急性甲状腺炎
satd(saturated)	飽和の
SB(sinus brady cardia)	洞徐脈
SB(soap bath)	石けん清拭
SB(spontaneous breathing)	自発呼吸
SB(stellate ganglion block)	星状神経節ブロック

SB

SB(stereotyped behavior)	常同(性)行動
SBC(serum bactericidal concentration)	血清殺菌濃度
SBC(sexual behavior center)	性行動中枢
SBC(solitary bone cyst)	単発性骨嚢腫
SBD(senile brain disease)	老人性脳疾患
SBE(self-breast examination)	乳房自己検査法
SBE(subacute bacterial endocarditis)	亜急性細菌性心内膜炎
SBO(small bowel obstruction)	小腸閉塞症
SBP(spontaneous bacterial peritonitis)	特(自)発性細菌性腹膜炎
SBP(systolic blood pressure)	最大(収縮期)血圧
SBR(small bowel massive resection)	小腸大量切除術
SBS(sick building syndrome)	シックビル症候群
SBS(spino-bulbo-spinal reflex)	脊髄延髄脊髄反射
SB tube(Sengstaken-Blakemore tube)	ゼングスターケン・ブレークモア・チューブ
Sc(scapula)	肩甲骨
SC, sc(subcutaneous injection)	皮下(注射) 参照 静脈内注射：i.v. 筋肉内注射：I.m. 皮内注射：Hypo
SCA(selective celiac arteriography)	選択的腹腔動脈造影
SCA(sickle cell anemia)	鎌状赤血球貧血
SCA(subclavian artery)	鎖骨下動脈＝ arteria subclavia 対 鎖骨下静脈：SV
SCA(sudden cardiac arrest)	心臓突然死
SCA(superior cerebellar artery)	上小脳動脈
scab	痂皮、かさぶた
scabies	疥癬
scald	熱傷
scale	鱗屑
scar	瘢痕
scarlet fever	猩紅熱
SCC(small cell carcinoma)	小細胞癌

SCC (squamous cell carcinoma)	扁平上皮癌
	参照 腺癌：AC
SCD (sickle cell disease)	鎌状赤血球症＝sickle syndrome
SCD (spinal-cerebellar degeneration)	脊髄小脳変性症
schizoaffective disorder	統合失調性感情障害
schizoid personality disorder	統合失調性人格障害
schizotypal personality disorder	統合失調性人格障害
school period	学童期
sciatic nerve	坐骨神経
SCID (severe combined immunodeficiency disease)	重症複合免疫不全症
scintigram	シンチグラム
scintigraphy	シンチグラフィー
SCIS (severe combined immunodeficiency syndrome)	重症複合免疫不全症候群
SCJ (squamocolumnar junction)	扁平円柱上皮境界
SCK (serum creatine kinase)	血清クレアチンキナーゼ
SCL (soft contact lens)	ソフトコンタクトレンズ
SCLC (small cell lung cancer)	小細胞肺癌
SCLE (subacute cutaneous lupus erythematosus)	亜急性皮膚(型)エリテマトーデス
Sclero (endoscopic sclerotherapy)	内視鏡的硬化療法
SCM (sternocleidomastoid muscle)	胸鎖乳突筋
SCN (suprachiasmatic nucleus)	視交叉上核
SCN (supra clavicular lymph node)	鎖骨上リンパ節
scoliosis	脊柱側弯症、側弯(症)
SCR (serum creatinine)	血清クレアチニン
scratch	掻く
scratches	かすり傷、ひっかき傷
screw-home movement	ねじ込み運動
SCT (sentence completion test)	文章完成法
scurf	ふけ
SCV (sensory nerve conduction velocity)	知覚神経伝導速度

SD

SD(scleroderma)	強皮症
SD(senile dementia)	老年痴呆
SD(spondylosis deformans)	変形性脊椎症
SD(standard deviation)	標準偏差
SD(sudden deafness)	突発性難聴
SDAT(senile dementia of Alzheimer type)	アルツハイマー型老年痴呆
SDB(superficial dermal burn)	真皮浅層熱傷
SDE(subdural effusion)	硬膜下水腫
SDH(subdural hematoma)	硬膜下血腫(サブドラ)
SDH(subdural hemorrhage)	硬膜下出血
SDHD(sudden death heart disease)	心臓突然死
SDMD(senile disciform macular degeneration)	老人性円板状黄斑変性症
SDR(simple diabetic retinopathy)	単純型糖尿病性網膜症
SDS(Self-Rating Depression scale)	うつ病自己評価尺度
SDS(Shy-Drager syndrome)	シャイ・ドレーガー症候群
SE(saline enema)	石けん浣腸
SE(standard error)	標準誤差
SE(status epilepticus)	てんかん重積状態
sebum	皮脂
seclusion room	隔離室
secondary teeth	永久歯 ◀関連▶乳歯：primary teeth
SED(spondyloepiphyseal dysplasia)	脊椎骨端異形成(症)
sedation	鎮静剤などによる(鎮静)
SEDC(spondyloepiphyseal dysplasia congenita)	先天性脊椎・骨端異形成症
Sed rate(sedimentation rate)	沈降率
SEF(staphylococcal enterotoxin-F)	ブドウ球菌性腸毒素F
SEH(subependymal hemorrhage)	脳室上衣下出血＝SHE
seizure	ひきつけ、発作
Seldinger	セルディンガー法(脳血管撮影)
SEMI(subendocardial myocardial infarction)	心内膜下心筋梗塞
semi-comatous	半昏睡状態
senile	高齢の、老衰した

senile dementia	老人性痴呆症
senility	老衰
sensory aphasia	感覚性失語
	参照 運動性失語： motor aphasia
sensory disturbance	知覚異常
SEP(somatosensory evoked potential)	体性感覚誘発電位
sepsis	敗血症
septic wound	膿創
sequester	腐骨
serum	血清、血清剤、漿液
sesamoid	種子骨
severe mental retardation	重症精神遅滞
sexual dysfunction	性機能不全
sexual perversion	性倒錯
SF(scarlet fever)	猩紅熱＝scarlatina
SF(seizure frequency)	発作頻度
SF(sigmoidofiberscope)	S状結腸内視鏡検査
SF(synovial fluid)	滑液
SFD (small for dates) infant	不当軽量児
SFH(schizophrenia family history)	統合失調症家族歴
SFR(split function ratio)	分腎機能比
SFR(stroke with full recovery)	完全寛解した脳卒中
SG(skin graft)	皮膚移植
SG(specific gravity)	比重
S-G(Swan-Ganz catheter)	スワン・ガンツカテーテル
SGA(short gastric artery)	短胃動脈
SGA(small for gestational age)	発育遅延児
SGC(Swan-Ganz catheter)	スワン・ガンツカテーテル
SGE(secondary generalized epilepsy)	二次性全般化てんかん
SGO(surgery gynecology and obstetrics)	外科、産婦人科
Sgt(Schwangerschaft)	妊娠
SGV(small granule vesicle)	小顆粒小胞
SH(serum hepatitis)	血清肝炎

SH

SH(steroid hormone)	ステロイドホルモン
shadow	陰影
SHE(subependymal hemorrhage)	脳室上衣下出血＝SEH
Sheehan syndrome	シーハン症候群
shelf operation	棚つくり手術
SHH(syndrome of hyporeninemic hypoaldosteronism)	低レニン血症性低アルドステロン症
shiver-chills	悪寒戦慄
SHN(spontaneous hemorrhagic necrosis)	突発性出血性壊死
shock therapy	ショック療法
short run	連発
short term dynamic psychotherapy	短期力動精神療法
short term supportive psychotherapy	短期支持精神療法
shoulder joint	肩関節
SHP(Schönlein-Henoch purpura)	シェーンライン・ヘノッホ紫斑病
SHP(silver health plan)	シルバーヘルスプラン
SHS(Schönlein-Henoch syndrome)	シェーンライン・ヘノッホ症候群
SHS(supine hypotensive syndrome)	仰臥位低血圧症候群
SI(smear index)	腟スメア指数
SI(stroke index)	1回心拍出係数
SIADH(syndrome of inappropriate secretion of ADH)	抗利尿ホルモン分泌異常症候群
sickle cell	鎌状赤血球(異常赤血球)
SICU(surgical intensive care unit)	外科集中治療室
side effect	副作用 ◀関連▶ 主作用：principal effect
SIDS(sudden infant death syndrome)	乳児突然死症候群
sig(sigmoidoscopy)	S状結腸鏡検査
signs	他覚症状
silent	無症状性の、潜在性の

simian line	猿線
simple drunkenness	病的酩酊
simple renal cyst	単純性腎嚢胞
simple type	単純型(統合失調症)
SIMV(synchronized intermittent mandatory ventilation)	同期式間欠的強制換気法
single nephron	単一ネフロン
shingles	帯状疱疹
singultus	吃逆、しゃっくり
SIRS (systemic inflammatory response syndrome)	全身炎症性反応症候群
SISI test (short increment sensitivity index test)	短時間増強感覚指数テスト
SIT(Stanford Intelligence Test)	スタンフォード知能テスト
SJS(Sjögren syndrome)	シェーグレン病
SK(senile keratosis)	老人性角化症
SK(streptokinase)	ストレプトキナーゼ
skeletal traction	直達牽引
SKl(skin metastasis)	皮膚転移
SL(saccharum lactis)	乳糖
SL(sensation level)	感覚レベル
SL(sensus luminous)	光覚
SL(Sublingual)	舌下
SLB(short leg brace)	短下肢装具
SLC(short leg cast)	短下肢ギプス包帯
SLE(systemic lupus erythematosus)	全身性エリテマトーデス
sleep apnea syndrome	睡眠時無呼吸症候群
sleeplessness	不眠
slipped disk	椎間板ヘルニア
SLK(superior limbic keratoconjunctivitis)	上輪部角結膜炎
slough	痂皮、かさぶた
slow virus infection	遅発性ウイルス感染症
slow VT(slow ventricular tachycardia)	徐脈性心室性頻拍
SLR(straight leg raising test)	伸展下肢挙上テスト

•SL

SLTA(standard language test of aphasia)	標準失語症検査
SM(streptomycin)	ストレプトマイシン
sm(submucosal)	粘膜下
SM(systolic murmur)	収縮期雑音
SMA(spinal muscular atrophy)	脊髄性筋萎縮
SMA(superior mesenteric artery)	上腸間膜動脈
smallpox	天然痘、疱瘡
SMAO (superior mesenteric artery obstruction)	上腸間膜動脈閉塞症
SMAS(superior mesenteric artery syndrome)	上腸間膜動脈症候群
SMBG(self monitoring of blood glucose)	血糖自己測定(患者による)
SMC(self mamma control)	自己乳房管理
SMC(smooth muscle cell)	平滑筋細胞
SMD(spina malleolar distance)	腸骨前上棘・果部間距離
SMDS(sudden manhood death syndrome)	成人突然死症候群
SME, SMEI(severe myoclonic epilepsy in infancy)	乳児重症ミオクローヌスてんかん
SMI(silent myocardial ischemia)	無症候性心筋虚血
SMON(subacute myelo-optico neuropathy)	スモン、亜急性脊髄視神経症
SMR(somnolent metabolic rate)	睡眠代謝率
SMR(standard metabolic rate)	標準代謝率
SMR(standard mortality ratio)	標準化死亡比
SMR(submucosal resection of nasal septum)	粘膜下鼻中隔切除(術)
SMT(submucosal tumor)	粘膜下腫瘍
SMV(selbstmord versuch)	自殺企図
SMV(superior mesenteric vein)	上腸間膜静脈
sm癌(submucosa)	粘膜下層までの癌(壁深達度)
SN(sinus node)	洞結節
SN(spontaneous nystagmus)	自発眼振
snapping finger	ばね指
SND(striato-nigral degeneration)	線条体黒質変性症
SNE(subacute necrotizing encephalomyelopathy)	亜急性壊死性脳脊髄症
sneeze	くしゃみ

sniffles	鼻風邪、鼻づまり
snivel	鼻水
SNMC(Stronger Neo-Minophagen-C)	強力ネオミノファーゲンC
snore	鼾
SNRT(sinus node recovery time)	洞回復時間
SNS(sympathetic nervous system)	交感神経系
	◀関連▶ 副交感神経系：PNS
SO(superior oblique muscle)	上斜筋
s/o(suspicion of)	疑い
SO₂(oxygen saturation)	酸素飽和濃度
SOAP (subjective, objective, assessment, plan)	主観的、客観的、評価、計画
SOB(shortness of breath)	息切れ
sodomy	同性愛、少年愛、獣姦
Sol(solutio)	溶液
SOL(space occupying lesion)	占拠性病変
SOMI(sternal occiput mandibular immobilization)	ソーミーブレス（胸骨、後頭骨、下顎骨固定術）
somnolence	傾眠
somnolent	傾眠状態
SON(supraoptic nucleus)	視索上核
Sones's method	ソーンズ法（冠動脈造影検査の１つ）
S-O-R(stimulus-organism-reaction)	刺激生体反応
sore throat	咽頭痛
Sos(si opus sit)	必要ある時
SoU(solar urticaria)	日光蕁麻疹
Sp(senile plaque)	老人斑
SP(serum protein)	血清蛋白
SP, sP(simultaneous perception)	両眼同時認知
Sp(Species)	種、分析種
SP(spinal)	脊椎（の）
Sp(spinal anesthesia)	脊椎麻酔
SP(spine line)	坐骨棘線

・sp・

sp (sputum)	痰
SP (standardized patient, simulated patient)	標準(模擬)患者
SP (substance P)	サブスタンスP
S-P shunt (subdural peritoneal shunt)	硬膜下腹腔短絡術
SPA (suprapubic aspiration)	恥骨上膀胱穿刺術
SpAb (spontaneous abortion)	自然流産
spasmodic cough	発作性咳
spasticity	痙縮
spastic palsy	痙性麻痺
s-PBC (symptomatic primary biliary cirrhosis)	症候性原発性胆汁性肝硬変
SPE (septic pulmonary)	敗血症性肺水腫
SPECT (single photon emission CT)	シングルフォトンエミッションCT
speed traction	介達牽引(スピードトラック)
SPHG (stomal polypoid hypertrophic gastritis)	吻合部ポリープ状肥厚性胃炎
SPIDDM (slowly progressive insulin depended diabetes mellitus)	低進行性インスリン依存性糖尿病
spina bifida cystica	嚢胞状二分脊椎
spina bifida occulta	潜在性二分脊椎
spinal canal	脊柱管
spinal canal stenosis	脊柱管狭窄症
spinal cord	脊髄
spinal cord injury	脊髄損傷
spinal fluid	髄液
spinal palsy	脊髄麻痺
spine	脊椎
spirometry	スパイロメトリー
spit	吐く
spitting	喀痰
SPK (superficial punctate keratopathy)	点状表層角膜症
SPL (sound pressure)	音圧レベル
SPL (status praesens localis)	局所所見
splay foot	開張足=spread foot

splint	副子
SPMA(spinal progressive muscular atrophy)	脊髄性進行性筋萎縮症
SPMSQ(Short Portable Mental Status Questionnaire)	短縮携帯型精神状態質問表
SPO(stimulated pepsin output)	刺激後ペプシン分泌量
SpO2(oxygen saturation of arterial blood measured〔by pulse oximeter〕)	(パルスオキシメーターによる)動脈血酸素飽和度
spondylolisthesis	脊椎すべり症
spondylolysis	脊椎分離症
spondylosis deformans	変形性脊椎症
spondylotic myelopathy	脊椎症性脊髄症
sponge kidney	海綿腎
spontaneous delivery	自然分娩
spot	しみ、斑点、面皰
Sppc(sinusitis paranasalias purulenta chronica)	慢性化膿性副鼻腔炎
sprain	捻挫
spread food	開帳足＝splay foot
SPS(simple partial seizure)	単純部分発作　◀関連▶複雑部分発作：CPS
SPS(social performance schedule)	社会遂行能面接基準
SPT(soft part tumor)	軟部腫瘍
spur	骨棘
sputum	喀痰、痰＝SP
SPV(selective proximal vagotomy)	選択的近位迷走神経切断術
SQ(social maturity quotient)	社会成熟指数
sq(squamous cell carcinoma)	扁平上皮癌
squatting position	しゃがみこみ、胸膝位
squint	斜視
SR(saturation recovery)	飽和回復法
SR(schizophrenic reaction)	統合失調症反応
SR(sex-linked recessive inheritance)	伴性劣性遺伝
SR(sigmoidectomy)	S状結腸切除術
SR(sinus rhythm)	洞調律
SR(speech range)	話声域

SR

SR(spontaneous respiration)	自発呼吸
SR(stapedius reflex)	あぶみ骨筋反射
SR(stretch reflex)	伸展反射
SR(sutures removed)	抜糸
SR(system review)	病歴要約
SRA(superior rectal artery)	上直腸動脈
SRC(scleroderma renal crisis)	強皮症腎クリーゼ
SRCA(specific red cell adherence test)	特異的赤血球吸着試験
SRRD(sleep related respiratory disturbance)	睡眠関連呼吸障害
SRS(schizophrenic residual state)	統合失調症残存状態
SRS-A(slow-reacting substance of anaphylaxis)	アナフィラキシー遅発反応物質
SRT(speech reception threshold)	語音聴取閾値
SRV(single right ventricle)	単右心室
SS(Schwangerschaft)	妊娠
SS(scleral spur)	強膜棘突起
ss(semis)	半分、半分の
SS(sickle cell)	鎌状赤血球
S-s(sinusitis sphenoidalis)	蝶形骨洞炎、蝶骨洞炎
SS(Sjögren's syndrome)	シェーグレン症候群
SS(sterile solution)	無菌溶液
ss(subserosal layer)	漿膜下層
SS(systemic sclerosis)	全身性硬化症
SSE(soap solution enema)	石けん水浣腸
SSE(subacute spongiform encephalopathy)	亜急性海綿状脳症
SSI(surgical site infection)	手術部位感染
SSL(skin surface lipid)	表皮脂質
SSLE(subacute sclerosing leukoencephalitis)	亜急性硬化性白質脳炎
SSM(specific substance Maruyama)	丸山ワクチン
SSM(superficial spreading melanoma)	表在性黒色腫
SSP(spinal spastic paralysis)	脊髄性痙性麻痺
SSPE(subacute sclerosing panencephalitis)	亜急性硬化性全脳炎
SSPL(saturation sound pressure level)	最大出力音圧レベル
SSS(sick sinus syndrome)	洞結節不全症候群

SSS(superior sagittal sinus)	上矢状静脈洞
SSSS(staphylococcal scalded skin syndrome)	ブドウ球菌性熱傷様皮膚症候群
SSST(superior sagittal sinus thrombosis)	上矢状静脈洞血栓(症)
SST(social skills training)	社会技能訓練
ss癌(subserosa)	漿膜下層までの癌(壁深達度)
ST(speech therapist)	言語療法士
	◀関連▶ 理学療法士：PT
	作業療法士：OT
ST(esotropia)	内斜視 ◀対▶ 外斜視：XT
ST(Schiötz tonometry)	シェッツ眼圧測定計
ST(sclerotherapy)	硬化療法
ST(sinus tachycardia)	洞〔性〕頻拍(脈)＝simple tachycardia
ST(skin test)	皮膚試験
ST(speech therapy)	言語療法
ST(supportive psychotherapy)	支持的精神療法
STA(superficial temporal artery)	浅側頭動脈
Stage A(active stage)	活動期(胃潰瘍)
Stage H(healing stage)	治癒過程期(胃潰瘍)
Stage S(scarred stage)	瘢痕期(胃潰瘍)
Staph(staphylococcus)	ブドウ球菌
stat(statim)	直ちに、至急
status asthmaticus	気管支喘息発作重積状態
status epilepticus	痙攣（てんかん）重積状態
STD(sexually transmitted disease)	性行為感染症
ST depression	ST低下
S-TEN(staphylococcal toxic epidermal necrolysis)	ブドウ球菌性中毒性表皮壊死性融解症
ST elevation	ST上昇
stenosis	狭窄
Stereo(stereotaxic neurosurgery)	定位脳手術
stereo(X-ray stereography)	立体撮影
stereotypy	常同症

·st·

sterility	不妊(症)
sternoclavicular joint	胸鎖関節
STG(split-thickness graft)	分層植皮術＝STSG
STH(simple total hysterectomy)	子宮単純全摘術
STH(somatotropic hormone)	成長ホルモン
STI(systolic time interval)	収縮時間
stiffness	こわばり、硬直、肩こり
stillbirth	死産
stimulation test	刺激試験
STM(short-team memory)	短期記憶
	◀関連▶ 長期記憶：LTM
STNI(subtotal nodal irradiation)	亜全リンパ節照射
STNR(symmetrical tonic neck reflex)	対称性緊張性頚反射
strabismus	斜視
strained back	ぎっくり腰
strawberry tongue	苺状舌
Strept(streptococcus)	連鎖球菌
stress fracture	疲労骨折
stridor	喘鳴、狭窄音
STS(serologic tests for syphilis)	梅毒血清反応
STSG(split-thickness skin graft)	中間層皮膚移植、分層植皮術
STT(serial thrombin time)	連続トロンビン時間
stunned myocardium	気絶心筋
stupor	昏迷
stuporous	昏迷状態
STV(short term variability)	短期変動性
SU(sulfonyl urea)	スルホニル尿素剤
SUA(single umbilical cord artery)	単一臍帯動脈
subacute	亜急性
	参照 急性：acute
	慢性：choronic
subacute thyroiditis	亜急性甲状腺炎
subcu, subcut(subcutaneous)	皮下の
subcutaneous emphysema	皮下気腫

• su

Subdura (subdural hematoma)	硬膜下血腫
subendocardial infarction	心内膜下梗塞
subject symptom	自覚症状
	参照 他覚症状
	：object symptom
sublimation	昇華、代理形成
subtalar joint	距骨下関節
subtotal thyroidectomy	甲状腺亜全摘
sub-Q (subcutaneous)	皮下
sucking reflex	吸啜反射
SUD (single use device)	単回使用医療器材、ディスポ器材
SUD (sudden unexpected natural death)	内因性急死
sudamina	汗疹、あせも
sudden deafness	突発性難聴
suffocation	窒息
SUI (stress urinary incontinence)	腹圧性尿失禁
	参照 切迫性尿失禁：UI
suicide	自殺
SUN (serum urina nitrogen)	血清尿素窒素
sunstroke	日射病
SUP (superior)	上(へ)
superego	超自我
superior sulcus	肺尖
supine position	仰臥位＝dorsal position
	◀関連▶ 腹臥位：proneness
	側臥位：lateral recumbent position
Supp (suppositorium)	坐薬
suppression	抑制
suppression test	抑制試験
surfactant	サーファクタント、表面活性物質
suspension traction	懸吊牽引

su

sut(sutura)	縫合（単数）
sutt(suturae)	縫合（複数）
suture	縫合
suture removal	抜糸
SUUD (sudden unexpected and unexplained death)	原因不明の突然死
SUZI(subzonal insemination)	透明帯精子注入法
Suzuki-Binet intelligence scale	鈴木・ビネー式知能検査
SV(selective vagotomy)	選択的胃迷走神経切離術
SV(single ventricle)	単心室
SV(sinus venosus)	静脈洞
SV(splenic vein)	脾静脈　**対** 脾動脈：SA
SV(Spontaneous ventilation)	自発呼吸、自発換気
SV(stroke volume)	１回拍出量
SV(subclavian vein)	鎖骨下静脈
SVA(selective visceral angiography)	選択的臓器動脈造影
SVBG(saphenous vein bypass graft)	伏在静脈バイパス移植
SVC(superior vena cava)	上大静脈　**対** 下大静脈：IVC
SVC(supraventricular contraction)	上室性期外収縮＝SVPC
SVCG(superior vena cavagraphy)	上大静脈造影
SVCS(superior vena cava syndrome)	上大静脈症候群
SVD(sinus venous defect)	静脈洞欠損症
SVD(spontaneous vaginal delivery)	自然腟分娩
SVI(slow virus infection)	遅発性ウイルス感染症候群
SVI(stroke volume index)	１回拍出係数
SVPC(supra ventricular premature contraction)	上室性期外収縮＝SVC
SVR(systemic vascular resistance)	全末梢血管抵抗
SVT(supraventricular tachycardia)	上室性頻拍
SW(social worker)	ソーシャルワーカー
Swan-Ganz's catheter	スワン・ガンツカテーテル
sweating	発汗

SWG(standard wire gauge)	標準注射針ゲージ
SWI(stroke work index)	１回仕事係数
SWR(serum Wasserman reaction)	血清ワッセルマン反応
SWS(slow wave sleep)	徐波睡眠
Sx(symptoms)	症状
sycosis	毛瘡
syncope	失神
syndactyly	合指症
synovitis	滑膜炎
syphilis	梅毒
systematic desensitization	系統的脱感作
SZ(schizophrenia)	統合失調症

T

T(primary tumor)	原発腫瘍の大きさ(TNM分類)
T(temperature)	体温
T(temporal)	側頭部の
	◀関連▶ 前頭部の：F
	後頭部の：O
T(Termin)	分娩予定日
T(Thomsen-phenomenon)	トムゼン現象
T(thoracic spine)	胸椎
T(thorax)	胸部、胸郭
T(Thymus derived lymphocyte)	Tリンパ球、胸腺由来リンパ球
T(transformation zone)	移行帯
T(transverse colon)	横行結腸
	◀関連▶ 上行結腸：A
	下行結腸：D
	S状結腸：S
T1, T2, T3,… T12(thoracic vertebrae first, second, third, … twelfth)	第1(2、3、…12)胸椎
T3(triiodothyronine)	トリヨードサイロニン
T4(thyroxine)	サイロキシン
TA(temporal arteritis)	側頭動脈炎
TA(threatened abortion)	切迫流産
TA(tibialis anterior muscle)	前脛骨筋
T & A(tonsillectomy and adenoidectomy)	扁桃摘出(術)とアデノイド切除(術)
TA(toxin-antitoxin)	毒素、抗毒素＝TAT
TA(transactional analysis)	交流分析
TA(transplantation antigen)	移植抗原
TA(tricuspid atresia)	三尖弁閉鎖症
TA(truncus arteriosus)	総動脈幹症
T antigen(tumor antigen)	T抗原
TA(typhus abdominalis)	腸チフス
TAA(thoracic aortic aneurysm)	胸部大動脈瘤

TA

TAA(tumor associated antigen)	腫瘍関連抗原
Tab(tablet)	錠剤、タブレット
TAB(therapeutic abortion)	治療的流産
TAC(transplant aspiration cytology)	移殖臓器穿刺吸引細胞診
tachy(tachycardia)	頻脈　対　徐脈：brady (bradycardia)
tachypnea	呼吸促迫
TAD(transient acantholytic dermatosis)	一過性棘融解性皮膚症
TAE(transcatheter arterial embolization)	経カテーテル肝動脈塞栓術
TAF(tumor angiogenic factor)	腫瘍血管新生因子
tages	1日血糖(ターゲス)
TA-GVHD(transfusion associated graft versus host disease)	輸血関連移殖片対宿主病
TAH(total abdominal hysterectomy)	腹式子宮全摘出術
TAH(total artificial heart)	完全人工心臓
TAI(transhepatic arterial infusion)	肝動脈注入療法
TAL(tendon Achilles lengthening)	アキレス腱延長
talipes valgus	外反足
talipes varus	内反足
talocrural joint	距腿関節
TAM(transient abnormal myelopoiesis)	一過性類白血病状態
TAN(total ammonia nitrogen)	総アンモニア窒素
TAO(thoracic aortic occlusion)	胸部大動脈遮断
TAO(thromboangiitis obliterans)	閉塞性血栓〔性〕脈管炎＝TO
TAP(tricuspid annuloplasty)	三尖弁弁輪形成術
TAPVC(total anomalous pulmonary venous connection)	総肺静脈還流異常症
TAPVD (total anomalous pulmonary venous drainage)	総肺静脈還流異常症
TAPVR (total anomalous pulmonary venous return)	総肺静脈還流異常症
TAR (thrombocytopenia-absent radius syndrome)	血小板減少橈骨欠損症候群(常染色体性劣性遺伝)

・TA・

TAR(total ankle replacement)	人工足関節置換術
tardy palsy	遅発麻痺
tarry stool	タール便、血便
tarsal tunnel	足根管
tarsometatarsal joint	足根中足関節
TASA(tumor associated surface antigen)	腫瘍関連表面抗原
TAT(thematic apperception test)	絵画統覚検査
TAT(toxin-antitoxin)	毒素、抗毒素＝TA
Tb(biological half time)	生物学的半減期
TB(total bilirubin)	総ビリルビン
TB(tub bathing)	沐浴
TB(tubercle bacillus)	結核菌
TB(tuberculosis)	結核
T-Bil(total bilirubin)	総ビリルビン
TBA(total bile acid)	総胆汁酸
TBG(thyroid binding globulin)	甲状腺ホルモン結合蛋白
TBI(total body irradiation)	放射線全身照射
TBL(tracheobronchial lavage)	気管支洗浄
TBLB(transbronchial lung biopsy)	経気管支肺生検
TBLU(term birth living infant)	満期産生存児
TBM(tubular basement membrane)	尿細管基底膜
TBP(thyroxine binding protein)	サイロシン結合淡白
TBSA(total body surface area)	総体表面積
TBT(tracheobronchial toilet)	気管気管支内洗浄
TBV(total blood volume)	全血液量
TBW(total body water)	体内総水分(量)
TC(cytotoxic T lymphocyte)	細胞障害性Tリンパ球
TC(Tetracycline)	テトラサイクリン
TC(total cholesterol)	総コレステロール
TC(true conjugate)	真結合線
TCA(tricyclic antidepressant)	三環系抗うつ薬
TCC(transitional cell carcinoma)	移行上皮癌
TCD(transcranial Doppler)	経頭蓋超音波ドップラー
TCF(total coronary flow)	全冠動脈血液量

TCIA(transient cerebral ischemic attack)	一過性脳虚血(乏血)発作
TcPCO₂ (transcutaneous carbon dioxide tension)	経皮的炭酸ガス分圧
TCR(T-cell receptor)	T細胞受容体
TCs(tetracyclines)	テトラサイクリン系抗生物質
TCT(thrombin clotting time)	トロンビン凝固時間
TD(tardive dyskinesia)	遅発ジスキネジア
TD(tic douloureux)	疼痛性チック
TDA(therapeutic drug assay)	血中薬物濃度測定
TDD(thoracic duct drainage)	胸管ドレナージ
TDL(thoracic duct lymphocyte)	胸管リンパ球
TDM(therapeutic drug monitoring)	治療薬物モニタリング
TdP(Tanzen der patella)	膝蓋跳動
Tds(ter die sumendus)	1日3回
TEA(thromboendarterectomy)	血栓内膜摘除術
TEACH(treatment and education of autistic and related communication handicapped)	自閉症ならびに関連コミュニケーション障害
TEC(total〔blood〕eosinophil count)	総血中好酸球数
TEC(transluminal extraction catheter)	経管吸引カテーテル
TEE(transesophageal echocardiography)	経食道心エコー法
TEEH (total elemental enteral hyperalimentation)	完全経腸成分栄養
TEF(tracheoesophageal fistula)	気管食道瘻
Teff(effective half life)	有効半減期
TEM (transanal endoscopic microsurgery)	経肛門的内視鏡下マイクロサージャリー
temp(temperature)	温度、体温
temperament	気質
temporal syndrome	側頭葉症候群
temporary	一時的な
TEN(toxic epidermal necrolysis)	中毒性表皮壊死症
TENS (transcutaneous electrical nerve stimulation)	経皮的電気的神経刺激
tension band wiring	引き寄せ締結法

•TE•

TEP(tracheoesophageal puncture)	気管食道穿刺
teratogen	催奇形物質
teratoma	奇形腫
TEshunt(tracheo-esophageal shunt)	気管食道短絡
TEST(tubal embryo-stage transplantation)	卵管内胚移殖
testicular tumor	精巣腫瘍
testosterone	テストステロン
TET(treadmill test)	トレッドミル〔運動〕負荷試験
tetanus	破傷風
tetany	テタニー
tetra(tetraplegia)	四肢麻痺
TEV(talipes equinovarus)	内反尖足
TF, T/F(tetralogy of Fallot)	ファロー四徴症（右心室肥大、大動脈右方転位、心室中隔欠損、肺動脈狭窄症）
TF(tissue factor)	組織因子
TF(total flow)	全流量
TF(tube feeding)	経管栄養
TF(tubular fluid)	尿細管腔液
TFI(tumor free interval)	無腫瘍期
TFR(total fertility rate)	合計特殊出生率
TFS(testicular feminization syndrome)	精巣性女性化症候群（男性偽半陰陽精巣を有するが外観は女性。X染色体連鎖劣性遺伝）
TG(tendon graft)	腱移植
TG(total gastrectomy)	胃全摘術
TG(triglyceride)	中性脂肪（トリグリセリド）
TGA(transient global amnesia)	一過性全健忘症
TGA(transposition of great arteries)	大血管転位＝TGV
TGC(truncus gastrocolicus)	胃結腸幹
TGF(therapeutic gain factor)	治療増強因子
TGF(tumor growth factor)	腫瘍成長因子
TGV(thoracic gas volume)	胸腔内ガス容量

TGV(transposition of great vessel)	大血管転位(症)＝TGA
Th(helper T lymphocyte〔cell〕)	ヘルパーTリンパ球
TH(thalamic hemorrhage)	視床(内側)出血
Th(thoracic)	胸部の、胸椎の、胸髄の
TH(thyroid hormone)	甲状腺ホルモン
	◀関連▶副甲状腺ホルモン：PTH
TH(total hysterectomy)	子宮全摘術
THA(terminal hepatic arteriole)	終末肝動脈枝
THA(total hip arthroplasty)	(人工)股関節全置換術＝THR
thalamic syndrome	視床症候群
THARIES(total hip articular replacement by internal eccentric shells)	股関節表面全置換術
thermohypesthesia	温度覚鈍麻
thinking	思考
thirsty	口渇
thoracentesis	胸腔穿刺
thoracic	胸郭の
thoracic duct	胸管
thoracic outlet syndrome	胸郭出口症候群
thoracoplasty	胸郭形成術
thoracoscopic surgery	胸腔鏡下手術
thoracotomy	開胸法
thought blocking	思考途絶
thought broad casting	思考伝播
thought inhibition	思考制止
thought insertion	思考吹入
thought withdrawal	思考奪取
THP(Total Health Promotion Plan)	トータルヘルスプロモーションプラン
THR(total hip replacement)	人工股関節全置換術＝THA
threatened abortion	切迫流産
threatened premature delivery	切迫早産

• th

three-day measles	風疹、三日はしか
three vessel disease	冠動脈三枝病変
thrush	口腔カンジダ症、鵞口瘡
thumb	親指
Thy(thymocyte)	胸腺細胞
thymoma	胸腺腫
thymus	胸腺
thyroid gland	甲状腺
	◀関連▶ 副甲状腺：parathyroid gland
thyroid hormone	甲状腺ホルモン
thyrotoxicosis	甲状腺中毒症
THYSA(thymus specific antigen)	T細胞特異抗原
TI(inversion time)	反復時間
TI(therapeutic index)	治療指数
TI(tricuspid insufficiency)	三尖弁閉鎖不全症
TI(tunnel infection)	皮下トンネル感染
TIA(transient cerebral ischemic attack)	一過性脳虚血発作
TIBC(total iron binding capacity)	総鉄結合能
tibiofibular joint	脛腓関節
TICO (thrombolysis in acute coronary occlusion)	急性冠動脈閉塞の血栓溶解
t.i.d.(s.)(ter in die〔sumendum〕)	1日3回(服用)
	参照 1日2回：b.d.
	1日4回：q.i.d.
TIG(tetanus immune globulin〔human〕)	破傷風免疫グロブリン
TIL(tumor infiltrating lymphocytes)	腫瘍浸潤リンパ球
TIN(tubulo-interstitial nephritis)	尿細管間質性腎炎
TINU(tubulo-interstitial nephritis and uveitis〔syndrome〕)	間質性腎炎ぶどう膜炎症候群
TIO(trans-ileocolic obliteration〔of esophageal varices〕)	経回腸結腸静脈(食道動脈瘤)塞栓術
TIPS(transjugular intrahepatic portosystemic shunt)	経頚静脈的経肝内門脈静脈短絡(シャント)術

Tis(tumor in situ)	上皮内癌
TIT(total ischemic timetake)	総虚血時間
TIU(tyroid iodine uptake ratio)	甲状腺ヨウ素摂取率
TIUV(total intrauterine volume)	子宮内総容積
TIVA(total intravenous anesthesia)	完全静脈麻酔
TJ(triceps jerk)	上腕三頭筋腱反射
TJR(total joint prosthesis)	関節全置換術
TK(killer T cell)	キラーT細胞
TKA(total knee arthroplasty)	(人工)膝関節全置換術
TKR(total knee replacement)	(人工)膝関節全置換術
TLA(translumbar aortography)	経腰大動脈造影法
TLC(total lung capacity)	全肺気量
TLC(total lymphocyte count)	全リンパ球数
TLE(temporal lobe epilepsy)	側頭葉てんかん
TLI(total lymphoid irradiation)	全リンパ組織照射(法)
TLR(tonic labyrinthine reflex)	緊張性迷路反射
TLV(total lung volume)	全肺容量
T-lymphocyte(thymus derived lymphocyte)	Tリンパ球、胸腺由来リンパ球
Tm(maximum capacity of tubular transport)	尿細管最大輸送量
TM(tumor marker)	腫瘍マーカー
TM(tympanic membrane)	鼓膜
TMA(thrombotic microangiopathy)	血栓性微小血管障害
TMD(temporomandibular disorder)	顎機能障害(顎関節症)＝arthrous of temporomandibular joint
TMF(transmitral flow velocity)	僧帽弁口血流速波形
TmG(maximum tubular reabsorption mass of glucose)	尿細管糖再吸収極量
TMJ(temporomandibular joint)	顎関節
TM line(tuber maxillae line)	上顎結節線
TmPAH(tubular excretory mass of para-aminohippurate)	パラアミノ馬尿酸塩の尿細管排泄極量
TNC(thymic nurse cell)	胸腺栄養細胞
TND(term normal delivery)	満期正常分娩

TN

TNF(tumor necrosis factor)	腫瘍壊死因子
TNG(trinitroglycerin)	トリニトログリセリン
TNI(total nodal irradiation)	全リンパ節照射法
TNM分類 (tumor node metastasis classification)	癌の進行度の国際的分類
TNR(tonic neck reflex)	緊張性頚反射
TO(thromboangiitis obliterans)	閉塞性血栓(性)脈管炎＝TAO
TO(tonus oculi)	眼圧
TO(total obstruction)	完全閉塞
TOB(tobramycin)	トブラマイシン
Tod(tension of oculus dexter)	右眼眼圧
	◀関連▶左眼眼圧：Tos
TOF, T/F(tetralogy of Fallot)	ファロー四徴症＝TF
tomo(tomography)	断層撮影
tongue tie	短舌、小舌
tonsillitis	扁桃炎
TOP(the association areas of the temporal, occipital and parietal lobes of the cerebral hemisphere)	側頭、後頭、頭頂葉連合野
TOPV(trivalent oral poliovirus vaccine)	経口ポリオワクチン
Torsade de Pointes	トルサード・ド・ポアンツ
torsion	捻転
Tos(tension of oculus sinister)	左眼眼圧
	◀関連▶右眼眼圧：Tod
total amnesia	完全健忘
	◀関連▶部分健忘：partial amnesia
Total G(total gastrectomy)	胃全摘術
toxemia of pregnancy	妊娠中毒症
toxicity	毒性
toxicoderma	中毒疹
toxic symptom	中毒症状
Tp(physical half life)	物理学的半減期

TP

TP(tibialis posterior muscle)	後脛骨筋
TP(tinea pedis)	足白癬
TP(total pancreatectomy)	膵全摘出術
TP(total protein)	総蛋白
TP(Treponema pallidum)	梅毒トレポネーマ
t-PA(tissue plasminogen activator)	組織プラスミノゲンアクチベータ
TPA(total parenteral alimentation)	完全静脈栄養＝TPN
TPC(therapeutic patient club)	治療的患者クラブ
TPCF (Treponema pallidum complement fixation)	梅毒トレポネーマ補体結合テスト、TPCFテスト
TPD(tip palmar distance)	指尖手掌間距離
TPD test(two point discrimination test)	二点識別テスト
TPE(therapeutic plasma exchange)	治療的血漿交換
TPE(tropical pulmonary eosinophilia)	熱帯性肺好酸球増多症
TPH, TPHA (total parenteral hyperalimentation)	完全静脈栄養法＝TRN
TPHA(Treponema pallidum hemagglutination assay)	梅毒トレポネーマ血球凝集反応
TPHA(treponema pallidum hemagglutination test)	梅毒トレポネーマ・パリダム感作血球凝集テスト
TPL(threatened premature labor)	切迫分娩
TPL(total pelvic exenteration)	全骨髄除臓〔術〕(骨盤内臓器全摘出と尿管腸吻合、人工肛門形成を含む)
TPM(temporary pacemaker)	一時的ペースメーカー
TPN(total parenteral nutrition)	完全静脈栄養法＝TPH, TPHA
TPO(thrombopoietin)	トロンボポエチン
TPP(thrombocytopenic purpura)	血小板減少性紫斑〔病〕
TPP(tidal plasma protein)	循環血漿蛋白
TPP(true precocious puberty)	真性早熟
TPR(temperature-pulse- respiration)	体温、脈拍、呼吸
TPR(total peripheral vascular resistance)	全末梢血管抵抗
TPR(total pulmonary resistance)	全肺血管抵抗＝TPVR

TP

TPV(total plasma volume)	全血漿量
TPVR(total pulmonary vascular resistance)	全肺血管抵抗＝TPR
TR(therapeutic radiology)	放射線治療学
TR(therapeutic ratio)	治療可能比
tr(traction)	牽引 参照 直達牽引：skeletal traction
Tr(treatment)	治療、処置
TR(tricuspid regurgitation)	三尖弁閉鎖不全
TR(tuberculin reaction)	ツベルクリン反応
trachea	気管
tracheal	気管の
tracheo-bronchomalacia	気管・気管支軟化症
traction response	引き起こし反射
TRALI(transfusion related acute lung injury)	輸血関連性肺障害
tranquilizer	鎮静薬
transference	転移
transient hyperglycemia of newborn	新生児一過性高血糖症
transmit	伝播する、媒介する、遺伝させる
transsphenoidal adenomectomy	経蝶形骨洞下垂体腺腫摘出術
trauma	外傷、心的外傷、トラウマ
traumatic arthritis	外傷性関節炎
traumatic dislocation	外傷性脱臼
TRBF(total renal blood flow)	全腎血流量
TRCV(total red cell volume)	全赤血球量
TRD(traction retinal detachment)	牽引性網膜剥離
treadmill	トレッドミル
Trep(Treponema)	トレポネーマ
TRF(thyrotropin releasing factor)	甲状腺刺激ホルモン放出因子
TRFR(tubular rejection fraction rate)	尿細管排泄率

TRH(thyrotropin releasing hormone)	甲状腺刺激ホルモン放出ホルモン
TRI(total red cell iron)	全赤血球鉄
TRIC(trachoma-inclusion conjunctivitis)	トラコーマ封入体結膜炎
trichotillomania	抜毛癖
Tri/F(trilogy of Fallot)	ファロー3徴症
trigeminal N	Ⅴ三叉神経
trigger finger	ばね指
triggered activity	激発電位
tring(trigeminy)	三段脈
trismus	咬痙、開口障害
TRM(transplantation related mortality)	移殖関連死亡
tRNA(transfer ribonucleic acid)	トランスファーRNA、転移リボ核酸
TRNB(transrectal needle biopsy)	経直腸的針生検
trochlear N(nerve)	Ⅳ滑車神経
TRP(tubular reabsorption of phosphate)	尿細管無機リン再吸収量
TRPF(total renal plasma flow)	全腎血流量
TRUS(transrectal ultrasonography)	経直腸的超音波断層(法)
TS(teaching strategy)	教授法
TS(terminal sensation)	末端感覚
TS(thoracic surgery)	胸部外科
TS(tricuspid stenosis)	三尖弁狭窄症
TS(tuberous sclerosis)	結節性硬化症
TSA(tumor specific antigen)	腫瘍特異抗原
TSB(total serum bilirubin)	総血清ビリルビン
TSB(total spinal block)	全脊椎麻酔(法)
TSE(transmissible spongiform encephalopathy)	伝染性海綿上脳症
TSH(thyroid stimulating hormone)	甲状腺刺激ホルモン
TSI(thyroid-stimulating immunoglobulin)	甲状腺刺激免疫グロブリン
TSLS(toxic shock like syndrome)	中毒様症候群
TSP(tropical spastic paraparesis)	熱帯性痙性不全対麻痺
TSPR(total systemic peripheral resistance)	全末梢(血管)抵抗＝TSVR

TS

TSS(toxic shock syndrome)	毒素性ショック症候群
TSSA(tumor specific surface antigen)	腫瘍特異性表面抗原
TSST (toxic shock syndrome associated toxin)	中毒性ショック症候群毒素
TSTA (tumor specific transplantation antigen)	腫瘍特異性移殖抗原
TSVR(total systemic vascular resistance)	全末梢(血管)抵抗＝TSPR
TT(thrombin time)	トロンビン時間
TT(thrombo test)	トロンボテスト
TTA(transtracheal aspiration)	経気管吸引
TTA(tumor transplantation antigen)	腫瘍移殖抗原
TTH(tension-type-headache)	筋緊張性頭痛
TTH(thyrotropic hormone)	甲状腺刺激ホルモン
TTN, TTNB (transient tachypnea of newborn)	新生児一過性多呼吸
TTP(thrombotic thrombocytopenic purpura)	血栓性血小板減少性紫斑病
TTR(triceps tendon reflex)	上腕三頭筋腱反射
TTS(temporary threshold shift)	一過性閾値変動
TTS(transdermal therapeutic system)	経皮的吸収治療システム
TTTS(twin-to-twin transfusion syndrome)	双胎間輸血症候群
TTX(Tetrodotoxin)	テトロドトキシン(トラフグの毒)
TU(toxic unit)	中毒単位
tub(tubular adenocarcinoma)	管状腺癌
tuberculosis	結核＝TB
tuberculous arthritis	結核性関節炎
tubular proteinuria	尿細管性蛋白尿
tubulitis	尿細管炎
tubuloglomerular feedback	尿細管糸球体フィードバック
tubulointerstitial nephritis	尿細管間質性腎炎
TUC(transurethral coagulation)	経尿道的凝固(術)
TUE(transurethral electro-coagulation)	経尿道的電気凝固術
TUF(transurethral fulguration)	経尿道的焼灼(術)
TUL(transurethral lithotomy)	経尿道的砕石術
TUL(transurethral ultrasonic lithotomy)	経尿道的超音波砕石術

ty

TULIP(transurethral ultrasound-guided laser-induced prostatectomy)	超音波ガイド下経尿道的レーザー前立腺切除(術)
TUR(transurethral resection)	経尿道的切除(術)
TUR-Bt(transurethral resection of the bladder tumor)	経尿道的膀胱腫瘍切除術
TUR-P(transurethral resection of the prostate)	経尿道的前立腺切除術
TUU(transureteroureterostomy)	経尿管吻合術
TUV(total urine volume)	全24時間尿量
TV(Trichomonas vaginalis)	腟トリコモナス
TV(tricuspid valve)	三尖弁
	◀関連▶僧帽弁：MV
TV(truncal vagotomy)	幹迷走神経切離(術)
TV, Vt(tidal volume)	１回換気量
TVC(timed vital capacity)	時間肺活量
TVD(trans vaginal delivery)	経腟分娩
TVD(triple vessel disease)	三枝病変
TVH(total vaginal hysterectomy)	腟式子宮全摘出(術)
TVP(tricuspid prolapse)	三尖弁逸脱
TVP(tricuspids valvuloplasty)	三尖弁形成(術)
TVR(total vascular resistance)	全血管抵抗
TVR(tricuspid valve replacement)	三尖弁置換術
twilight state	もうろう状態
tx(traction)	牽引
TX(transplantation)	移植
Tx(treatment)	治療
TXT(docetaxel)	ドセタキセル
typhoid	チフス

U

U(unit)	単位
U(urea)	尿素
U(uric acid)	尿酸
UA(umbilical artery)	臍動脈
UA, UAP(unstable angina pectoris)	不安定狭心症 参照 安定性狭心症：SA
UA(uric acid)	尿酸
UA(urine analysis , urinalysis)	検尿
UAB(under arm brace)	アンダーアームブレース(脊柱側弯症用装具)
UAC(umbilical artery catheter)	臍動脈カテーテル
UB(unconjugated bilirubin)	非抱合ビリルビン
UB(uric blood)	尿潜血
UB(urinary bladder)	膀胱
UBF(uterine blood flow)	子宮血流
UC(ulcerative colitis)	潰瘍性大腸炎
uc(unclassified)	分類不能腫瘍
UC(uterine contraction)	子宮収縮
UCC(urgent care center)	緊急治療センター
UCF(unsatisfactory colposcopic findings)	不適例
UCG(ultrasonic cardiogram)	心臓超音波検査(心エコー図)
UCG(urethrocystography)	尿道膀胱造影法
UCHD(usual childhood disease)	一般小児病
UCR(unconditioned reflex)	無条件反射＝inborn reflex
UCS(unconditioned stimulus)	無条件刺激(ある反射を起こし得る自然刺激)
UCT(ultrasonic cardiotomogram)	心断層エコー図
UCTD (undifferentiated connective tissue disease)	不全型(分類困難な)膠原病
U-D(ulcus duodeni)	十二指腸潰瘍
ud(undifferentiated carcinoma)	未分化癌
UDT(undescended testicle)	停留睾丸

UES(upper esophageal sphincter)	上部食道括約部
UFA(unesterified fatty acid)	遊離脂肪酸
UFR(ultrafiltration rate)	限外濾過率
Ug(unguentum)	軟膏＝Ung
UG(urethrography)	尿道造影法
UGAA(urethritis gonorrhoica anterior acuta)	急性淋菌性前部尿道炎
UGI(S)(upper gastrointestinal〔series〕)	上部消化管（撮影）
UGPA (urethritis gonorrhoica posterior acuta)	急性淋菌性後部尿道炎
UHD(unstable hemoglobin disease)	不安定ヘモグロビン症
UHL (unilateral hilar lymphonodi enlargement)	片側性肺門リンパ節腫大
UI(urgent incontinence)	切迫性尿失禁
	参照 腹圧性尿失禁：SUI
UIBC(unsaturated iron-binding capacity)	不飽和鉄結合能
UIC(uninhibited contraction)	無抑制収縮
UIP(usual interstitial pneumonia)	通常型間質性肺炎
UK(urokinase)	ウロキナーゼ
ULBW(ultra low birth weight)	極端な低出生体重
ulcer	潰瘍
ULN(upper limits of normal)	正常値の最高
ulnar nerve	尺骨神経
	◀関連▶橈骨神経： radial nerve 正中神経： median nerve
ulnar tunnel	尺骨管
uls(ulcer scar)	潰瘍瘢痕
ultrasonic diagnosis	超音波診断法
umbilical cord	臍帯
uMDD(unipolar major depressive disorder)	単極性うつ病
UMN(upper motor neuron)	上位運動ニューロン
UN(ulnar nerve)	尺骨神経＝nervus ulnaris
UN(urea nitrogen)	尿素窒素

un

unconscious	意識不明の、無意識
uncovertebral joint	椎鉤関節
undifferentiated type	未分化型（統合失調症）
unfavorable prognosis	予後不良
Ung(unguentum)	軟膏＝Ug
unproductive cough	乾性咳
unruptured aneurysm	未破裂動脈瘤
unstable angina	不安定狭心症
UO(urinary output)	尿量
UP(umbilical portion)	門脈臍部
UP(urinal protein)	尿蛋白
U/P(urine/plasma〔ratio〕)	尿／血漿濃度比
UPC(unknown primary carcinoma)	原発不明癌
UPI(uteroplacental insufficiency)	子宮胎盤機能不全
UPJ(uretero-pelvic junction)	尿管腎盂結合部
upper extremity	上肢＝upper limb
	対 下肢：lower extremity
upper GI series	上部消化管X線造影検査
upper lung field	上肺野
UPPP(uvulopalatopharyngoplasty)	口蓋軟口蓋咽頭形成（術）
UPT(unknown primary tumor)	原発不明腫瘍
UQ(urine quantity)	尿量
uremia	尿毒症
ureter	尿管
ureteral ectopia	異所性尿管
ureteral stone	尿管結石
urethral indwelling catheter	留置カテーテル
urethritis	尿道炎
URF(uterine relaxing factor)	子宮弛緩因子
urge incontinence	切迫性尿失禁
URI(upper respiratory infection)	上気道感染症
urinary disturbance	排尿障害
urinary incontinence	尿失禁
urinary retention	尿閉

UV

urinary sediment	尿沈渣
urinalysis	検尿＝urine analysis
urination	排尿
urine	尿
Uro(urology)	泌尿器科、泌尿器科学
urogram	尿路造影図
urolithiasis, urinary stones	尿路結石症
URT(upper respiratory tract)	上気道
URTI(upper respiratory tract infection)	上気道感染症
urticaria	蕁麻疹
US(ultrasonography)	超音波検査
US(ultrasound)	超音波
US(urinal sugar)	尿糖
USB(unstable bladder)	不安定膀胱
USI(urinary stress incontinence)	緊張性尿失禁、ストレス性尿失禁
USL(ultrasonic lithotripsy)	超音波砕石術
USN(ultrasonic nebulizer)	超音波ネブライザー
UST(ultrasonographic tomography)	超音波断層法
USWT(usual weight)	通常体重
ut(upper thoracic esophagus)	胸部上部食道
UT(urinary tract)	尿路
UTC(uterine cancer)	子宮癌
Ut ca(cancer of uterus)	子宮癌
uterine	子宮の
uterine fundus	子宮底
uterine tube	卵管
uterus	子宮
UTI(urinary tract infection)	尿路感染症
UTJ(utero-tubal junction)	子宮卵管境界
UTM(urinary tract malformation)	尿路奇形
UTS(urinary tract stone)	尿路結石
UU(urine urobilinogen)	尿ウロビリノーゲン
UV(ulcus ventriculi)	胃潰瘍

UV

UV(ultraviolet light)	紫外線=ultraviolet rays
UV(umbilical vein)	臍静脈
UV(urine volume)	尿量
UVA(ultraviolet A)	長波長紫外線
UVB(ultraviolet B)	中波長紫外線
UVC(ultraviolet C)	短波長紫外線
UVC(umbilical vein catheter)	臍静脈カテーテル
uveitis	ぶどう膜炎
UVJ(uretero-vesico junction)	尿管膀胱結合部

V(vein)	静脈 **対** 動脈：A
V(venous)	静脈血 **対** 動脈血：a
V-A(venoarterial bypass)	静脈動脈バイパス(法)
VA(ventricular aneurysma)	心室瘤
Va(verdacht auf 〜)	〜の疑い
VA(vertebral artery)	椎骨動脈
VA(visual acuity)	視力
VAB(venous- arterial bypass)	動脈静脈バイパス
vaccination	種痘、予防接種
vaccine	ワクチン
VAD(ventricular assist device)	補助心臓
VAG(vertebral angiography)	椎骨動脈造影(法)
vagina	腟
vaginal discharge	おりもの、腟分泌物
vaginal portion	子宮腟部
vagus N	迷走神経
VAHS (virus associated hemophagocytic syndrome)	ウイルス感染に伴う血球貪食症候群
VAIN(vaginal intraepithelial neoplasia)	腟上皮内癌
valgus	外反
valvular	心臓弁膜の
valvular heat disease	心臓弁膜症
VAP(variant angina pectoris)	異型狭心症(発作時ST上昇を起こす攣縮性狭心症) ＝Prinzmetal's angina
VAP(ventilator associated pneumonia)	人工呼吸器関連性肺炎
Va/Q(ventilation/perfusion ratio)	換気血流比
VA-PICA(vertebral artery posterior inferior cerebellar artery aneurysm)	椎骨後下小脳動脈分岐部動脈瘤
variable deceleration	変動性一過性徐脈
variant form angina	異型狭心症＝VAP
varicella	水痘

va

varix	静脈瘤
VAS(ventricular assist system)	補助人工心臓
VAS(ventricular- atrial shunt)	脳室心房シャント
VAS(visual analog scale)	視覚アナログ尺度
vascular anastomosis	血管吻合
vascular shadow	血管陰影
vasculitis	血管炎
V-A shunt(ventriculo-atrial shunt)	脳室心房短絡術
vasoconstrictor	血管収縮薬
vasodilator	血管拡張薬＝VD
vasopressin	バソプレシン(抗利尿ホルモン)
vasospastic angina	冠攣縮性狭心症＝VSA
VAST(vibro-acoustic stimulation test)	胎児振動音刺激試験
VAT(ventricle atrium trigger)	P波同期型ペーシング
VAT(ventricular activation time)	心室興奮伝達時間
VATS(video-assisted thoracic surgery)	胸腔鏡下手術
VAZ(vena azygos)	奇静脈
VB(venous blood)	静脈血
VB(vitamin-B)	ビタミンB
VBA(vertebrobasilar artery)	椎骨脳底動脈
VBI(vertebrobasilar insufficiency)	椎骨脳底動脈循環不全
VBNS (transvaginal bladder-neck suspension)	経腟的膀胱頸部吊り上げ術
VBP(venous blood pressure)	静脈血圧
	対 動脈圧：ABP
VC(vena cava)	大静脈
VC(vital capacity)	肺活量
VC(vitamin-C)	ビタミンC
VC(vocal cord)	声帯＝plica vocalis
VCD(vena colica dextra)	右結腸静脈
Vcf (velocity of circumferential fiber shortening)	心筋(左心室)円周短縮速度
VCG(vectorcardiogram)	ベクトル心電図
VCG(voiding cystography)	排尿時膀胱造影

VCM(vena colica media)	中結腸静脈
VCR(vasoconstriction rate)	血管収縮率
VCS(vena cava superior)	上大静脈
VD(vascular dementia)	脳血管性痴呆
VD(vasodilator)	血管拡張神経、血管拡張薬
VD(venereal disease)	性病
V. d.(visus dexter)	右眼視力
	◀関連▶左眼視力：V.s.
VD(volume of dead space gas)	死腔換気量
VDA(visual discriminatory acuity)	視覚識別正確度
VDD(ventricle double double〔pacing〕)	心室抑制心房同期型ペーシング
vdE(vor dem Essen)	(毎)食前
	参照 (毎)食後：ndE
VDG(venereal disease gonorrhoea)	淋病
VDH(valvular disease of heart)	心臓弁膜症
VDM(vasodepressor material)	血管拡張物質
VDRL (Venereal Disease Research Laboratory test)	(アメリカ)性病研究所梅毒検査法、ガラス板法
VDS(venereal disease syphilis)	梅毒
vds(vor dem schlafgehen)	就寝前
V. d. s.(von den Schlafen)	眠前服用
VDT/I(ventricle-double-trigger/inhibit)	心房同期型心室ペーシング
VE(minute volume of ventilation)	分時換気量
VE(vacuum extraction)	吸引分娩
VE(vaginal examination)	腟内診
vector	媒介者
VEDP(ventricular end-diastolic pressure)	心室拡張終期圧
VEDV(ventricular end-diastolic volume)	心室拡張終期容積
vegetable state	植物状態
vena cava	大静脈＝VC
ventilation	換気、呼吸
ventilator	人工呼吸器
ventricular aneurysm	心室瘤

VE

VEP(visually evoked potential)	視覚誘発電位
verbosity	冗長
vermiform appendix	虫垂
vernix caseosa	胎脂
verruca	いぼ
vertical immunization	垂直免疫
vertigo	めまい
vesicourethral junction	膀胱尿道移行部
vesicular breathing	肺胞呼吸音
vesicular mole	胞状奇胎
VF(ventilatory failure)	換気不全
Vf(ventricular fibrillation)	心室細動
VF(ventricular flutter)	心室粗動
VF(visual field)	視野
VF(vocal fremitus)	声音振盪
VG(ventriculography)	脳室撮影
VGED(vena gastroepiploica dextra)	右胃大静脈
VH(vaginal hysterectomy)	腟式子宮摘出術
VH(viral hepatitis)	ウイルス性肝炎
VHD(valvular heart disease)	心弁膜疾患
VHDL(very high-density lipoprotein)	超高比重リポ蛋白
VHF(viral hemorrhagic fever)	ウイルス性出血熱
VI(inspired volume)	呼気量
VI(vagina irrigation)	腟内洗浄
VI(venous incompetence)	静脈弁不全
VIA(virus inactivating agent)	ウイルス不活性薬
VIG(varicella immune globulin)	水痘免疫グロブリン
villus	絨毛
VIN(vulvar intraepithelial neoplasia)	外陰上(表)皮内腫瘍
VIP(vasoactive intestinal polypeptide)	血管作働性腸管ポリペプチド
VIP(very important person)	重要人物
VISA(vancomycin insensitive resistant staphylococcus aureus)	バンコマイシン低感受性黄色ブドウ球菌
viscosity	粘性

visual hallucination	幻視
Vit(vitamin)	ビタミン
VKH(Vogt-Koyanagi-Harada disease)	フォークトー小柳ー原田病
VKM(vall kuh Milch)	全乳
VLAP(visual laser ablation of the prostate, visual laser assisted prostatectomy)	直視下レーザー前立腺切除術
VLBW(very low birth weight〔infant〕)	極小未熟児
VLCD(very low caloric diet)	超低カロリー食
VLDL(very low density lipoprotein)	超低比重リポ蛋白
VLG(venereal lymphogranuloma)	性病性リンパ肉芽腫
VLM(visceral larva migrans)	内臓幼虫移行症
VL thalamotomy (ventrolateral thalamotomy)	視床腹外側核破壊術
VMA(vanillylmandelic acid)	バニリルマンデル酸
Vmax(maximal expiratory flow)	最大呼気流量
Vmax(maximum velocity of shortening)	最大短縮速度
VMR(vasomotor rhinitis)	血管運動性鼻炎
VMS(visual memory span)	視覚記憶スパン
VN(vestibular neuronitis)	前庭神経炎
VO(verbal order)	口頭指示
VO_2(oxygen consumption)	酸素消費量
VOD(various organ disorder)	多臓器不全
VOD(veno-occlusive disease)	肝中心静脈閉塞症
Vol(volume)	容積
vomiting	嘔吐
VOR(vestibulo-ocular reflex)	前庭眼反射
voyeurism	窃視癖
VP(vasopressin)	バソプレシン
VP(vena portae)	門脈
VP(venous pressure)	静脈圧
	対 動脈圧：VP
VP(ventricular pressure)	脳室圧
VP(Vibrio parahaemolyticus)	腸炎ビブリオ
VPB(ventricular premature beat)	心室性期外収縮＝VPC

VP

VPC(ventricular premature contraction)	心室性期外収縮＝VPB
V-P shunt(ventriculo-peritoneal shunt)	脳室腹腔短絡術
VR(vascular resistance)	血管抵抗
VR(ventilation reserve)	換気予備率
VR(vocal resonance)	声帯共鳴
VRD(viral respiratory disease)	ウイルス性呼吸器疾患＝VRI
VRE(vancomycin resistant Enterococcus)	バンコマイシン耐性腸球菌
VRI(viral respiratory infection)	ウイルス性呼吸器疾患＝VRD
VS(vaginal smear)	腟内容塗布
VS(ventricular septum)	心室中隔
V. s.(visus sinister)	左眼視力
	◀関連▶ 左眼視力：V.d.
VSA(vasospastic angina)	冠攣縮性狭心症
VSC(voluntary surgical contraception)	自発的手術の避妊
VSD(ventricular septal defect)	心室中隔欠損症
VSP(ventricular septal perforation)	心室中隔穿孔
VSR(ventricular septal rupture)	心室中隔破裂
VSS(visual sexual stimulation)	視覚性的刺激
VSV(vesicular stomatitis virus)	水疱性口〔内〕炎ウイルス＝VS virus
VT(tidal volume)	１回換気量
VT(vasotocin)	バソトシン
VT(ventricular tachycardia)	心室性頻拍
VTEC(verotoxin producing Escherichia coil)	ベロ毒素産生性大腸菌
VTH(vaginal total hysterectomy)	腟式子宮全摘出術
VUG(voiding upto urethrography)	排尿時膀胱尿道造影(法)
VUJ(vesico-ureter junction)	膀胱尿管結合部
VUR(vesico-ureteral reflux)	膀胱尿管逆流現象
vv(verruca vulgaris)	尋常性疣贅
Vv(voided volume)	排尿量
VW(vessel wall)	血管壁
VW(von Willebrand's disease)	フォン・ウィルブランド病
VWF(vibration white finger)	白蝋病

VZ

VZIG(varicella-zoster immune globulin) 水痘帯状疱疹免疫グロブリン

VZV(varicella-zoster virus) 水痘帯状疱疹ウイルス

W(white epithelium)	白色上皮
WAIS(Wechsler adult intelligence scale)	ウェクスラー成人知能検査
WAIS-R(Wechsler adult intelligence scale-Revised)	ウェクスラー成人知能検査改訂版
wale	みみず腫れ
walk on heel	踵歩行
wandering kidney	遊走腎
Wa-R(Wassermann reaction)	ワッセルマン反応
wart	いぼ
washout ratio	洗い出し率
watery feces	水様便
water deprivation test	水制限試験
WB(whole blood)	全血
WB-F(whole-blood fresh)	新鮮保存血
WBC(white blood cell〔count〕)	白血球(数)
	◀関連▶赤血球：RBC
WC(wheel chair)	車いす
WD(well-developed)	発育良好
WD(wet dressing)	湿布、罨法
WD(withdrawal dyskinesia)	ジスキネジアを伴わない
WDHAS(watery diarrhea, hypokalemia, and achlorhydria syndrome)	WDHA症候群(水様性下痢低K血症無酸症)ヴァーナー・モリソン症候群、膵コレラ
WDLL(well-differentiated lymphocytic lymphoma)	高分化型小球性悪性リンパ腫
WD syndrome(withdrawal syndrome)	離脱症候群
Wd-syndrome (withdrawal syndrome)	離脱症候群＝abstinence syndrome
weakness	脱力
weaning	離乳
Wegener's granulomatosis	ウェグナー肉芽腫瘍＝WG

WR

Wernicke's aphasia	ウェルニッケ失語
	参照 感覚性失語：
	sensory aphasia
Wernicke's syndrome	ウェルニッケ症候群
WF(warfarin)	ワーファリン
WG(Wegener's granulomatosis)	ウェゲナー肉芽腫症
W/H(waist/hip)	腹部周囲／殿囲比
WHD (Werdnig-Hoffmann disease)	ウェルドニッヒ・ホフマン病（家族性遺伝性脊髄性筋萎縮）
wheeze	喘鳴
whiplash injury	むち打ち損傷
white coat	白苔
white coat hypertension	白衣高血圧
WHO(World Health Organization)	世界保健機関
whooping cough	百日咳
WHVP(wedged hepatic venous pressure)	閉塞肝静脈圧
Willis circle	ウィリス動脈輪
Wilms tumor	ウィルムス腫瘍（腎芽細胞腫）＝WT
WISC(Wechsler intelligence scale for children)	ウェクスラー児童知能検査
withdrawal	禁断症、自閉症、離脱症
WK(Wernicke-Korsakoff syndrome)	ウェルニッケ・コルサコフ症候群
WMS(Wilson-Mikity syndrome)	ウィルソン・ミキティ症候群＝bronchopulmonary dysplasia
W／N(well nourished)	栄養状態良好な
WN(well-nourished)	栄養状態良好
WNL(within normal limits)	正常範囲
WO(written order)	指示票
work therapy	働き療法
wound toilet	デブリードマン
WPPSI(Wechsler preschool and primary scale of intelligence)	ウェクスラー小児知能検査
WPW(Wolff-Parkinson-White syndrome)	WPW症候群
WR(Wassermann reaction)	ワッセルマン反応

WR

WRC(washed red cells)	洗浄赤血球
WRD(work related disease)	作業関連疾患
WRIPT (wide range intelligence and personality test)	広範囲知能人格検査
wrist joint	手関節
wryneck	斜頚
WS(Wallenberg syndrome)	ワレンベルグ症候群
Wt(weight)	体重　**関連** 身長：Ht
WT(Wilms tumor)	ウィルムス腫瘍

X

Xan(xanthine)	キサンチン
Xanth(xanthomatosis)	黄色腫症
xanthoma	黄色腫
xenophobia	外人恐怖
xerostomia	口腔乾燥症
XGP(xanthogranulomatous pyelonephritis)	黄色肉芽腫性腎盂腎炎
XIP(X-ray in plaster〔examination〕)	ギプス固定のままのX線写真
XLI(X-linked ichthyosis)	伴性遺伝性魚鱗癬
XOP(X-ray out of plaster)	ギプスを外した状態でのX線写真
XP(exophoria)	外斜位
XP(xeroderma pigmentosum)	色素性乾皮症
X-P(X-ray photograph)	X線写真
XSCID(X-linked severe combined immunodeficiency)	X連鎖重症複合免疫不全症
XT(exotropia)	外斜視　**対** 内斜視：XT
XU(excretory urography)	排泄性尿路造影
XYY syndrome(Klinefelter syndrome)	クラインフェルター症候群

Y

YAM(young adult mean)	若年成人平均値

yawn	欠伸
yellow fever	黄熱病
Y-G test (Yatabe-Guilford test)	矢田部・ギルフォード性格検査
yolk sac	卵黄嚢(包)
Yr (year)	年
YS (yellow spot retina)	網膜黄斑
YST (yolk sac tumor)	卵巣包囊腫瘍

Z

ZEEP (zero end-expiratory pressure breathing)	ゼロ呼息終期圧呼吸
ZES (Zollinger-Ellison syndrome)	ゾリンジャー・エリソン症候群
ZIFT (zygote intrafallopian transfer)	接合子卵管内移植
ZIG (zoster immune globulin)	帯状疱疹免疫グロブリン
ZIG-v (zoster immune globulin〔venous〕)	静注用帯状疱疹免疫グロブリン
ZIP (zoster immune plasma)	帯状疱疹免疫血清
ZK (Zervixkrebs) (独)	子宮頚癌
ZKS (zentrale koordinations storung)	中枢性協調障害
Z line (zigzag line)	食道噴門接合部
Zn (zu nehmen)	服用
ZNS (zentralnervensystem)	中枢神経系
	対 末梢神経系:PNS
zoonosis	人畜共通伝染病
zoophilia	動物嗜愛
ZPG (zero population growth)	ゼロ人口成長
ZST (zinc sulfate turbidity)	硫酸亜鉛混濁試験
Zung depression scale	ツングうつ病自己評価尺度
zwdE (zwischen den Essen)	食間に
	参照 (毎)食前:vdE
	(毎)食後:ndE
zygoite	受精卵、接合体

各科の頻出病名

診療科（病棟）	略語・単語	疾患名
ICU	ARDS	成人呼吸窮迫症候群
	burn	熱傷
	CPAOA	到着時心肺停止
	DIC	播種性血管内凝固症候群
	MOF	多臓器不全
	esophageal varix	食道静脈瘤
	HI	頭部外傷
	LOC	意識障害
	ICH	脳内出血
	SAH	クモ膜下出血
CCU 循環器内科	AMI	急性心筋梗塞
	AP	狭心症
	AAA	腹部大動脈瘤
	DAA	解離性大動脈瘤
	AR	大動脈弁閉鎖不全症
	AS	大動脈弁狭窄症
	MR	僧帽弁閉鎖不全症
	MS	僧帽弁狭窄症
	HCM	肥大型心筋症
	HF	心不全
脳神経外科 神経内科	IVH	脳出血
	SDH	硬膜下血腫（サブドラ）
	EDH	硬膜外血腫
	CVD	脳血管疾患、脳血管障害
	BT	脳腫瘍
	CI	脳梗塞
	LOC	意識消失
	PD	パーキンソン病
	AD	アルツハイマー病
	ALS	筋萎縮性側索硬化症

診療科（病棟）	略語・単語	疾患名
消化器科	EC，Eca	食道癌
	GU	胃潰瘍
	MK	胃癌
	PK	膵臓癌
	HCC	肝細胞癌
	CCC	胆管細胞癌
	RK	直腸癌
	DM	糖尿病
	LC	肝硬変
	FHF	劇症肝炎
血液内科	ALL	急性リンパ球性白血病
	CLL	慢性リンパ球性白血病
	AML	急性骨髄性白血病
	CML	慢性骨髄性白血病
	ATL	成人T細胞リンパ腫
	MDS	骨髄異形性症候群
	ML	悪性リンパ腫
	MM	多発性骨髄腫
	HD	ホジキン病
	IDA	鉄欠乏性貧血
呼吸器科	AB	喘息性気管支炎
	BE	気管支拡張症
	LC	肺癌
	PE	肺気腫（pulmonary emphaysema） 肺水腫（pulmonary edema） 肺塞栓症（pulmonary embolsm）
	PP	肺結核
	Pn	肺炎
	Pnx	気胸
	empyema	膿胸
	RF	呼吸不全
	BC	気管支癌

診療科(病棟)	略語・単語	疾患名
腎臓内科 内分泌科	RCC	腎癌
	RF	腎不全
	RVH	腎血管性高血圧症
	NS	ネフローゼ症候群
	PN	腎盂腎炎
	NDI	腎性尿崩症
	CD	膠原病
	SLE	全身性エリテマトーデス
	LN	ループス腎炎
	PKD	多発性嚢胞腎
泌尿器科	PC, Pca	前立腺癌
	BT	膀胱腫瘍
	ED	勃起障害
	UTM	尿路奇形
	UTI	尿路感染症
	BPH	前立腺肥大症
	DI	尿崩症
	STD	性行為感染症
	VDG	淋病
	VDS	梅毒
整形外科	Fx	骨折
	FNF	大腿骨頚部骨折
	osteo	骨髄炎
	OS	骨肉腫
	DIS	脱臼
	OA	変形性関節症
	OI	骨形成不全症
	OM	骨軟化症
	PID	椎間板ヘルニア
	SMA	脊髄性筋萎縮

診療科（病棟）	略語・単語	疾患名
産婦人科	BT	乳房腫瘍
	EUP	子宮外妊娠
	UTC	子宮癌
	OVC	卵巣癌
	TV	膣トリコモナス
	GDM	妊娠糖尿病
	YST	卵巣包（嚢）腫瘍
	PMS	月経前症候群
	IVF	体外受精
	IUGR	子宮内胎児発育不全
小児科 NICU	AD	アトピー性皮膚炎
	CP	脳性（小児）麻痺、口蓋裂
	CB	クループ性気管支炎
	Sb（strabismus）	斜視
	TOF	ファロー4徴症
	FC	熱性痙攣
	SIDS	乳児突然死症候群
	MR	麻疹
	INE	乳児壊死性脳脊髄障害
	VSD	心室中隔欠損症
精神科	MD	躁うつ病、精神発達遅延
	SZ	統合失調症、シゾ
	PTSD	外傷性ストレス障害
	ASD	急性ストレス障害
	ADHD	注意欠陥多動障害
	MR	精神薄弱、精神遅滞
	PD	人格障害（personality disorder） パニック障害（panic disorder）
	PDD	広汎性発達障害
	GID	性同一性障害
	MSBP	代理ミュンヒハウゼン症候群

頻用カタカナ用語

ア

アーテリー	動脈（arteryまたは、Artivie）。
アイエム	筋肉注射（i.m.：intramuscular）。
アイシーエイチ	頭内出血 （ICH：Intracranial Hemorrhage）。
アイシーピー	頭蓋内圧（ICP：Intracranial Pressure）。
アイテル	膿（Eiter）。
アイデンティティ	他人とは異なる自分。同一性（identity）。
アイブイ	静脈内注射（i.v.：intravenous）。
アイブイエイチ	中心静脈栄養（高カロリー輸液）。 （IVH：Intravenous Hyperelimentation）。
アイブイチューブ	点滴の管（IV tube）。
アイブイドリップ	静脈持続点滴注入法（intravenous drip）。
アウゲ	眼、眼科（Auge：独語）。
アウス	搔破（Auskratzung）。人工妊娠中絶のこと。
アオルタ	大動脈（aorta）。
アカウンタビリティ	説明責任（義務）（accountability）。
アカシジア	静座不能 （acathisiaまたは、Akathisie）。 錐体外路障害の症状の1つ。
アクア	水。溶液（aqua）。
アゴニスト	作用薬（agonist）。
アサーティブネス	説得力と配慮のある意見の主張 （assertiveness）。
アシドーシス	動脈血のpHが低下する方向に変動する病的過程（acidosis）。（⇔alkalosis：アルカローシス）。
アス	乱視（As：astigmatism）。
アストマ	喘息（Asthma）。
アスピレーション	吸引（Aspiration）。
アセスメント	主観的・客観的情報を収集して問題点を明らかにすること（assessment）。

アタック	発作のこと。心臓発作や喘息発作など（attack）。
アッペ	虫垂炎（appendicitis）。
アディクション	中毒。嗜癖（addiction）。
アディポ	脂肪過多（adipositas）。
アテトーシス	無定位運動症（athetosis）。
アテレク	無気肺（atelectasisまたはAtelektase）。肺の一部に空気が入らない状態。
アドヒアランス	患者が治療に自ら能動的に係わり、粘り強くセルフケアを実践していくこと（adherence）。
アトピー	アトピー（atopy）。アトピー体質、アトピー性皮膚炎、アトピー素因。遺伝・家族的要因の強い即時型過敏状態。
アドボケイト	（患者の権利の）擁護者（advocate）。
アドミッション	入院（admission）。
アナフィラキシー	即時型過敏症（anaphylaxis）。アナフィラキシー・ショック。
アナムネ	既往歴。アナムネーゼ（Anamnese：独語）の略。患者本人や関係者から入院までの経過を聴取すること。
アニソコ	瞳孔不同（アニソコリア Anisocoria）。脳ヘルニアの所見。
アノレキシア	無食欲。拒食症（anorexia）。
アパタイト	食欲（appetite）。
アビュース	虐待。乱用（abuse）。
アブサンス	失神、欠損（absence）。
アフタ	小潰瘍（aptha）、アフタ性口内炎（aphthous stomatitis）。
アプニア、アプネア	呼吸停止、無呼吸（apnea）。
アプラ	再生不良性貧血（aplastic anemia）。
アポ、アポプレキシー、アポる	脳卒中（米では現在、stroke【ストローク】を使っている）（apoplexy）。
アルコールハビット	飲酒癖。

アルコリカ	常習飲酒家（Alkoholica：独語）。
アルス	二次救命処置（ALS：advanced life support）。
アルツ	アルツハイマー病（Alzheimer's）。
アレスト	心停止（arrest）。
アンギオ	血管造影（angiography）。
アンギナ	狭心症（angina：アンジャイナ、Angina：独語）。
アンビュー	送気バッグ（ambu bag）。人工呼吸に用いる器具。
アンプタ	切断（amputation）。
アンプル	注射用薬剤（ampule）（の入れ物）。ガラス瓶状のものをアンプル（A）という。

イ・ウ

イーシージー	心電図（ECG：Electrocardiogram）。
イバリュエーション	（看護過程の最終段階としての）評価（evaluation）。
イリガートル	イリガートル、灌注器（irrigator）。洗浄台（irrigator stand）。
イリゲーション	洗腸（irrigation）。
イレウス	腸閉塞（ileus）。
イン・ビイボ、イン・ビトロ	試験管内／体内（in vivo／in vitro）。
インキュベーション	潜伏期（incubation）。インキュベーション・ステージ（incubation stage）。
インセン	陰部洗浄。
インソムニア	不眠症（insomnia）。
インターバル	間隔（interval）。（月経の）周期。
インターベンション	介入（intervention）。ナーシング・インターベンション：看護介入。
インバギ	腸重積（invagination）。
インフェクション	感染（infection）。

インフォームドコンセント	説明と同意（informed consent）。
インフュージョン	注入（infusion）。
ウイニング	離脱（weaning）。人工呼吸から自発呼吸に戻ること。一般には（治療的に）呼吸器を外すこと。
ウロ、ウロロジー	泌尿器科（urology）。
ウロストミー	人工排尿口（urostomy）。膀胱や尿道に障害がある患者の腹部に作った排尿口。

エ

エアウェイ	気道（airway）。舌根沈下患者の舌根を挙上し、気道を確保する器具。
エー	動脈（A：artery）。
エーカーゲー	心電図。EKGの独語読み。
エーライン	動脈ライン（arterial line）。
エオジノ	好酸球（eosinocyte）。
エクスレイ	X線。レントゲン（X-ray）。
エクトピー	転移（ectopy）。 子宮外妊娠（ectopypregnancy）。
エコ	生態。生態系（eco）。 エコロジー（ecology）。
エコー	超音波検査（echo）。
エスエス	妊娠（Schwangerschaft）。
エスシー	皮下注射（SC：subcut-aneous）。
エスビー	ゼングスターケン・ブレークモアチューブ（S-B：Sengstaken-Blakemore tube）。
エッセン	食事（Essen：独語）。
エッチアー	A型肝炎（HA：hepatitis A）。
エッチシー	C型肝炎（HC：hepatitis C）。
エッチビー	B型肝炎（HB：hepatitis B）。
エデーマ、エデマる	水腫、浮腫、むくみ（edema）。
エヌピーオー	禁飲食（NPO：non per os）。

エピ、エピレプシー	てんかん（epilepsy）。
エピドラ	硬膜外麻酔（epidural anesthesia）。
エピソード	発作、症状の発現（episode）。てんかんのエピソード。
エビデンス	証拠。根拠（evidence）。
エビデンス・ベイスト・メディスン（EBM）	証拠（根拠）に基づく医療（Evidence-Based Medicine）。
エフエフピー	新鮮凍結血漿（FFP：fresh frozen plasma）。
エマージェンシー	緊急事態、非常事態（emergency）。
エム	MRSA。保菌者を指すこともある。「患者からエムが出た」などと使う。
エムティ	マーゲンチューブ（MT：Magenschlauch／stomach tube）、胃管。
エルブレ	嘔吐（Erbrechen：独語）。
エンセファロパシー	脳症（encephalopathy）。
エンゼルセット	死後処置セット。
エンテロトキシン	腸管毒（enterotoxin）。
エント、エントラッセン	退院（独語）。「ENT」と記載される。
エンパワメント	力や能力、権力を与えること（empowerment）。
エンベロープ	エンベロープ（envelop）。ウイルスの外殻。
エンボリ	塞栓術（embolization）。動脈瘤や腫瘍のある血管にコイルやエタノールなどをつめる治療方法。

オ

オウビサティ	（病的な）肥満（obesity）。
オージオメトリー	聴力検査、聴力測定（audiometry）。
オースキュルテーション	聴診（auscultation）。

オートノミー	自律性(autonomy)。
オートプシー	解剖。病理解剖(autopsy)。
オープン	開放性の(open)。オープンフラクチャー：開放骨折。
オカズ	薬剤。点滴内に入れる薬剤をまとめて「おかず」とよんだりする。
オカルト（ブラッド）	潜血(occult blood)。
オステオ、オステオポローシス	骨粗鬆症(osteoporosis)。
オト	耳鼻咽喉科(otorhinolaryngology)。
オブザベーション	観察(observation)。
オプトメーター	眼計測計(optometer)。
オペ	手術。オペレーション(operation)の略。
オルターナティブ	代替となるもの。代わりに取りうる方法(alternative)。
オルターナティブメディスン	代替医療(alternative medicine)。
オルト	整形外科(orthopaedics)。
オンコール	呼び出し。手術(検査)の開始時間が不定の場合、手術室から呼び出しがかかる(on call)。

カ

ガーグルベイスン	膿盆(gargle basin)。ガーグルはうがいのこと。
ガーレ	胆汁(Galle)。吐物が緑色をしていると「ガーレ様」と表現される。
カイザー	帝王切開(Kaiserschnitt)。
ガイニン	子宮外妊娠。
カウンターショック	電気的除細動器。重症不整脈を治療する機器(countershock)。
ガス	おなら(gas)。

頻用カタカナ用語

ガストロ		ガストロボタン（ボタン型胃瘻チューブ）、もしくは消化管造影（剤）、ガストログラフィン（gastrographin）。
ガット		腹。腸（gut）。
カテ、カテーテル		カテーテル（catheter）、カテーテル法（catheterization）。
カニューレーション		カニューレ挿入（cannulation）。
カニューレ、カヌラ		酸素吸入器具。鼻腔に装着するタイプのもの（canula）。カニューレーション：カニューレ挿入（cannulation）。
カマ		酸化マグネシウム。下剤。「化」と「マ」をとってカマという。
ガム		歯肉。歯茎（gums）。
カリフラワー（癌）		cauliflower（cancer）。カリフラワーのような外観に増殖する腫瘍。
カリョウ		化学療法。ケモと同じ。
カルチ		癌、悪性腫瘍（carcinoma）。カルテには「Ca」と記載される。
ガングリオン		包腫。ゼリー状の内容物を含む包腫（ganglion）。
ガンツ		スワン・ガンツカテーテル。
カンファ		カンファレンス、打ち合わせ、会議（室）（conference）。

キ

キープ	維持（keep）。通常「キープで」と言われたら、指示量を24時間かけて注入する。点滴ルートを確保する時にも使う。
キザミ食	副食の形態。咀嚼困難の場合や嚥下しやすいように、おかずが刻んである。
キセツ	気管切開。
ギネ	婦人科（gynecology）。
キャスト	ギブス。包帯（cast）。

ギャストロ(ガストロ)・カメラ	胃カメラ(gastrocamera)。
ギャストロ(ガストロ)・ファイバースコープ	胃電子内視鏡(gastrofiberscope)。
キャリア	保菌者(carrier)。
キュア	治療(cure)。
キュウガイ	救急外来。
キュウヘン	急変。患者の状態が急に悪化してショック状態に陥ること。
キューレット	掻爬器、有窓鋭匙(curette kurette：独語)。
キョクマ	局所麻酔。
キルシュナー	牽引用の鋼線(Kirschner)。
キント	子ども、小児科(Kind)。

ク

クーリング	冷却(cooling)。
クール	治療単位(course)。
クオリティ・オブ・ライフ	生活の質。生命の質(Quality Of Life(QOL))。クオリティ・ケア：質の高い看護。
クベース	保育器(incubator)。
クライエント	対等の立場で相談目的に来る人のこと。来談者。患者(client)。
グラニューロ	顆粒球(granulocyte)。
クランケ	患者(Kranke)。
クランプ	鉗子(clamp)または鉗子でドレーン類をはさんで流出を一時的に止めること。
クリアランス	浄化値、清掃率(clearance)。血漿クリアランス。
グリカン	グリセリン浣腸。「GE」と記載される。60mLや120mLなど各種あるので注意。
クリティカル・シンキング	批判的思考。客観的思考(critical thinking)。

頻用カタカナ用語

クリティカル・パス	入院指導、検査、治療、退院指導など一連の手順を標準化し、時系列にまとめたもの。クリニカル・パスともいう（critical path）。	
グルオン、グル音	腸蠕動音。「gul音」と記載される。	
クレブス	癌（Krebs）。	
クレンメ	点滴ルートなどに付いている調節器具。「ローラークランプ」ともいう。滴下を調節し速度を合わせる。	
クローン	クローン（clone）。免疫学的特異性がすでに決定された1つのリンパ球から由来した細胞の総称。複製生物。無性生殖的に作られた遺伝的に同一の個体（clone）。	
クロスマッチ	輸血血液と患者の血液の適合を調べること（cross matching）。	
クロット	凝塊（clot）。	
クロニック	慢性の（chronic）。	

ケ

ケアマネ、ケアマネジャー	介護支援専門員（care manager）。
ケアリング	患者の身体面、情緒面に対する気遣いを示す目的でとる看護師の行動や態度（caring）。
ケイカン	経管栄養。
ケツガス、血ガス	血液ガスのこと。
ケッサン	血球算定。
ゲノム	ゲノム、全遺伝情報（genome）。
ケモ	化学療法（chemotherapy）。主に抗癌薬を指す。
ケモラジ	化学療法＋放射線療法（chemo＋radiation）。

ケンタイ	検体（術中やバイオプシーなどで摘出した組織・腫瘤・腫瘍のことで、病理検査部に提出し悪性所見を調べる）、もしくは献体（大学病院などで死亡後に今後の医療のために役立ててほしいと解剖登録すること。またはその身体）。

コ

コアグラ、コアグる	凝固（coagulation）。排液などに血塊が混入している場合に「コアグってる」と表現する。
コート	便（独語）。「kot」と記載される。
コーピング	打開。対処。対処能力（coping）。ストレスコーピング：ストレス対処
コーマ	昏睡状態（coma）。
ゴールストーン	胆石（gall stone）。
コスメティック	美容的な、見た目の（cosmetic）。
コット	乳児を寝かせるベッド。
コッヘル	鈎つき鉗子。
コメディカル	医師と一緒に治療にかかわる職種（co-medical）。
コラボレーション	連携。共働（collaboration）。
コレステロール・リーディング	コレステロール値（cholesterol reading）。
コロストミー	人工肛門（colostomy）。人工肛門形成（術）（colostomy）。
コロナリーケアユニット	冠疾患集中治療室（coronary care unit）。
コロン	大腸（colon）。大腸癌を指す場合も多い。
コンサルテーション	診察。相談（consultation）。
コンスタント	不断の（constant）。constant pain：絶え間ない痛み。
コンセント・フォーム	同意書（consent form）。

コンタミ、コンタミネーション	汚染（contamination）。
コンプライアンス	弾性。指示に従うこと（conpliance）。指示に従わないことは「ノン・コンプライアンス」。
コンプレイント	患者の訴え（complaint）。

サ

ザ・ピル	経口避妊薬（the pill）。
ザー、サバラ	クモ膜下出血（subarachnoid hemorrhage）。「SAH」と記載される。
サーフロー	静脈留置針。
サーベイランス	疾病監視（surveillance）。HIV surveillance。
ザール	手術室（Operationssaal）。「ザールイン」などと使用する。
サイケデリック	サイケデリックな、幻覚発動薬（psychedelic）。
サイコソマティック	心身の（psychosomatic）。
サイド・イフェクト	副作用（side effect）。
サイナス	正常調律（sinus rhythm）。心電図での正常調律（リズム）を表す。
サイレント	無症候性の（silent）。
サイレントストーン	無症候性結石（silent stone）。
サクション	吸引（suction）。サクションチューブは、吸引に使用する細い管（suction tube）。
サチュレーション	動脈血酸素飽和度（arterial oxygen saturation）。
サッキング	吸引（sucking）。
サニタリー	衛生的な（sanitary）。
サブドラ	硬膜下血腫（subdural hemorrhage）。頭を打って硬膜下に出血したもの。
サポ	坐剤。「sup」と記載される（suppository）。

サマリー	看護要約(summary)。転院する際に先方の病院に宛てて患者の状態を報告すること。
サルコイド	類肉腫(sarcoid)。
サンカツ	三方活栓。点滴ルートの途中に入れる器具。

シ

ジーイー	グリセリン浣腸(GE：glycerine enema)。
シーネ	副子固定の道具。骨折した際に患肢の安静を保つために固定する板状の道具。
シーピーアール	心肺蘇生法(CPR：Cardio-Pulmonary Resuscitation)。
シーブイ	中心静脈(ライン)(CV：Central Venous〔line〕)、中心静脈栄養(intravenous hyperalimentation)(＝IVH)。
ジーン	遺伝子(gene)。
ジーンセラピー	遺伝子治療(gene therapy)。
シェーマ	図表(schema)。
ジギ	①ジギタリス(digitalis)。 ②(直腸)指診。
システミック	全身性の(systemic)。
シゾ	統合失調症(schizophreniaまたは、Schizophrenie)。
シャーカステン	レントゲンを見るための器具。
ジャクソンリース	送気バッグ。挿管している時に使う用手的人工換気器具。ジャクソン。
シャンゲる、シュワンゲる	妊娠する(Schwangerschaft：独語)。
シャント	短絡術(shunt)。水頭症の治療法。
シュード	偽膜(pseudomembrane)。
ジョウショク	普通食。

シリンジ	注射器（syringe）。ガラスの注射器のこと。使い捨ての注射器はディスポとよぶことが多い。
シンカテ	心臓のカテーテル検査（catheter）。
シンチレーション	閃光（scintillation）。
シンマ	心臓マッサージ。

ス

スイサイド	自殺（suicide）。自殺未遂の意味でも使用される。
スカル	頭蓋（skull）。
スカルボーン	頭蓋骨（skull bone）。
スキャンニング	画像走査（scanning）。
スクリーニング	選別法（screening）。
スタイレット	気管内チューブを挿入する時、チューブの中に入れて誘導する細い針金状の器具（stylet）。
スティグマ	徴候（stigma）。
ステージ	段階（stage）。初期（early stage：アーリー・ステージ）。（initial stage：イニシャル・ステージ）。末期（end stage：エンド・ステージ）。終末期（terminal stage：ターミナル・ステージ）。
ステート	聴診器（stethoscope）。
ステる、ステルベン	死亡（Sterben：独語）。「ステる」「ステった」などと表現される。
ストーマ	人工肛門（stoma）。
ストーン	結石（stone）
ストマック	胃（stomach）。独語ではマーゲン。
ストレッサー	ストレスの原因となる刺激（stressor）。
スパイナル	脊髄（spinal）。
スパズム	発作、痙攣（spasm）。
スプーター	痰（sputum）。「sp」と記載される。

スプリーン	脾臓（spleen）。
スプレイン	捻挫（sprain）。
スペシフィック、ノンスペシフィック	特異的な／非特異的な（specific／nonspecific）
スペシメン	検体（specimen）。
ズポ	坐剤（suppository）。サポと同義語。
スミア	塗抹（smear）。
スモークフリー	禁煙（smoke-free）。
スライディング	スライディングスケールの略（sliding）。BSの値によって指示されたインスリンを投与し、血糖コントロールをする。
スロー	ゆるやかな（slow）。遅反応性物質（slow reacting substance：スロー・リアクティング・サブスタンス）。遅発性ウイルス感染（slow virus infection：スロー・ヴァイラス・インフェクション）。

セ

セイカ	生化学検査。
セカンドオピニオン	別の医師の意見（second opinion）。
セカンドハンド・スモーキング	間接喫煙（second-hand smoking）。
セキソン	脊髄損傷。
ゼク、ゼクチオン	解剖（Sektion：独語）。
セクレート（セクリーション）	分泌物（secrete、secretion）。
セデーション	不穏や疼痛コントロールなどのために、眠剤や鎮静剤で患者を眠らせること（sedation）。「癌性疼痛コントロール不良で本人の苦痛も著しく、本人と家族の希望によりセデーションをかける方針となった」などと使う。
ゼネラル	全身麻酔（general anesthesia）。
ゼプシス	敗血症（sepsis）。

セル	細胞(cell)。
ゼンガユ	全粥。主食がお粥の食事。

ソ

ソウカン	気管内挿管。呼吸を維持するため気管内に管を留置すること。
ソセアタ	ソセゴン(sosegon)、アタラックスP(Atarax-P)の両薬剤の合成語。鎮静、術前前投薬。
ソセイ	蘇生。
ソセチュウ	ペンタジン(＝ソセゴン)中毒。
ソッカン	側管。三方活栓や注入用の栓から注入すること。「別ルートで」と指示されたら、側管から注入せずに新たに静脈を確保する。
ソルトフリー	塩分抜き(salt-free)。
ゾンデ	管の総称(Sonde)。

タ

ターゲス	血糖値日内変動(tages)。各食前、各食後2時間、寝る前に血糖値を測定する検査。
ターゲット	標的(target)。
ターミナル	終末期(terminal)。末期癌患者などに使われる。
ターミナルケア	終末期医療(terminal care)。
ターミネーション	産科的早産(termination)。
タール	タール(tar：黒い粘着性物質)の様な。tarry stool(タール便)。
ダイアビーティス	糖尿病(diabetes)。
タイム・フリー	時間不定(time-free)。手術(検査)の開始時間が不定の場合、手術室から呼び出しがかかること。

タキる	頻脈(tachycardia)。
ダクト	導管。管(duct)。
タップ	穿刺(tap)。
ダブルチェック	投薬、処置などを看護師、医師など2人で確認すること(double check)。
ダブルルーメン	内腔が二重になった管(double lumen)。
ダンポウ	弾性包帯。
タンポナーデ	タンポン法(tamponade)。心タンポナーデ(cardiac tamponade)。

チ・ツ

チアノーゼ	血液中の酸素が欠乏して皮膚や粘膜が青色になること(Zyanose:独語、cyanosis:英語)。
チーフ・コンプレイント	主訴(chief complaint)。
チック	随意筋の不随意運動(tic)。
チュウケン	中央検査室。
チュウチョウ	注腸造影。
チュートリアル	個人指導。チューターによる少人数指導(tutorial)。
チューマー	腫瘍(tumor)。
ツァンゲ	鉗子分娩(Zange Entbindung)。
ツッカー	ブドウ糖(Zucker:独語)。さまざまな濃度(5、20、50%など)のものがあり、5%なら「5プロツッカー」という。
ツモール	腫瘍(tumor)。

テ

ディアベ	糖尿病(DM:diabetes mellitus)。
ティーアイエー	一過性脳虚血発作(TIA:transient ischemic attack)。

ディーエヌアール	蘇生せず（DNR：Do Not Resuscitate）。臨死の際に無理な蘇生を行わないこと。
ディーエム	糖尿病（DM：Diabetes Mellitus）。
ディーオーエー	来院時死亡（DOA：Dead on arrival）。来院時すでに死亡していること。
ディーシー	除細動（DC：defibrillation）。カウンターショックの別名。
ディジタル	指の（digital）。
ディスオリエンテーション	見当識障害（disorientation）。
ディスチャージ	退院（discharge）。ディスチャージガイダンス：退院指導。
ディスポ	使い捨て。ディスポーザブル（disposable）の略。
ディプレション	うつ病（depression）。
ディペンダンス	依存（dependence）。
ディメンツ、デメる、デメンツ	認知症（症状）（Demenz）。
テーベー	肺結核（tuberculosis）。
デクビ	褥瘡（Decubitus）。
デコる	代償不全（decompensation）。肝不全や過剰輸液で心不全になった時などに「デコった」などと使う。
デブる、デブリートマン、デブリードメント	創面を切除すること（de´bridement：仏語）。褥瘡の壊死した部分を切除する場合を「デブる」と言う。
デリバリー	分娩（delivery）。デリバリールーム：分娩室。
デルマ	皮膚科（dermatology）。
テレ	遠隔の（tele）。
テレメディシン	遠隔医療（telemedicine）。
テンション	緊張（tension）。
デンタルカリエス	う食。虫歯（dental caries）。
デンチャー	義歯（denture）。

ト

トーヌス	緊張(tonus)。
トクショク	治療食。特別食の略で、特別食事箋が必要となる。
ドナー	臓器を提供する人、部位(donor)。
トラウマ	(精神的)外傷(trauma)。
トラケア	気管(trachea)。
ドラッグハビット	薬物乱用。
トランキライザー	精神安定剤(tranquilizer)。
トランス、トランスファー	移す(患者をベッドから車いす、ストレッチャーからベッドへと移すこと)、転院(transfer)。
トリガー	引きがね(trigger)。トリガーゾーン(引きがね帯：trigger zone)
トリガーレベル	人工呼吸器の吸気を引き起こす水準(trigger level)。
ドレッシング	包帯など皮膚保護に用いる絆創膏類(dressing)。
ドレナージ	排液法(drainage)。排液管を「ドレーン」という。
トレマー	振戦(tremor)。
トロンボ	血小板(thrombo)。
トンボ	翼状針。

ナ

ナート	縫合(Naht)。創傷部を縫い合わせること。
ナウゼア	吐き気、悪心(nausea)。
ナチュラル・コース	自然死。終末期の患者に対して無理な蘇生は行わないこと(natural course)。
ナトカリ	ナトリウム(Na)とカリウム(K)のこと。
ナルコる	ナルコーシスになること。もしくは過眠症(居眠り病)になること(narcosis)。

ニ・ネ

ニッシェ	陰影欠損(Nische)。
ニトロ	ニトログリセリン(nitroglycerin)。
ニボー	鏡面像(空気と液体の境界)(Niveau)。
ニューモニア	肺炎(pneumonia)。
ネーザル	鼻(nasal)。
ネーザル・チューブ	鼻管。鼻からの酸素吸入用の管(nasal tube：英語、Nasal Kanule：独語)。
ネクる	壊死(necrosis)。褥瘡部が壊死して黒くなった時などに「ネクロってる」などと言う。
ネッパツ	発熱。
ネブライザー、ネブ	吸入。吸入器(nebulizer)。
ネラトン	ネラトンカテーテル。導尿の時などに用いるカテーテル。

ノ

ノイトロ	好中球(neutrocyte)。
ノーシーピーアール	No CPR。延命治療を行わない。
ノクターナル	夜間の(nocturnal)。
ノクターナルペイン	夜間痛。
ノルアド、ノルアドレナリン	昇圧薬(noradrenalin)。
ノンコンペティティブ	非競合的(noncompetitive)。
ノンサージカル	非外科的(nonsurgical)。
ノンスペシフィック	非特異性(nonspecific)。
ノンファット・ミルク	脱脂乳(nonfat milk)。
ノンプロティーン	非蛋白性の(nonprotein)。

ハ

バージョン、カルジオバージョン	電気的除細動器(cardioversion)。カウンターショックの別名。

バースコントロール	受胎調節 (birth control)。
ハート・インフュージョン	心浸出液 (heart infusion)。
ハートマーマー	心雑音 (heart murmur)。
ハーベー	ヘモグロビン (Hb：hemoglobin)。
バーン	熱傷 (burn)。
バイアル	注射用薬剤の容器 (vial)。
バイオアッセイ	生物検定法 (bioassay、biological assay)。
バイオケミカル・サイクル	生化学的周期 (biochemical cycle)。
バイオプシー	病理生検 (biopsy)。
バイオプシー・スペシメン	生検材料 (biopsy specimen)。
ハイカリ	高カロリー輸液、もしくはカリウム値が高いこと。
ハイティー	高血圧 (HT：hypertension)。
ハイドロ	水 (hydro-)。水頭症や水腎症など水のつく疾患の前置詞で、そのまま疾患の略語になる。
ハイパー	高カロリー輸液。もしくは高い (高血圧)、過剰 (hyper-)。
ハイポ、ヒポ	低い、過少 (hypo-)。「ヒポ症状」という場合、おおむね低血糖症状を指す。
バイラス	ウイルス (virus)。
パターナリズム	父権主義。保護主義 (paternalism)。
バッキング	咳嗽反射 (bucking)。一般には呼吸器装着中に咳嗽反射によって人工呼吸と不調和を起こす状態。
バッシ	抜糸。縫合した糸を抜き取ること。
パッシブスモーキング	受動喫煙 (passive smoking)。
ハトキ	破傷風トキソイド (toxoid)。
パラノイア	偏執症、妄想症 (paranoia)。
パリアティブケア	緩和ケア (palliative care)。

頻用カタカナ用語

バリアフリー	障壁を取り除いた生活空間（barrier-free）。
バリックス	食道静脈瘤（varix）。
パルス、プルス	脈（pulse）。
ハルン	尿（Harn）。「Hr」と記載される。
バルン、バルンカテーテル	膀胱留置カテーテル（baloon cathter）。
パンクチャー、プンク	穿刺（puncture）。
パンゲ	一般消化器外科。

ヒ

ビーエス	血糖（blood sugar または BZ）。
ビーティー	脳腫瘍（BT：brain tumor）。
ピーティー	患者（Pt.：patient）。
ビーナス	静脈の（venous）。
ピオ	緑膿菌（pseudomonas aeruginosa）。創面や褥瘡に感染しやすく、感染すると緑色になる。
ピギ	「ピギで」と言われたら、通常、薬剤を生理食塩水100mLに溶いて注入する。
ヒストリー	現病歴・既往歴（hisotry）。
ピル	丸薬（pill）。
ピンホール	瞳孔が、針で突いた小さい孔程に縮瞳した状態（pinhole）。

フ

ファイティング	人工呼吸と自発呼吸が合わずに不調和を起こしている状態。
ファイバー	（気管支）ファイバースコープ（fiberscope）。
ファントム	幻覚、幻想（phantom）。
ブイ、ブイライン	静脈（vein）。

フィードバック	フィードバック、帰還(feed-back)。
フィールチェアー	車いす(wheelchair)。
フィステル	瘻孔(fistula、Fistel：独語)。
ブースター	追加免疫(booster)。
フォビア	恐怖症(phobia)。
プシコ	精神病(psychiatry)。
プステル	膿疱(pustule、Pustel：独語)。
フットバス	足浴(foot bath)。
プライマリ	初期の、最初の(primary)。プライマリケアは初期治療のこと。
フラクチャー	骨折(fracture)。略語で「FX」などと記載される。
プラクティショナー	専門職の開業者(practitioner)。
プラシーボ、プラセボ	偽薬(placebo)。新薬の開発の段階で、新薬と同じ形状の全く効果のない薬を投与して、効果を比較するテスト。一般臨床では、薬としての効果はないが暗示効果を期待して与薬する薬剤をいう。
プラズマ	血漿(plasma)。
プラセンタ	胎盤(placenta)。
フラッシュ	点滴ルートの側管から直接薬剤を静脈注射すること(flash)。
フラッシュバック	再燃現象。薬物依存の患者が使用をやめた後にも突然幻覚が現れるなど、使用時の精神体験が再現されること(flashback)。
フラット	心電図モニターの心拍数・呼吸数がゼロになること(flat)。
ブラッドサンプル	血液検体(blood sample)。
ブラディ	徐脈(bradycardia)。「タキ」の逆。
フリー・エア	遊離ガス(free air)。消化管穿孔の際に腹腔内に生じるガス像(X線)のこと。
フリッカー	ちらつき(flicker)。フリッカー値。
プリミ、プリミパラ	初妊・初産(primigravida)。プリミパラ(primipara)は、初産婦のこと。

フルーイッド	液体（fluid）。
ブルート	血液（Blut：独語、blood：英語）。
フルコース	急変時に延命行為をすべて行うこと。
プルス	脈拍（Pulse：独語、pulse：英語【パルス】）。
フレ、フレンチ	フレンチ（Fr）。カテーテルのサイズ。
ブレード	喉頭鏡。気管内挿管の際に使用する器具。
プレート	血小板（platelet）。
ブレーンウェイブ	脳波（brain wave）。
プレメデ、プレメディ	（手術などの）前投薬、予備与薬（premedication）。
プレメディケーション	前投薬（premedication）。
フローチャート	項目別に変化の流れを簡潔に図表に表す看護記録（flow chart）。
プローブ	消息子（probe）。
フローラ	植物相（flora）。
プロセスレコード	対人関係の一場面の経過（言動）を記録する方法（process record）。
プロパー	製薬会社の営業マンのこと。最近ではMRとよばれている。
ブロンコ	気管支鏡、気管支ファイバースコープ（bronchoscopy）。
プンク	穿刺（puncture）。

へ

ペアレンティング	親役割（parenting）。
ペアン	鉤なし鉗子。
ペインキラー	痛み止め。鎮痛剤（pain killer）。
ペースメーカー	脈拍調整器（pacemaker）。
ベースン	洗面器（basin、wash basin）。
ベジ、ベジタブル	植物状態（vegetable）。
ヘッドナース	看護師長（head nurse）。

ベッドレスト	床上安静（bed rest）。
ベネセク	静脈切開。
ヘパセイ	ヘパリン加生理食塩水。ヘパロックを行うためのヘパリンと生理食塩液の混合液。
ヘパタイティス	肝炎（hepatitis）。
ヘパロック	ルートの閉鎖。三方活栓や専用のアダプターよりヘパリン入り生理食塩液を注入し、ルート内で血液凝固が起こらないようにして三方活栓から留置針までを患者に残す。
ヘマト	ヘマトクリット（hematocrit）。
ヘモ	痔核（hemorrhoid）。「血液」の意味もある。
ヘルスプロモーション	健康増進（health promotion）。
ヘルツ	心臓（Herz）。心臓病を指す場合も多い。
ベンチレーター	人工呼吸器（ventilator）、レスピレーター。

ホ

ホウカン	訪問看護。
ホウコウ	包帯交換。
ボウセン	膀胱洗浄。
ポー	服薬（po）。
ボディフルイド	体液（body fluid）。
ボディメカニクス	人間の姿勢や動作時の各系統間の力学的相互関係（body mechanics）。
ボトル	点滴薬（bottle）。
ポリペクトミー	内視鏡治療（polypectomy）。
ボリューム	容積（volume）。ボリュームを上げる、下げるといったら、おおむね輸液量のこと。
ホルター（ホルター心電図）	長時間心電図（Holter electrocardiogram：ECG）。

マ

マーゲン	胃（Magen）。独語だがストマックより常用されている。
マーサ	メチシリン耐性黄色ブドウ球菌（MRSA：methicillin resistant staphylococcus aureus）。
マーマー	雑音（murmur）。
マスキング	遮蔽（masking）。
マタニティブルーズ	分娩後の軽症の情動混乱（maternity blues）。
マッキントッシュ	喉頭鏡の名前。
マップ	輸血（MAP：mannitol adenine phosphate solution）。
マリグナント	悪性（⇔ベナイン）（malignant）。
マルク	骨髄（穿刺）（Mark）。
マンシェット	血圧測定用の圧迫帯（manschette）。
マンマ	乳房、乳癌（Mamma, mammary cancer）。
マンモ、マンモグラフィ	乳房X線撮影法（mammography）。

ミ・ム

ミエロパシー	脊髄病（myelopathy）。
ミオパシー	筋障害（myopathy）。
ミルキング	搾取法（milking）。
ムルチ	経産。
ムンテラ	病状説明（Mund Therapie）。医師が患者やその家族に病状を説明すること。
ムンプス	流行性耳下腺炎（mumps）。

メ・モ

メタ	転移（metastasis）。腫瘍が転移していること。

メディケーション	与薬。投薬（medication）。
メラノーシス	黒色症（melanosis）。
メランコリー	抑うつ症（melancholia）。
メレナ	下血（melana）。
メンタルパワー	知力（mental power）。
モーション	動き。便通（motion）。
モチベーション	動機（motivation）。患者が治療や闘病に対して前向きな姿勢をもっているかどうかということ。
モニター	患者監視装置（monitor）。心電図モニターに代表されるME機器のこと。

ユ・ヨ

ユーリン	尿（urine）。
ヨウマ	腰椎麻酔。

ラ

ライフサイエンス	生命科学（life science）。
ライン	管（line）。点滴の管のこと。ルート。
ラウンド	病棟・病室内の見回り、もしくは回診（round）。
ラジ、ラジエーション	放射線治療（radiation）。
ラスト	放射性アレルギー吸着試験。
ラド	放射線治療（radiation）。
ラプチャー	破裂（rupture）。
ラボ	検査室、研究室（laboratory）。
ラング	肺（lung）。

リ

リーク	漏れ（leak）。主に、呼吸関係で使われる。
リーディング	測定値（reading）。

リオペ	創部が化膿して再手術（reoperation）になること。
リカバリー ルーム	回復室（recovery room）。
リキッド	液体（liquid）。
リキッドダイエット	流動食（liquid diet）。
リコール	髄液（liquor）。
リスクマネージメント	危機管理（risk management）。
リストカット	手首を切る自傷行為（wrist cut）。
リハ	リハビリテーション（rehabilitation）。機能訓練。
リペレント	忌避剤（repellent）。
リラクセーション	精神や神経、筋肉などの緊張状態を緩めること（relaxation）。

ル・レ・ロ

ルート	管（route）。点滴の管のこと。ライン。
ルンゲ	肺（Lunge：独語）。
ルンバール	腰椎穿刺（lumbar puncture）。腰椎麻酔（lumbar anesthesia）の意味もある。
レアギン	感作抗体（reagin）。
レイバールーム	陣痛室（labor room）。
レーベル	肝臓（Leber）。
レギュラー	規則正しいこと（regular）⇔イレギュラー：irregular
レジ	レジデント（resident）。研修医。
レジスタンス	抵抗（resistance）。
レシピエント	臓器をもらう人、受領者（recipient）。
レスキュー	救助（rescue）。レスキュー・チューブ（rescue tube）。
レストレス	不穏状態（restless）。暴れている状態。
レスピ	呼吸器（respirator）。レスピレーターのこと。
レセプタ	受容体、受容器（receptor）。

レディネス	学習するうえで、身体的にも心理認知的にも適応できる準備状態にあること（readiness）。
レファレンス	紹介状。参考（reference）。
レプレッサー	抑制因子（repressor）。
ロイケ、ロイケミー、ロイコ	白血病（Leukamie）。
ローカル	局部的。局所的（local）。
ローテ	赤血球（Rotes Blutkorperchen）。

ワ

ワイセ	白血球（Weisen Blutkorperchen）。
ワッサー	蒸留水（destillertes Wasser：独語、distilled water：英語）。
ワッセルマン、ワッセルマン反応	梅毒血清反応（Wassermann's reaction）。
ワン・ショット	静脈注射。少量の薬剤を静脈内に三方活栓から1回で注入すること（one shot）。

第3章

難読漢字・難読病名

1画

一側性　いっそくせい

2画

七日熱　なぬかやみ

3画

三叉神経　さんさしんけい
三尖弁　さんせんべん
上擾　じょうじょう
大彎（弯）　だいわん
大脳鎌　だいのうかま
大菱形筋　だいりょうけいきん
子癇　しかん
小口病　おぐちびょう
小屑　しょうせつ
小菱形筋　しょうりょうけいきん
小彎（弯）　しょうわん
小人症　こびとしょう、しょうじんしょう
下縁　かえん
下外側　かがいそく
下角　かかく
下顎前突　かがくぜんとつ
下脚　かきゃく
下極下筋　かきょくかきん
下血　げけつ
下後鋸筋　かこうきょきん
下甲状腺動脈　かこうじょうせんどうみゃく
下行結腸　かこうけっちょう
下斜筋　かしゃきん
下焦　げしょう
下唇　かしん
下垂手　かすいしゅ
下垂体後葉　かすいたいこうよう
下膳　げぜん
下双子筋　かそうしきん
下足関節　かそくかんせつ
下直筋　かちょくきん
下殿　かでん
下鼻道　かびどう
下品　げほん
下壁梗塞　かへきこうそく
下矢状静脈洞　かしじょうじょうみゃくどう
下痢　げり
下疳　げかん
下瞼　したまぶた
丸剤　がんざい
弓下窩　きゅうかか
弓状核　きゅうじょうかく
弓倉症状　ゆみくらしょうじょう
口蓋帆挙筋　こうがいはんきょきん
口渇　こうかつ
口蹄疫　こうていえき

4画

王水　おうすい
犬吠　けんぼう
犬咬症　いぬこうしょう
内眥　ないし
内套　ないとう
円回内筋　えんかいないきん
円蓋　えんがい
円索　えんさく
円背　えんはい
片麻痺　かたまひ
欠伸　あくび
欠趾　けっし
切截　せっさい
切石位　せっせきい
毛囊　もうのう
亢進　こうしん
収斂　しゅうれん

心悸　しんき
心腔　しんくう
心嚢　しんのう
爪郭　そうかく
爪下皮　そうかひ
爪甲鉤弯症　そうこうこうわん
　しょう
天疱瘡　てんぽうそう
止咳薬　しがいやく
止瀉薬　ししゃやく
止痒　しよう
止痢薬　しりやく
巴布　ぱっぷ
反芻　はんすう
反肘　はんちゅう
日和見　ひよりみ
不感蒸泄　ふかんじょうせつ
幻暈　げんうん
毛瘡　もうそう
手掌　しゅしょう
手足口病　てあしくちびょう
手足煩熱　しゅそくはんねつ
手足蕨逆　しゅそくけつぎゃく
手袋状皮膚剥脱創　てぶくろじょ
　うひふはくだつそう
手白癬　てはくせん
不定愁訴　ふていしゅうそ
勾配　こうばい

5画

凹窩　おうか
圧痕　あっこん
圧挫　あつざ
圧痛　あっつう
圧排　あっぱい
外顆　がいか
外寒内熱　がいかんないねつ
外腔　がいくう
外鞘　がいしょう

外邪　がいじゃ
外旋　がいせん
外鼠径　がいそけい
外側上顆　がいそくじょうか
外反股　がいはんこ
外反膝　がいはんしつ
外反肘　がいはんちゅう
可撓　かとう
甲心　よろいしん
氷枕　ひょうちん
失外套　しつがいとう
包埋　ほうまい
冬瓜草　とうかそう
白湯　さゆ
白暈黒色腫　はくうんこくしょく
　しゅ
白癬　はくせん
白体　はくたい
白蝋病　はくろうびょう
半夏　はんげ
広濶　こうかつ
広汎性天疱瘡　こうはんせい
　てんぽうそう
母趾　ぼし
末梢　まっしょう
目瞼　がんけん
矢状面　しじょうめん
右脚　うきゃく
右心耳　うしんじ、みぎしんじ
右総頚動脈　うそうけいどうみ
　ゃく、みぎそうけいどうみゃく
右尿管　うにょうかん
右肺　うはい、みぎはい
右葉　（肝臓の）うよう
加虐嗜愛　かぎゃくしあい
加減方　かげんほう
加療　かりょう
加齢　かれい
牙関緊急　がかんきんきゅう

石綿沈着症　せきめんちんちゃくしょう
石綿肺　いしわたはい、せきめんはい
叩打　こうだ

6画

安息香酸　あんそくこうさん
安堵　あんど
会陰　えいん
会厭　ええん
合趾症　ごうししょう
汗孔角化症　かんこうかくか（かっか）しょう
汗疱　かんぽう
臼蓋形成　きゅうがいけいせい
臼歯　きゅうし
多趾　たし
仮骨　かこつ
仮肋　かろく
気腎法　きじんほう
汚穢　おわい
仰臥位　ぎょうがい
血漿　けっしょう
血痰　けったん
血乳糜尿　けつにゅうびにょう
血餅　けっぺい
米杉喘息　べいすぎぜんそく
弛緩　しかん
弛張熱　しちょうねつ
羊歯　しだ
充填　じゅうてん
吸啜　きゅうてつ
舌咽　ぜついん
舌口蓋筋　ぜつこうがいきん
舌苔　ぜったい
尖圭　せんけい
吐瀉　としゃ
肉牙　にくげ
肉芽　にくげ
肉荳蔻肝　にくずくかん
灰白　かいはく
帆状弁　はんじょうべん
汎　はん
汎下垂体　はんかすいたい
耳垢　じこう
耳茸　じじょう、みみたけ
耳鍼　じしん
耳朶　じだ
耳鼻咽喉科　じびいんこうか
耳痒　じよう
耳瘻　じろう
耳漏　じろう
有棘　ゆうきょく
有鉤　ゆうこう
有鞘　ゆうしょう
迂回状紅斑　うかいじょうこうはん
印環細胞（腺）癌　いんかんさいぼう（せん）がん
回旋枝　かいせんし
回旋性眼振　かいせんせいがんしん
回内運動　かいないうんどう
回盲弁　かいもうべん
自殺念慮　じさつねんりょ

7画

亜鈴状　あれいじょう
足趾　そくし
足蹠　そくしょ
杆体細胞　かんたいさいぼう
疔　ちょう
含嗽　がんそう
肘筋　ちゅうきん
肝円索　かんえんさく
肝鎌状間膜　かんかま（れん）じょうかんまく

肝憩室　かんけいしつ
肝充織　かんじゅうしき
肝蛭　かんてつ
肝庇護薬　かんひごやく
肘窩　ちゅうか
沈渣　ちんさ
呈味成分　ていみせいぶん
尿嚢　にょうのう
尿瘻　にょうろう
妊孕　にんよう
呑気症　どんきしょう
禿髪性毛嚢炎　とくはつせいもうのうえん
禿頭症　とくとうしょう
吻合　ふんごう
麦穂帯　ばくすいたい
沐浴　もくよく
卵管采　らんかんさい
佝僂病　くるびょう
囲繞麻酔　いにょうますい
忌避　きひ
克山病　こくざんびょう
児心音　じしんおん
児頭大　じとうだい
吹入　すいにゅう
折衷派　せっちゅうは
扼死　やくし

8画

盂　う
炙　しゃ
疝　せん
采　さい
乖離　かいり
青蒿　せいこう
軋歯　あっし
軋轢音　あつれきおん
兎唇　としん
兎糞　とふん
易感染　いかんせん
易疲労　えきひろう
季肋　きろく
果殻　かかく
苔癬　たいせん
昏迷　こんめい
昏蒙　こんもう
杯細胞　さかずきさいぼう
侏儒症　しゅじゅしょう
呻吟　しんぎん
咀嚼　そしゃく
空壺音性共鳴音　くうこおんせいきょうめいおん
直達牽引　ちょくたつけんいん
泥膏　でいこう
苦味　くみ
乳暈　にゅううん
乳糜　にゅうび
昇汞　しょうこう
披裂　ひれつ
拇指　ぼし
奔馬調　ほんばちょう
松果体　しょうかたい
味蕾　みらい
夜驚症　やきょうしょう
夜啼　やてい
芽細胞　がさいぼう
芽腫　がしゅ
芽殖弧虫　がしょくこちゅう
芽胞　がほう
茎状突起　けいじょうとっき
肩手症候群　かたてしょうこうぐん
肩峰腸稜示数　けんぽうちょうりょうしすう
肩峰幅　けんぽうふく
姑息的治療　こそくてきちりょう
拘急　こうきゅう
拘縮　こうしゅく

拘攣　こうれん
刺入　しにゅう
刺絡法　しらくほう
垂涎　すいぜん

9画

胡座　あぐら
紅暈　こううん
眉間　みけん
疣　ゆう、いぼ
疣痔　いぼじ
疣贅　ゆうぜい
胝　たこ
秋疫　あきやみ
脂漏性皮膚炎　しろうせいひふえん
按手　あんしゅ
按摩　あんま
胃角　いかく
胃気　いき
胃憩室　いけいしつ
胃軸捻　いじくねん
胃小窩　いしょうか
胃皺襞　いすうへき
胃体部　いたいぶ
胃中不和　いちゅうふわ
胃底部　いていぶ
胃反　いほん、いはん
胃瘻　いろう
疥癬　かいせん
疫痢　えきり
咽喉頭　いんこうとう
咽後膿瘍　いんこうのうよう、いんごのうよう
咽中炙臠　いんちゅうしゃれん
咽頭後膿瘍　いんとうこうのうよう
咽頭側索炎　いんとうそくさくえん

咽頭扁桃肥大症　いんとうへんとうひだいしょう
後嚢　こうのう
後鋸筋　こうきょきん
後彎　こうわん
後篩骨洞　こうしこつどう
後産　あとざん
後乳　あとにゅう
後産期陣痛　こうさんきじんつう
重篤　じゅうとく
風棘　ふうきょく
風癩　ふうらい
柑皮症　かんぴしょう
閂症状　かんぬきしょうじょう
茸状　じじょう
急峻型　きゅうしゅんがた
急奔性　きゅうはんせい
臥位　がい
臥床　がしょう
臥褥療法　がじょくりょうほう
限外濾過　げんがいろか
神経鞘腫　しんけいしょうしゅ
砂嚢　さのう
砒素　ひそ
咳嗽　がいそう
背臥　はいが
穿孔　せんこう
胎嚢　たいのう
胎芽　たいが
肺痿　はいい
肺紋理　はいもんり
発赤　ほっせき
発露　はつろ
飛蚊症　ひぶんしょう
飛沫　ひまつ
扁桃　へんとう
星膠腫　せいこうしゅ
星芒　せいぼう
前彎　ぜんわん

巻綿子　けんめんし
指趾　しし
屎尿　しにょう
歪視　わいし
海馬　かいば
海綿体　かいめんたい
咬筋痙攣　こうきんけいれん
咬合　こうごう
咬耗症　こうもうしょう
咬痙　こうけい
枯燥　こそう
枯草菌　こそうきん
狐惑病　こわくびょう
砕石位　さいせきい
柔痙　じゅうけい
信憑性　しんぴょうせい
泉熱　いずみねつ
泉門　せんもん
炭疽　たんそ
面疔　めんちょう
面皰　めんぽう
恍惚　こうこつ

10画

痂　か
痂皮　かひ
疼　とう
疳　かん
疽　そ
疱　ほう
皰　にきび
倚褥感　いじょくかん
疲憊期　ひはいき
恙虫　つつがむし
烏賊骨　うぞくこつ
烏口腕筋　うこうわんきん
烏啄下脱臼　うたくかだっきゅう
馬杉腎炎　ますぎじんえん
馬反足　ばはんそく
馬鼻疽菌　ばびそきん
補綴　ほてつ
起坐呼吸　きざこきゅう
套管針　とうかんしん
宦官症　かんがんしょう
記銘障害　きめいしょうがい
挙睾筋　きょこうきん
唇状瘻　しんじょうろう
珪肺　けいはい
原発疹　げんぱつしん
被嚢　ひのう
骨梁　こつりょう
骨稜　こつりょう
骨粗鬆症　こつそしょうしょう
骨釘　こってい
骨盤闊部　こつばんかつぶ
骨柩　こつきゅう
骨棘　こつきょく
粉瘤　ふんりゅう
索状　さくじょう
索痕　さくこん
莢膜　きゅうまく
残渣　ざんさ
洒渣　しゅさ
書痙　しょけい
浸潤　しんじゅん
浸煎剤　しんせんざい
脆弱　ぜいじゃく
脊索　せきさく
脊髄　せきずい
脊椎　せきつい
閃輝　せんき
造瘻　ぞうろう
帯下　たいげ
高安動脈炎　たかやすどうみゃくえん
凍瘡　とうそう
流涎　りゅうぜん
涙丘　るいきゅう

涙腺　るいせん
涙嚢　るいのう
涙瘻　るいろう
粃糠　ひこう
根尖部　こんせんぶ
這行　しゃこう
破瓜型　はかがた
剥離　はくり
挺子　ていし
恥垢菌　ちこうきん
破綻　はたん
被曝　ひばく
浮腫　ふしゅ
粉塵　ふんじん
振盪　しんとう
胼胝　べんち
紡錘状　ぼうすいじょう
娘染色体　じゅうせんしょくたい
胸膝位　きょうしつい
胸悶　きょうもん
胸下痞硬　きょうかひこう
胸骨柄　きょうこつへい
胸痺　きょうひ
眩暈　げんうん
破壺音　はこおん
留飲　りゅういん
留鍼　りゅうしん
益気　えっき
荻野式　おぎのしき
格子状角膜変性　こうしじょうかくまくへんせい
陥凹　かんおう
陥入爪　かんにゅうそう
陥没呼吸　かんぽつこきゅう
挫滅腎　ざめつじん
挫瘡　ざそう
狼瘡　ろうそう
紋画症　もんかくしょう

涎沫　ぜんまつ
痃癖　げんぺき
眥部眼瞼炎　しぶがんけんえん
翅脈　しみゃく
蚋刺症　ぶよししょう
蚯血　じくけつ

11画

痒　よう
痔　じ
球麻痺　きゅうまひ
萎黄病　いおうびょう
萎縮　いしゅく
黒子　ほくろ、こくし
黒苔　こくたい
視交叉　しこうさ
産湯　うぶゆ
産瘤　さんりゅう
産褥　さんじょく
陰萎　いんい
陰窩　いんか
陰虚　いんきょ
陰茎海綿体　いんけいかいめんたい
陰茎絞扼症　いんけいこうやくしょう
陰股部　いんこぶ
陰唇　いんしん
陰嚢　いんのう
陰嚢水瘤　いんのうすいりゅう
陰陽　いんよう
黄汗　おうかん
黄径　おうけい
黄色髄　おうしょくずい
黄体　おうたい
黄苔　おうたい
黄疸　おうだん
黄斑　おうはん

黄斑皺襞症　おうはんしゅうへきしょう
黄疸　おうげん
黄癬　おうせん
悪液質　あくえきしつ
悪寒戦慄　おかんせんりつ
悪心　おしん
悪阻　おそ
悪露　おろ
悪風　おふう
郭清　かくせい
偏倚現象　へんきげんしょう
脚気　かっけ
眼窩　がんか
眼白子症　がんしらこしょう
眼瞼縁炎　がんけんえんえん
眼瞼下垂　がんけんかすい
桿菌　かんきん
桿状　かんじょう
乾癬　かんせん
乾酪化　かんらくか
乾嘔　かんおう
黄靱帯　おうじんたい
黄癬　おうせん
剪刀　せんとう
偽脊髄癆　ぎせきずいろう
魚鱗癬様皮膚　ぎょりんせんようひふ
牽引　けんいん
衒奇　げんき
梗塞　こうそく
粗鬆　そしょう
匙状　さじじょう
痔瘻　じろう
悉無律　しつむりつ
羞明　しゅうめい
宿主　しゅくしゅ
視蓋　しがい
雀卵斑　じゃくらんはん

清拭　せいしき
剪断　せんだん
搔爬　そうは
搔破　そうは
搔痒　そうよう
側隙　そくげき
側彎　そくわん
躯幹　くかん
断綴　だんてつ
動悸　どうき
鳥媒　ちょうばい
貪食　どんしょく
梨状窩　りじょうか
軟膏　なんこう
猫喘　びょうぜん
粘稠　ねんちゅう
脳振盪　のうしんとう
脳穿通枝　のうせんつうし
脳梁　のうりょう
梯形筋　ていけいきん
絆創膏　ばんそうこう
菲薄　ひはく
菱形窩　りょうけいか
菱脳　りょうのう
眸　ぼう、む、ひとみ
笛声音　てきせいおん
娩出　べんしゅつ
萌出遅延　ほうしゅつちえん
焔状母斑　えんじょうぼはん
麻痺　まひ
野兎　やと
淋疾　りんしつ
異嗅症　いきゅうしょう
異所性　いしょせい
異味症　いみしょう
移植片対宿主病　いしょくへんついしゅくしゅびょう
渇感　かつかん
渇熱　かつねつ

難読漢字・難読病名

葛湯　くずゆ
葛藤　かっとう
亀甲帯　きっこうたい
虚言妄想　きょげんもうそう
虚煩　きょはん
虚無妄想　きょむもうそう
経緯　いきさつ、けいい
経絡　けいらく
混沌　こんとん
進捗　しんちょく
陳旧性　ちんきゅうせい
徘徊癖　はいかいへき
毫鍼　ごうしん

12画

項　うなじ、こう
項部硬直　こうぶこうちょく
痙　けい
痙咳　けいがい
痙攣　けいれん
痞塞　ひそく
痩身長躯　そうしんちょうく
痘瘡　とうそう
喀痰　かくたん
棍毛　こんもう
喘鳴　ぜんめい
喘ぎ　あえぎ
間代性　かんたいせい
間歇(欠)的　かんけつてき
集蔟　しゅうぞく
落屑　らくせつ
覚醒　かくせい
椎間板　ついかんばん
蛔虫　かいちゅう
粥腫　じゅくしゅ
粥状　じゅくじょう
硝子　しょうし
間隙　かんげき
間擦疹　かんさつしん

距骨　きょこつ
距踵　きょしょう
結紮　けっさつ
結痂　けつか
減感作　げんかんさ
腔内　くうない
腋窩　えきか
腓骨　ひこつ
脾腫　ひしゅ
犀角　さいかく
詐病　さびょう
軸索　じくさく
絞窄輪　こうさくりん
絞扼　こうやく
絨毛　じゅうもう
歯槽膿漏　しそうのうろう
猩紅熱　しょうこうねつ
舒筋　じょきん
遂娩　すいべん
過蓋咬合　かがいこうごう
過角化　かかくか
過強陣痛　かきょうじんつう
毳毛　ぜいもう
粟粒　ぞくりゅう
粟粒性丘疹状結核疹　ぞくりゅうせいきゅうしんじょうけっかくしん
粟粒性痘瘡　ぞくりゅうせいとうそう
短頸　たんけい
散腫　さんしゅ
散瞳　さんどう
掌蹠　しょうせき
掌蹠膿疱症　しょうせきのうほうしょう
貼付　ちょうふ
棘間　きょくかん
棘孔　きょくこう
棘突起　きょくとっき

無棘　むきょく
喃語　なんご
鈍匙　どんぴ
歯齦　しぎん
撥水音　はっすいおん
撥指　ばちゆび
嵌頓　かんとん
跛行　はこう
開咬　かいこう
開放隅角緑内障　かいほうぐうかくりょくないしょう
琺瑯質　ほうろうしつ
無鉤　むこう
揉捏法　じゅうねつほう
焼灼　しょうしゃく
裂溝窩洞　れっこうかどう
裂隙　れつげき
裂肛　れっこう
渙散　かんさん
腕尺関節　わんしゃくかんせつ
腕木　わんぼく
渦状癬　かじょうせん
運動野　うんどうや
営衛不和　えいえふわ
温覚　おんかく
温感四肢　おんかんしし
温浸　おんしん
温湯　おんとう
温病　うんびょう
温補剤　おんぽざい
温薬　おんやく
温罨法　おんあんぽう
温鍼　おんしん
割球　かっきゅう
割髄症　かつずいしょう
割創　かっそう
稀有　けう
尋常性乾癬　じんじょうせいかんせん
尋常性魚鱗癬　じんじょうせいぎょりんせん
尋常性白斑　じんじょうせいはくはん
尋常性毛瘡　じんじょうせいもうそう
尋常性狼瘡　じんじょうせいろうそう
尋常性疣贅　じんじょうせいゆうぜい
葡行性迂回状紅斑　ほこうせいうかいじょうこうはん
傀儡　かいらい
厥陰病　けっちんびょう
厥逆　けつぎゃく
厥冷　けつれい

13画

鉤　こう
鉗　かん
痺　ひ
瘙痒　そうよう
馴化　じゅんか
蜂窩織炎　ほうかしきえん
蜂巣　ほうそう
溢飲　いついん
溢血斑　いっけつはん
溢水状態　いっすいじょうたい
溢乳　いつにゅう
溢流尿失禁　いつりゅうにょうしっきん
暗紫　あんし
罨法　あんぽう
裏急後重　りきゅうこうじゅう
裏熱　りねつ
蓋膜　がいまく
頑癬　がんせん
楔　くさび
楔状　け(せ)つじょう

楔入圧　け(せ)つにゅうあつ
楔舟関節　けっしゅうかんせつ
楔状　けつじょう
楔状骨　けつじょうこつ、せつじょうこつ
較正　こうせい
腱鞘炎　けんしょうえん
腸絨毛　ちょうじゅうもう
腸嵌頓　ちょうかんとん
腮弓　さいきゅう
腺腫　せんしゅ
腹臥　ふくが
睫毛　しょうもう
解痙　かいけい
解毒　げどく
解熱・下熱　げねつ
解肌　げき
解表　かいひょう
触瘡　しょくそう
嗜愛　しあい
嗜眠　しみん
嗜癖　しへき
嗄声　させい
腫瘤　しゅりゅう
腎盂　じんう
腎髄質　じんずいしつ
腎瘻　じんろう
鼓桴状指　こふじょうし
蓄膿　ちくのう
溺液　できえき
殿　でん
鉛疝痛　えんせんつう
鉛毒性脳症　えんどくせいのうしょう
塗抹　とまつ
鼠径　そけい
煩渇多飲症　はんかつたいんしょう
煩驚　はんきょう

煩燥　はんそう
酩酊　めいてい
酪酸　らくさん
矮小　わいしょう
寛骨　かんこつ
猿手　さるて
遠点　えんてん
塊椎形成　かいついけいせい
隔世遺伝　かくせいいでん
滑液包　かつえきほう
滑車神経　かっしゃしんけい
滑脳回　かつのうかい
禁忌　きんき
催奇形性　さいきけいせい
催吐　さいと
愁訴　しゅうそ
槌指(趾)　つちゆび
槌状指(趾)　ついじょうし
頓挫　とんざ
嗚咽　おえつ
斟酌　しんしゃく
溲瓶　しびん

14画

皸　あかぎれ
窩　か
瘍　よう
綴　てつ、てい
厭世　えんせい
嘔気　おうき
誤嚥　ごえん
誤謬　ごびゅう
疑徴　ぎちょう
廓清　かくせい
関係念慮　かんけいねんりょ
睾丸　こうがん
酸石榴　さんせきりゅう
酸蝕症　さんしょくしょう
静臥　せいが

塵埃感染　じんあいかんせん
塵肺　じんぱい、じんはい
滲出　しんしゅつ
精嚢　せいのう
截石位　せっせきい
鼻茸　はなたけ
稗粒腫　ひりゅうしゅ
膀胱　ぼうこう
増悪　ぞうお
蜜蝋　みつろう
漏洩　ろうえい
漏斗　ろうと
蝋様　ろうよう
暦年齢　れきねんれい
演繹　えんえき
遮光　しゃこう
遮蔽　しゃへい
截石位　せっせきい
塹壕熱　ざんごうねつ

15画

瘤　りゅう
噎　いつ
槽　そう
踝　くるぶし
瘡　そう
瘢　はん、あと
瘢痕　はんこん
頬　ほお、きょう
頬骨弓幅　きょうこつきゅうふく
慧眼　けいがん
遺残　いざん
遺精　いせい
遺尿　いにょう
遺糞　いふん
遺屎　いし
遺伝性掌蹠角化症　いでんせいしょうせきかくか（かっか）しょう
遺伝性象牙質形成不全症　いでんせいぞうげしつけいせいふぜんしょう
遺伝性尋常性魚鱗癬　いでんせいじんじょうせいぎょりんせん
潰瘍　かいよう
蝸牛　かぎゅう
緘黙症　かんもくしょう
緩衝作用　かんしょうさよう
緩下剤　かんげざい
窮迫　きゅうはく
緊満　きんまん
緊縛法　きんばくほう
稽留　けいりゅう
漿液　しょうえき
漿膜　しょうまく
膠原病　こうげんびょう
膠様稗粒腫　こうようはいりゅうしゅ
緩下　かんか
膝蓋　しつがい
膝窩　しっか
膵臓　すいぞう
膵嚢　すいのう
皺襞　しゅうへき
皺曲　しゅうきょく
皺眉筋　しゅうびきん
蕁麻疹　じんましん
褥瘡　じょくそう
鋭性亀背　えいせいきはい
鋭匙　えいひ
蝶形動脈　ちょうけいどうみゃく
蝶番　ちょうつがい
蝶番運動　ちょうばんうんどう
糊化　こか
糊膏　ここう
播種　はしゅ
瞑眩　めんげん

範疇　はんちゅう
賦活　ふかつ
僻地医療　へきちいりょう
魯鈍　ろどん
鋤骨　じょこつ
褥婦　じょくふ
鞍関節　くらかんせつ、あんかんせつ
鞍鼻　あんび
暴露　ばくろ＝曝露（ばくろ）
横臥位　おうがい
横行結腸　おうこうけっちょう
横骨折　おうこっせつ
横指　おうし
横静脈洞　おうじょうみゃくどう
横線　おうせん
横中隔　おうちゅうかく
横紋筋　おうもんきん
億劫　おっくう
潜函病　せんかんびょう
遷延横位　せんえんおうい
憔悴　しょうすい

16画

頤　い、おとがい
頤前方　いぜんぽう
瘦　ろう
篩　ふるい
篩骨　しこつ
噯気　あいき
瘦孔　ろうこう
閾値　いきち
緻密質　ちみつしつ
謡人結節　ようじんけっせつ
諧謔　かいぎゃく
機序　きじょ
嘴管　しかん
嘴部　しぶ
頸髄　けいずい

踵　かかと
踵骨　しょうこつ
壊死　えし
壊疽　えそ
錆色　さびいろ
樽形　たるがた
橈骨　とうこつ
橈屈　とうくつ
鋸歯　きょし
鋸状縁　きょじょうえん
蹄状紋　ていじょうもん
憑依妄想　ひょういもうそう
輻輳　ふくそう
膨瘤　ぼうりゅう
罹患　りかん
燐脂質　りんししつ
蟒蛇　うわばみ
襁褓　おしめ
懈怠　けたい
衛気　えき
燕麦　えんばく
橋　きょう
橋出血　きょうしゅっけつ
錯綜　さくそう
錯味症　さくみしょう
錘体筋　すいたいきん
積聚　しゃくじゅ
噫気　あいき
縊死　いし
蹂躙　じゅうりん
霍乱　かくらん

17画

癆　ろう
鼾　いびき
膿漿　のうしょう
濶部　かつぶ
癌腫　がんしゅ
矯正　きょうせい

蹉跌　さてつ
趨勢　すうせい
瞳孔　どうこう
膿瘡　のうそう
膿盆　のうぼん
膿痂疹　のうかしん
膿疱　のうほう
鍼麻酔　はりますい
糜粥　びじゅく
糜爛　びらん
頻回　ひんかい
頻脈　ひんみゃく
朦朧　もうろう
螺旋　らせん
螺子　らし
鍍銀染色　とぎんせんしょく
翼突筋静脈叢　よくとっきんじょうみゃくそう
燥屎　そうし
邂逅　かいこう

18画

鬆　しょう
叢　そう
叢生　そうせい
嚢　のう
嚢疱　のうほう
燻蒸　くんじょう
癒す　いやす
癒合　ゆごう
癒合歯　ゆごうし
顔貌　がんぼう
顎補綴　がくほてつ
顎嚢胞　がくのうほう
観念奔逸　かんねんほんいつ
蟯虫　ぎょうちゅう
燻煙剤　くんえんざい
鎖肛　さこう
鎮痙　ちんきょう

鎮痒薬　ちんようやく
鎮痙薬　ちんけいやく
鎮咳薬　ちんがいやく
癜風　でんぷう
瀉下　しゃげ
瀉血　しゃけつ
覆髄法　ふくずいほう
臍　さい、へそ
臍囲　さいい
臍窩　さいか
臍帯　さいたい
臍傍悸　さいぼうき
瞼球癒着　けんきゅうゆちゃく
瞼板　けんばん
鞭虫　べんちゅう
鞭毛　べんもう
類宦官症　るいかんがんしょう
類洞　るいどう
類鼾音　るいびおん
類狼瘡　るいろうそう
鵞口創　がこうそう
鵞足炎　がそくえん

19画

嚥下　えんげ
蟹足腫　かいそくしゅ
蟻走感　ぎそうかん
髄鞘　ずいしょう
蹲踞　そんきょ
濾胞　ろほう
鶏状歩行　けいじょうほこう
蟾蜍皮膚　せんじょひふ
離被架　りひか

20画

譫言　うわごと
譫妄　せんもう
鰓管　さいかん
鰓嚢　さいのう

鰓弓　さいきゅう
霰粒腫　さんりゅうしゅ
灌流　かんりゅう
灌注膿瘍　かんちゅうのうよう
懸鉤　けんこう
懸吊　けんちょう
懸濁液　けんだくえき
蠕動　ぜんどう
蠕虫　ぜんちゅう
躁鬱　そううつ
瀰慢　びまん

21画

齧歯類　げっしるい
癩球　らいきゅう
癩腫癩　らいしゅらい
露蜂　ろほう
囈語　じご

22画

彎　わん
癬　せん
驚悸　きょうき
聾唖　ろうあ
轢創　れきそう
驕り　おごり

23画

癰　よう
黴　かび
鱗茎　りんけい
鱗屑　りんせつ
鱗翅　りんし
攣縮　れんしゅく
鷺皮反応　がひはんのう
鷲手　わして

24画

癲癇　てんかん

齲窩　うか
齲歯　うし
齲蝕　うしょく
鷹揚　おうよう

26画

鑷子　せっし

29画

鬱血　うっけつ
鬱結　うっけつ
鬱帯　うったい

逆引き

和文⇒略語

あ

数字、欧文

1音	SⅠ
1回換気量	TV、Vt、VT
1回仕事係数	SWI
1回心拍出係数	SI
1回拍出係数	SVI
1回拍出量	SV
1日2回(服用)	b.d.
1日3回(服用)	t.i.d.(s).、t.i.d.
1日4回(服用)	q.i.d.、quad id
1日最低必要量	MDR
1秒量	FEV1.0
2音	SⅡ
2時間ごと	Q2h
2相性喘息反応	DAR
2点同時刺激	DSS
2倍量	qdx
2弁置換	DVR
3音	SⅢ
4音	SⅣ
5-フルオロウラシル	5-FU
17-ヒドロキシコルチコステロイド	17-OHCS
α₁-アンチトリプシン欠損症	AAD
αフェトプロテイン(胎児性蛋白)	AFP
β溶血性連鎖球菌	βHS
γグロブリン血症欠乏症	AGG
ABO式血液型	ABO
A群溶連菌	GAS
A型肝炎	HA
A型肝炎ウイルス	HAV
A型肝炎抗原	HA-Ag
BCNU、シクロホスファミド、ナツラン、プレドニゾロン併用療法	BCPP
B群溶血性連鎖球菌	GBS
B群溶連菌感染症	GBS
B型肝炎	HB
B型肝炎e抗原	Hbe-Ag
B型肝炎ウイルス	HBV
B型肝炎コア抗原	HBc-Ag
B型肝炎表面抗原	HBs-Ag
B型慢性肝炎	CHB
B細胞急性リンパ芽球性白血病	BALL
B細胞慢性リンパ性白血病	B-CLL
CO拡散能	DLCO
Cペプチド	CPR
C型肝炎ウイルス	HCV
C型慢性肝炎	CHC
C反応性蛋白	CRP
D群溶連菌	GDS
FAB分類(急性白血病の分類)	FAB
HDLコレステロール	HDL-C
HTLV-1(ヒトT細胞白血病ウイルス1)関連脊髄症	HAM
IDカード	ID
NPHインスリン、中間型インスリン	NPH
PB型(耳下腺唾液)	PB
P波同期型ペーシング	VAT
Rh因子	Rh
S状結腸	S
S状結腸鏡検査	sig
S状結腸切除術	SR
S状結腸内視鏡検査	SF
S波	S
Tリンパ球	T
T抗原	T-antigen
T細胞受容体	TCR
T細胞特異抗原	THYSA
WDHA症候群	WDHAS
WPW症候群	WPW
X線写真	X-P
X連鎖重症複合免疫不全症	XSCID

あ

アイゼンメンゲル症候群	EM
亜急性壊死性脳脊髄症	SNE
亜急性海綿状脳症	SSE
亜急性甲状腺炎	SAT
亜急性硬化性全脳炎	SSPE
亜急性硬化性白質脳炎	SSLE
亜急性細菌性心内膜炎	SBE
亜急性心筋梗塞	RMI
亜急性皮膚(型)エリテマトーデス	SCLE
亜全リンパ節照射	STNI
アキレス腱延長	TAL

アキレス腱反射	AJ、ASR、ATR	アドリアマイシン、キロサイド、6-メルカプトプリン、プレドニン併用療法	ACMP
アキレス腱反射時間	ARZ	アドリアマイシン、シクロホスファミド、タモキシフェン併用療法	ACT
悪性の	M		
悪性リンパ腫	ML		
悪性関節リウマチ	MRA	アドリアマイシン、シクロホスファミド、メトトレキセート併用療法	ACM
悪性巨細胞腫	malignant GCT		
悪性血管内皮腫	MHE	アドリアマイシン、シクロホスファミド、メドロキシプロゲステロン併用療法	ACM
悪性高体温症、悪性高熱症	MH		
悪性黒子黒色腫	LMM		
悪性黒色腫	MM	アドリアマイシン、ビンクリスチン、プレドニゾロン併用療法	DdVP
悪性持続性頭位眩暈症	MPPV		
悪性腫瘍随伴性高カルシウム血症	MAHC	アドリアマイシン、ビンクリスチン、イホスファミド、プレドニゾロン併用療法	AVIP
悪性線維性組織球腫	MFH		
悪性組織球症	MH	アドリアマイシン、ブレオマイシン、ビンブラスチン、ダカルバジンの併用療法（ホジキン病の治療）	ABVD
悪性貧血	PA		
悪性末梢性神経鞘腫瘍	MPNST		
握力	GP		
朝のこわばり	MS	アドレナリン	AD
アシクロビル（ゾビラックス）	ACV	アトロピン昏睡療法	ACT
アスコルビン酸	AA	アナフィラキシー性紫斑病	AP
アスパラギン酸アミノトランスフェラーゼ	AST、GOT	アナフィラキシー遅発反応物質	SRS-A
		アプガー・スコア	APGAR score
アスピリン誘発喘息	AIA		
アスロー	ASLO	あぶみ骨筋反射	SR
アセスメント	a	アミロイドアンギオパチー	AA
アセチルコリン	ACh	アメーバ性髄膜脳炎	AME
アダムス・ストークス症候群	Ad-St	アラニンアミノトランスフェラーゼ	ALT、GPT
アダルト・チルドレン	AC		
圧	P	アリューシャン病	AD
圧維持換気法	PSV	アルカリホスファターゼ	ALP
圧・容積関係	PVR	アルコール依存症	alc
圧・容積指標	PVI	アルコール性肝炎	AH
圧・容積反応	PVR	アルコール性肝障害	ALD
圧力尿流試験	PFS	アルコール性膵炎	AIP
アデノイド切除・扁桃摘出術	A&T、ASN	アルコール精神病	A
		アルコール中毒性小脳変性	ACD
アデノシン三リン酸	ATP	アルツハイマー型認知症	DAT、AD、ATD
アテレクトミー、方向性冠状動脈粥腫切除	DCA	アルツハイマー型老年痴呆	SDAT、ASD
アテローム硬化性心血管疾患	ACVD		
アトピー性皮膚炎	AD	アルツハイマー病	AD

和文⇒略語

あ

アルブミン／グロブリン比	A/G ratio
アルブライト遺伝性骨形成異常症	AHO
アレルギー	A
アレルギー性気管支肺アスペルギルス症	ABPA
アレルギー性気管支肺真菌症	ABPM
アレルギー性湿疹状接触皮膚炎	AECD
アレルギー性接触性皮膚炎	ACD
アレルギー性肉芽腫性血管炎	AGA
アレルギー性鼻炎	AR
アンギオテンシンⅡ	A-Ⅱ
アンギオテンシン変換酵素	ACE
アンギオテンシン変換酵素阻害(抑制)薬	ACEI、ACE inhibitor
安静、冷却、圧迫、挙上（応急処置）	RICE
安静時狭心症	RA
安静時熱量消費量	REE
安静代謝量	RM
アンダーアームブレス（脊柱側弯症用装具）	UAB
安定性狭心症	SA
アンチトロンビンⅢ	AT-Ⅲ

い

家・樹木・人物画法	HTP
胃液	G
胃液検査	GA
胃炎	GS
胃下1/3	A1/3
胃潰瘍	GU、MG、UV
胃癌	MK、GCa、GC
息切れ	SOB
胃空腸吻合術	GJ stomy
異型移行形	AT
異型狭心症	VAP
異型血管	aV
異型上皮	ATP
異型腺腫過形成	AAH
異型乳管過形成	ADH
胃結腸幹	TGC
移行上皮癌	TCC
移行帯	T
胃後壁	post
胃酸分泌抑制ペプチド	GIP
胃酸分泌抑制ポリペプチド	GIP
医師、医学博士	MD
意識	cons
意識消失	LOC
意識障害	LC
胃十二指腸潰瘍	GDU
胃十二指腸動脈	GDA
萎縮	Atr
萎縮性結節性皮膚アミロイドーシス	ACNA
萎縮性鼻炎	AR
胃上部	C
胃食道逆流	GER
胃食道逆流性疾患	GERD
胃食道接合部	GEJ
異常（コルポスコープ）所見	ACF
異常性格性攻撃者	MDSO
異常糖負荷試験	AGTT
異常なし	n.p.、NB、NP、OB
異常不随意運動	AIM
異常不随意運動疾患	AIMD
胃小弯	Min
移植	TX
移植抗原	TA
移植片対宿主	GVH
移植片対宿主反応	GVHR
移植片対宿主病	GVHD
移殖関連死亡	TRM
移殖臓器穿刺吸引細胞診	TAC
胃切除術	MR
胃全摘術	TG、Total G
胃大弯	Maj
一次救命処置	BLS
一次循環救命処置	BCLS
一次求心性線維脱分極	PAD
一次性変性痴呆	PDD
一時的ペースメーカー	TPM
一日許容量	RDA

胃チューブ	GT、MT
一卵性双生児	MZ、EZ
一過性全健忘症	TGA
一過性脳虚血(乏血)発作	TCIA、TIA
一過性類白血病状態	TAM
一過性棘融解性皮膚症	TAD
一過性閾値変動	TTS
一酸化炭素	CO
一酸化窒素	NO
一般小児病	UCHD
胃-腸-膵内分泌系	GEP
胃腸の	GI
胃腸ファイバースコープ検査	GIF
遺伝性球状赤血球症	HS
遺伝性痙性対麻痺	HSP
遺伝性血管運動神経性浮腫	HANE
遺伝性楕円赤血球症	HE
胃透視	MDL
胃内視鏡、胃ファイバースコープ	GF、GFS、FGS
胃バイパス手術	GBS
胃壁細胞	GPC
イホスファミド、シスプラチン併用療法	IP
医用工学	ME
医用生体工学	BME
医用電子工学	ME
イリノテカン、シスプラチン併用療法	IP
医療ソーシャルワーカー	MSW
インスリン依存性糖尿病	IDDM
インスリン非依存性糖尿病	NIDDM
インスリン負荷試験	ITT
インスリン様成長因子	IGF
陰性	Neg
陰性症状評価尺度	SANS
陰性反応的中度	PVN
インターフェロン	IFN
インターフェロンβ、ニムスチンと放射線照射の併用療法	IAR
インターフェロンβ、ラニムスチンと放射線照射の併用療法	IMR
インターロイキン	IL
咽頭結膜熱	PCF
インドシアニングリーン試験	ICG test
インフォームド・コンセント	IC

う

右頤横位(胎位)	RMT
右頤後方位(胎位)	RMP
右頤前方位(胎位)	RMA
右胃大静脈	VGED
右胃大網動脈	RGE
右胃動脈	RGA
ウイルス感染に伴う血球貪食症候群	VAHS
ウイルス感染後疲労症候群	PVFS
ウイルス性呼吸器疾患	VRI
ウイルス性肝炎	VH
ウイルス性呼吸器疾患	RVD、VRD
ウイルス性出血熱	VHF
ウイルス不活性薬	VIA
ウィルソン・ミキティ症候群	WMS
ウイルムス腫瘍	WT
ウェクスラー小児知能テスト	WPPSI、WISC
ウェクスラー成人知能テスト	WAIS
ウェクスラー成人知能テスト改訂版	WAIS-R
ウェゲナー肉芽腫症	WG
植込み型除細動器	AICD、ICD
上(へ)	SUP
ウェルドニッヒ・ホフマン病(家族性遺伝性脊髄性筋萎縮)	WHD
ウェルニッケ・コルサコフ症候群	WK
右横前頭位(胎位)	RFT
右下行肺動脈	RDPA
右下腹部	RLQ
右冠状静脈洞	RCS
右冠尖	RCC
右冠動脈	RCA
右冠動脈主幹部病変	RMTD
右肝静脈	RHV
右肝動脈	RHA
右肝葉	RHL

う

和文	略語
右眼	Od、RE
右眼眼圧	Tod
右眼視力	RV、V.d.
右脚前枝ブロック	RAH
右脚ブロック	RBBB
右結腸静脈	VCD
右結腸動脈	RCA
烏口肩峰靱帯	CAL
右後斜位	RPO
右後前頭位(胎位)	RFA
右鎖骨下動脈	RSA
牛海綿状脳症(狂牛病)	BSE
右軸偏位	RAD
右室圧	RVP
右室一回仕事係数	RVSWI
右室一回仕事量	RVSW
右室拡張期圧	RVDP
右室梗塞	RV infarction、RVI
右室収縮期圧	RVSP
右室収縮時間	RVSTI
右室造影	RVG
右室肥大	RVH
右室不全	RVF
右室流出路	RV out
右斜位	RAO
右上肢	RUL
右上腹部	RUQ
右心カテーテル(法)	RHC
右心形成不全	HPRH
右心耳	RAA
右心室	RV
右心室拡大	RVE
右心室流出量	RVO
右心不全	RHF
右心負荷	RHS
右心房	RA
右心房圧	RAP
右心房肥大	RAH
右腎結核	NPD
右仙骨前位(胎位)	RSA
右前方後頭位(胎位)	ODA、ROA
右鼠径ヘルニア	RIH
疑い	s/o、Va
右中葉	RML
右腸骨窩	RIF
うっ血型心筋症	COCM、CCM
うっ血型心疾患	CGD
うっ血性右心不全	CRVF
うっ血性心不全	CHF、CCF
うつ病	D
うつ病自己評価尺度	SDS
右内胸動脈	RITA
右肺下葉	RLL
右肺上葉	RUL
右付属器摘出術	RSO
右葉後区域(肝)	P
右葉前区域(肝)	A
ウロキナーゼ	UK
運動、訓練	ex
運動指数	MI
運動時発作の呼吸困難	PDE
運動神経伝導速度	MCV、MNCV
運動制限	LOM
運動痛	POM
運動ニューロン疾患	MND
運動誘発性気管支喘息	EIA

え

和文	略語
エイズ関連症候群	ARC
エイズ関連痴呆	DART
栄養障害関連糖尿病	MRDM
栄養状態良好な	W/N
壊死性潰瘍性歯肉炎	NUG
壊死性気道粘膜炎	NTB
壊死性血管炎	NA
壊死性腸炎	NEC
壊死性遊走性紅斑	NME
エストラジオール	E2
エストリオール	E3
エストロン	E1
壊疽性膿皮症	PG
エチレンジアミン四酢酸(エデト酸)	EDTA

和文	略語
エトポシド、シスプラチン併用療法	EP
エトポシド、アドリアマイシン、シスプラチン併用療法	EAP
エトポシド、エノシタビン、ビンデシン併用療法	EVB
エトポシド、プレドニゾロン、ビンクリスチン、シクロホスファミド、ドキソルビシン併用療法	EPOCH
エトポシド、メチルプレドニゾロン、高用量シタラビン、シスプラチン併用療法	ESHAP
エトポシド、メトトレキセート、ダクノマイシン、シクロホスファミド、ビンクリスチン併用療法	EMA-CP
エネルギー代謝率	RMR
エノシタビン、ダウノマイシン、メチルプレドニン、プレドニゾロン併用療法	DMP
エピネフリン	E
エプスタイン・バー・ウイルス	EBV
エミッションCT	ECT
エリスロポエチン	EPO
遠位指(趾)節間関節	DIP joint
エンカウンターグループ	EG
遠隔転移（TNM分類）	M
塩基過剰	BE
塩基欠乏	BD
円形脱毛症	AA
塩酸ドパミン	DOA
塩酸ドブタミン	DOB
円周短縮速度	Vcf
円周短縮率	FS
炎症	Inf
炎症性腸疾患	IBD
延髄呼吸化学受容体	MRC
塩素	Cl
円柱上皮	C
エンドキサン、アドリアマイシン、オンコビン、プレドニゾロン併用療法	CHOP
円板状エリテマトーデス（円板状紅斑性狼瘡）	DLE

お

和文	略語
オープニングスナップ、僧帽弁開放音	OS
横隔膜	D
横行結腸	T
黄色腫症	Xanth
黄色肉芽腫性腎盂腎炎	XGP
黄色靱帯骨化(症)	OLF、OYL
悪心・嘔吐	N&V
黄体形成ホルモン	LH
黄体形成ホルモン放出ホルモン	LH-RH
黄体形成未破裂卵胞（症候群）	LUF(S)
黄体刺激ホルモン	LTH
黄疸指数	MG
横紋筋肉腫	RMS
大型顆粒リンパ球性白血病	LGL
オキシトシン	OT、OX、OXY
オキシトシン負荷テスト	OCT
オキシトシン分娩誘導	OI
同じ（処方箋などで前回と同じ内容の場合にdoと書く）	do
オリーブ橋小脳萎縮症	OPCA
オリーブ橋小脳皮質変性	OPCD
オルガスムス障害	OI
オルニチントランスカルバミラーゼ	OTC
音圧レベル	SPL
音階	PO
音声振盪	frem
温度、体温	temp

か

和文	略語
カーンズ・セイヤー症候群	KSS
外陰上(表)皮内腫瘍	VIN
外陰部単純ヘルペス	HSG
絵画・欲求不満テスト	PFT
絵画統覚検査	TAT
外眼筋	EOM
外眼筋運動	EOM
外径	OD
外頚－内頚動脈バイパス	EC-IC bypass
外頚動脈	ECA

か

和文	略語
外耳炎	OE
外耳道	EAM、EAC
外斜位	XP（exophoria）
外斜視	XT
外傷後健忘	PTA
外傷重症度スコア	ISS
外傷性ストレス障害	PTSD
外傷性脳障害	CCI
開心術、直視下心臓手術	OHS
外旋	ER
外側視床下部	LHA
外側側副靱帯	LCL、FCL
外側半月	LM
咳嗽反射	CR
外転	ABD、Abd
回腸	I
回腸S状結腸吻合術	I-S stomy
回腸結腸動脈	ICA
回腸直腸吻合術	IRA
回腸肛門吻合術	IAA
外腸骨動脈	EIA
解凍濃厚赤血球液	FTRC
外反母趾	HV
開腹（術）	lap
回復室	RR
解剖学的死腔	ADS、Vdan
開放点滴	OD
回盲部切除術	ICR
外用	ad.us.ext.
潰瘍性大腸炎	UC
潰瘍瘢痕	uls
外来患者	OP
外来診療部門	OPD
外来用薬局	OPD
解離性胸部大動脈瘤	DTAA
解離性大動脈瘤	DAA
下咽頭	Ph
カオリン凝固時間	KCT
化学の酸素必要量	COD
下顎反射	JJ
化学療法	CT
過換気症候群	HVS
下眼瞼	LL
可逆性虚血性神経脱落症状	RIND
芽球増加性不応性貧血	RAEB
蝸牛内直流電位	EP
核医学脳血管撮影	RNCA
角化上皮	K
顎間固定	IMF
顎関節	TMJ
顎機能障害（顎関節症）	TMD
核磁気共鳴	NMR
隔日に	QOD
学習障害	LD
学習能力障害	ASD
拡張期血圧	DBP
拡張期充満	DFP
拡張期心雑音	DM
拡張期弁後退速度	DDR
拡張型心筋症	DCM
拡張末期圧	EDP
拡張末期容量	EDV
角膜後面沈着物	KP
下行結腸	D
下斜筋	IO
過剰投与	OD
仮診断、暫定診断	PD
下垂体後葉ホルモン	PPH
下垂体腺腫	PA
下垂体前葉ホルモン	APH
下垂体副腎皮質系	PAS
仮性球麻痺	PBP
仮性早熟	PPP
下前腸骨棘	AIIS
画像収集通信解析システム	PACS
家族	fa
家族性アミロイドポリニューロパチー	FAP
家族性血球貪食性組織球症	FHL
家族性複合型高脂血症	FCHL
家庭内暴力	DV
家族歴	FH
下腿切断	BK amp
下大静脈	IVC
下腸間膜静脈	IMV

か

下腸間膜動脈	IMA
下直腸動脈	IRA
滑液	SF
褐色細胞腫	PC
活性化凝固時間	ACT
活性化部分トロンボプラスチン時間	APTT
カッツ法	KAS
活動期（胃潰瘍）	Stage A
活動性慢性肝炎	ACH
活動療法	AT
カテーテル出口部感染	ESI
カテーテル尿	CSU
カテーテル肺血症	CRS
カテコールアミン	CA
果糖（フルクトース）	Fru
過粘稠度症候群	HVS
下肺動脈	PAI
下肺葉	LL
過敏性結腸症候群	ICS
過敏性腸管症候群	IBS
ガフキー度表	G
下部食道括約筋	LES
下部直腸	Rb
カポジ肉腫	KS
鎌状赤血球貧血	SCA、SS
鎌状赤血球症	SCD
ガラクトース	Gal
カリウム	K
カリフォルニア心理検査	CPI
顆粒球コロニー刺激因子	G-CSF
顆粒細胞腫	GCT
過量吸引症候群	MAS
カルシウム	Ca
カルシトニン	CT
加齢性黄斑変性	AMD、ARMD
カロリー	C / kal
川崎病、急性熱性皮膚粘膜リンパ節症候群	MCLS
癌	ca.
眼圧	IOP、OT、TO
簡易式外傷指数	AIS
簡易式熱傷重傷度指数	ABSI
肝右葉切除術	rHL
肝炎関連抗原	HAA
肝外胆道閉鎖症	EBA
肝外門脈閉塞症	EHO
眼科学	Ophth
感覚神経伝導速度	SAP
感覚性失語	SA
感覚レベル	SL
肝癌細胞	HTC
肝癌占拠率を示す記号	E1-4
換血流比	Va / Q
肝機能検査	LFT
換気不全	VF
眼球運動	EOM
換気予備率	VR
換気予備量	BR
換気亢進、呼吸亢進（過呼吸）	HV
管腔内超音波検査法	IDUS
間欠性陰圧呼吸	INPB
間欠性跛行	IC
間欠の陰圧換気	INPV
間欠の強制換気法	IMV
間欠的強制呼吸	IDV
間欠的腹膜透析	IPD
間欠的陽圧換気法	IPPV
間欠的陽圧呼吸	IPPB
間欠的陽陰圧換気	IPNPV
間欠的陽陰圧呼吸	IPNPB
冠血流量	CBF
肝血流量	HBF
肝硬変	LC
肝細胞癌	HCC、Lcc
冠疾患集中治療室	CCU
間質性腎炎ぶどう膜炎症候群	TINU
間質性肺炎	IP
間質性肺気腫	PIE
間質性肺疾患	ILD
患者	Pt、pt
患者の状況によって	prn
患者管理問題	PMP
患者血清	PS
癌腫	CA
緩衝塩基	BB
感情障害ならびに統合失調症面接基準	SADS

か

和文	略語
肝静脈	HV
冠静脈洞	CS
管状腺癌	tub
環状鉄芽球を伴う不応性貧血	RARS
冠状動脈下行枝	PD
眼振	Ny
癌神経周囲浸潤	PNI
関心領域	ROI
肝膵頭十二指腸切除	HPD
眼精神身体症	OPD
眼精疲労	Asth
関節運動の最大域	FRJM
関節可動域	ROM
関節可動域テスト	ROMT
関節可動域訓練	ROME
関節(全)置換術	TJR
関節内	IA
関節軟骨石灰化症	ACC
関節リウマチ	RA
関節リウマチ赤血球凝集(試験)	RAHA
完全右脚ブロック	CRBBB
完全寛解	CR
完全寛解した脳卒中	SFR
完全型心内膜床欠損症	complete ECD
完全経腸成分栄養	TEEH
感染後糸球体腎炎	PIGN
完全左脚ブロック	CLBBB
完全人工心臓	TAH
完全静脈栄養	TPA
完全静脈栄養高カロリー輸液	TPN
完全静脈麻酔	TIVA
乾癬性関節炎	PA
感染性心内膜炎	IE
乾癬病巣範囲重症度指数	PASI
完全閉塞	TO
完全房室ブロック	CABB、CHB
肝臓	H
癌胎児性抗原	CEA
肝中心静脈閉塞症	VOD
浣腸	E
環軸椎亜脱臼	AAS
環軸椎脱臼	A-A dislocation
環椎歯突起間距離	ADI
環軸椎の	AA
眼底	Fds、FO
眼底血圧計	ODN
眼底血圧測定	ODM、ODG
肝転移	HEP
冠動脈	CA
肝動脈	HA
眼動脈圧	OAP
肝動脈血流量	HAF、HABF
肝動脈塞栓術	TAE
肝動脈持続動注療法	CHAI
肝動脈注入療法	TAI
冠動脈バイパス	CAB
冠動脈バイパス手術	CABS
冠動脈回旋枝	CX
冠動脈硬化症	CS
冠動脈硬化性心疾患	CAHD
冠動脈疾患	CAD
冠動脈性心疾患	CHD
冠動脈造影法	CAG
冠動脈バイパス術	CABG
冠動脈内血栓溶解療法	ICT
冠動脈閉塞	CAO
冠動脈閉塞性疾患	CAOD
肝特異抗原	LSA
眼内コンタクトレンズ	ICL
肝内胆管	IHD
肝内胆汁	C bile
肝内胆汁うっ滞	IHC
肝内門脈圧	IPP
肝内門脈圧亢進	IHPH
眼内レンズ	IOL
眼軟膏	EO
鑑別診断	DD
感冒	CC
陥没骨折	DF
幹迷走神経切離(術)	TV
顔面神経麻痺	FP
顔面播種状粟粒性狼瘡	LMDF
肝門脈	HPV
緩和ケア病棟	PCU

き

キース・ワグナーの分類	KW
キーゼルバッハ部位	LK
既往歴	PH
期外収縮	PB
機械的人工換気	MV
気管気管支内洗浄	TBT
気管支	br
気管支ファイバースコープ	BFS
気管支拡張症	BE
気管支拡張薬	BD
気管支関連リンパ組織	BALT
気管支癌	BC
気管支鏡検査	BRO
気管支洗浄	BL、TBL、BT
気管支造影	BG
気管支動脈	BrA
気管支動脈塞栓術	BAE
気管支動脈造影	BAG
気管支動脈注入	BAI
気管支動脈閉塞症	BAE
気管支肺異形成	BPD
気管支肺胞洗浄	BAL
気管支喘息	BA
気管食道穿刺	TEP
気管食道短絡	T-E shunt
気管食道瘻	TEF
気管内エアウェイ	ETA
気管内挿管チューブ	ETT
気胸	Pnx、PTX、Px
器具による日常生活動作	IADL
キサンチン	Xan
器質性心疾患	OHD
器質性精神疾患	OMD
器質性脳疾患	OBD
気縦隔(症)	PM
奇静脈	A-V、VAZ
寄生虫密度	PD
偽性副甲状腺機能低下症	PHP、PPHP
基節骨	PP
季節性感情障害	SAD
基礎エネルギー消費量	BEE
規則的	reg
基礎酸分泌量	BAO
基礎体温曲線	BBT
基礎胎児心拍数	BFHR
基礎代謝率	BMR
基礎培地	BM
基礎分泌最高酸濃度	BAC
基礎分泌量	BSV
基礎ペプシン分泌量	BPO
気体amp圧計	PTG
基底細胞癌	BCC
基底細胞上皮腫	BCE
気道、エアウェイ	AW、AC
気道圧開放換気	APRV
気道確保、人工呼吸、閉胸式心マッサージ	ABC
気道感染	RTI
気導骨導差	AB gap
気道抵抗	Raw
気道内圧	Paw
危篤状態	CC
偽妊娠	PSp
気脳撮影	PEG
気脳室撮影	PVG
偽脳腫瘍	PC
機能性心雑音	FM
機能的残気量	FRC
機能的不応期	FRP
ギプス	Gips
ギプスを外した状態でのX線写真	XOP
ギプス固定のままのX線写真	XIP
逆受身皮膚アナフィラキシー	RPCA
客観的情報	O
逆行性腎盂造影法	REP、RP
逆行性電気ショック療法	REST
逆浸透	RO
逆説睡眠	PS
逆転写酵素阻害薬	RTI
脚ブロック	BBB
逆流性腎症	RN
吸引生検細胞診	ABC
吸引分娩	VE

和文⇔略語

307

き

語	略語
白蓋指数	AI
吸気	Insp
吸気時間/呼気時間	I/E
吸気肺活量	IVC
救急医療システム	EMS
救急外来室	ER
救急救命士	ELST
救急心処理、心臓急迫症管理	ECC
救急部	ED
吸収不良症候群	MA syndrome、MAS
急性アレルギー性脳炎	AAE
急性胃腸炎	AGE
急性胃粘膜病変	AGML
急性ウイルス性肝炎	AVH
急性壊死性膵炎	ANP
急性炎症性多発ニューロパチー	AIP、AIDP
急性横断性ミエロパチー	ATM
急性灰白髄炎(ポリオ)	polio
急性肝炎	AH
急性間欠性ポルフィリン症	AIP
急性間質性腎炎	AIN
急性間質性肺炎	AIP
急性感染性心内膜炎	AIE
急性冠動脈梗塞	ACI
急性冠動脈症候群	ACS
急性冠動脈不全	ACI
急性冠動脈閉塞の血栓溶解	TICO
急性冠動脈閉塞症	ACO
急性肝不全	ALF
急性期	AP
急性局所性脳浮腫	AFCE
急性後極部多発性鱗状網膜色素上皮症	APMPPE
急性硬膜下血腫	ASDH
急性硬膜外血腫	AEDH
急性呼吸器疾患	ARD
急性呼吸窮迫症候群	ARDS
急性呼吸不全	ARF
急性骨髄芽球性白血病	AML
急性骨髄性白血病	AML
急性骨髄単球性白血病	AMMoL
急性細菌性心内膜炎	ABE
急性細菌性前立腺炎	ABP
急性錯乱状態	ACS
急性散在性脳脊髄膜炎	ADEM
急性糸球体腎炎	AGN
急性十二指腸粘膜病変	ADML
急性出血性結膜炎	AHC
急性出血性腸炎	AHC
急性出血性膵炎、劇症膵炎	AHP
急性腎盂腎炎	APN
急性心筋梗塞	AMI
急性心疾患	AHD
急性心不全	AHF
急性腎不全	ARF
急性ストレス障害	ASD
急性前骨髄性白血病	AProL、APL
急性全身性エリテマトーデス	ASLE
急性単球性白血病	AML、AMOL、AMoL
急性中耳炎	AOM
急性転化	BC
急性伝染病	AID
急性動脈閉塞症時にみられる症候の6つのP	PPPPPP
急性特発性心膜炎	AIP
急性尿細管壊死	ATN
急性尿細管間質性腎炎	ATN
急性熱性呼吸器疾患	AFRD
急性脳症候群	ABS
急性播種性脳脊髄膜炎	ADE
急性播種性表皮壊死	ADEN
急性破壊性股関節症	RDC
急性肺炎	AP
急性肺障害	ALI
急性白血病	AL
急性皮膚エリテマトーデス	ACLE
急性非分類型性白血病	AUL
急性非リンパ性白血病	ANLL
急性不安大発作	AAA
急性閉塞性化膿性胆管炎	AOSC
急性閉塞性胆管炎	AOC
急性放射線症候群	ARS
急性免疫性多発神経炎	AIMP
急性網膜壊死	ARN

き

急性溶連菌感染後糸球体腎炎	APSGN
急性リウマチ熱	ARF
急性顆粒球性白血病	AGL
急性淋菌性後部尿道炎	UGPA
急性淋菌性前部尿道炎	UGAA
急性リンパ芽球性白血病	ALbL
急性リンパ性白血病	ALL
急速充満期	RF
急速進行性糸球体腎炎	RPGN
嗅電図	EOG
吸入気酸素濃度	FIO_2
吸入療法	IT
牛乳	KM
橋・延髄歩行誘発野	P-BLR
境界型ブドウ糖負荷試験	BGTT
境界性人格障害	BPD
仰臥位低血圧症候群	SHS
胸管ドレナージ	TDD
胸管リンパ球	TDL
胸腔鏡下手術	VATS
胸腔鏡下交感神経遮断術	ETS
胸腔内ガス容量	TGV
胸腔内圧	ITP
胸骨下部左縁	LLSB
胸骨左縁	LSB
胸骨中線	MSL
胸鎖乳突筋	SCM
胸式呼吸	cost resp
教授法	TS
狭心症	AP、AG
強制分時換気量	MMV
強制利尿	FD
胸腺栄養細胞	TNC
胸腺細胞	Thy
胸腺由来リンパ球	T-lymphocyte
橋中心髄鞘崩壊症	CPM
強直性脊椎炎	AS
強直性脊椎骨増殖症	ASH
胸椎	BW、T
胸痛	CP
共通性急性リンパ球性白血病	CALL
共通房室弁口	CAVC
強迫性障害	OCD
強迫性人格障害	OCPD
強皮症	SD
強皮症腎クリーゼ	SRC
胸部、胸郭	T
胸部の、胸椎の、胸髄の	Th
胸部下部食道	Ei、Lt
胸部外科	TS
胸部上部食道	Iu、ut
胸部大動脈遮断	TAO
胸部大動脈瘤	TAA
胸部中部食道	Im、Mt
峡部膨大部境界	IAJ
胸壁外心〔臓〕圧迫	ECC
胸膜、肋膜	pl
強膜棘突起	SS
胸膜転移	PLE
強力ネオミノファーゲンC	SNMC
強力抗ウイルス薬多剤併用療法	HAART
巨核球	Mgk
極小未熟児	VLBW
局所所見	SPL
局所心筋血流量	rMBF
局所脳血流	rCBF
局所ヘパリン化	RH
局所麻酔	LA
極端な低出生体重	ULBW
虚血性急性腎不全	IARF
虚血性後部視神経ニューロパチー	PION
虚血性心筋障害	IMD
虚血性心疾患	IHD
虚血性大腸炎	IC
巨細胞性間質性肺炎	GIP
巨細胞性封入体病	CMID
巨赤芽球貧血	MA
巨大細胞腫	GCT
許容摂取量	ADI
キラーT細胞	TK
キラー細胞	K cell
ギラン・バレー症候群	GBS、AIDP
起立性蛋白尿	OA
起立性調節障害	OD
起立性低血圧症	OH
近医、開業医	LMD

き

近位曲尿細管	PCT
近位筋緊張性筋障害	PROMM
近位指節間関節	PIP joint、PIPJ
筋萎縮性小脳形成不全	ACH
筋萎縮性側索硬化症	ALS
禁飲食	NPO
緊急開胸	ERT
緊急集中治療室	CCU
緊急生命維持装置	ELSS
緊急治療センター	UCC
筋緊張性ジストロフィー	MD、MMD、MyD
筋緊張性頭痛	MCH、TTH
近視	My
筋ジストロフィー	MD
菌状息肉腫	MF
筋腎代謝性症候群	MNMS
禁断症候群	WD syndrome
緊張性頚反射	TNR
緊張性尿失禁、ストレス性尿失禁	USI
緊張性迷路反射	TLR
緊張部	PT
筋電図	EMG
筋肉(筋肉内注射)	IM、im
筋肉内注射	l.m.
筋肉皮弁	M-C flap

く

空気注腸造影	ACBE
空腸再建術	JPD
空腹時(朝食前)血糖	FBS、FBG
空腹時血糖値	FAP
クエッケンシュテット検査	Q-test
駆出時間	ET
駆出性収縮期雑音	ESM
駆出率	EF
屈曲	fl
クモ膜下出血	SAH
クラインフェルター症候群	47XXY
	syndrome、XYY syndrome
グラスゴー・コーマ・スケール	GCS
グラム陰性桿菌	GNB
グラム陰性球菌	GNC
グラム陽性桿菌	GPB
グラム陽性球菌	GPC
グリセオフルビン	GF
グリセリン浣腸	GE
グルコース・インスリン療法	GI
グルコース・インスリン・カリウム療法	GIK
グルタミン酸オキサロ酢酸トランスアミナーゼ	GOT、AST
グルタミン酸ピルビン酸トランスアミナーゼ	GPT、ALT
クループ性気管支炎	CB
車いす	WC
クレアチニン・クリアランス	Ccr
クレアチン	Cr
クレアチンキナーゼ	CK
クレアチンホスホキナーゼ MB	CPK-MB
クレアチンリン酸酵素(クレアチンホスホキナーゼ)	CPK
クロイツフェルト・ヤコブ病	CJD
グローバル診断法	GAS
クローン病	CD
クローン病活動指数	CDAI

け

形質細胞異常症	PCD
慶応式臨床知能検査	KIP
経回腸結腸静脈(食道動脈瘤)塞栓術	TIO
経過記録	PN
計画	P
頚管	EC
経管栄養	TF
経管吸引カテーテル	TEC
頚管粘液(検査)	CM(T)
経気管吸引	TTA
経気管支肺生検	TBLB
経頚静脈的肝内門脈静脈	TIPS

け

短絡術	
蛍光眼底血管造影	FFA
経口経静脈胆嚢胆管造影	OC-DIC
経口血糖降下薬	OHA
蛍光(眼底)血管造影	FAG
経口摂取不可、禁食	NBM
経口胆管鏡検査	PCS
経口胆嚢造影(法)	OCG
経口的	O
経口的(口から摂取する)	POpo
経口的膵管鏡検査	POPS
経口避妊ホルモン	OCH
経口避妊薬	OC、BCP
経口ブドウ糖負荷試験	OGTT
経口ポリオワクチン	OPV、TOPV
経口輸液療法	ORT
経肛門的内視鏡下マイクロサージャリー	TEM
経産	MP
経産回数	P
芸術療法	AT
経静脈的胆嚢造影	IVC
頸静脈怒張	JVD
頸静脈波	Jug.
経食道心エコー法	TEE
携帯型自動血圧計、24時間血圧測定	ABPM
経腟自然分娩	NSD
経腟の膀胱頚部吊り上げ術	VBNS
経腟分娩	TVD
経腸栄養	EN
経直腸的針生検	TRNB
経直腸的超音波断層(法)	TRUS
頸椎	C、CS
頸椎の、頸髄の	C
頸椎症性脊髄症	CSM
頸椎椎間板ヘルニア	CDH
経頭蓋超音波ドップラー	TCD
系統的多臓器不全	MSOF
頸動脈海綿静脈洞瘻	CCF、C-C fistula
頸動脈造影法	CAG
頸動脈波	Car.
経尿管吻合術	TUU
経尿道的凝固(術)	TUC
経尿道的焼灼(術)	TUF
経尿道的切除(術)	TUR
経尿道的砕石術	TUL
経尿道的前立腺切除術	TUR-P
経尿道的電気凝固術	TUE
経尿道的超音波砕石術	TUL
経尿道的膀胱腫瘍切除術	TUR-Bt
経妊回数	G
経皮経肝肝膿瘍ドレナージ	PTAD
経皮経肝食道静脈瘤塞栓術	PTO
経皮経肝胆道ドレナージ	PTBD
経皮経肝胆道鏡検査	PTCS
経皮経肝胆道造影	PTC
経皮経肝胆嚢ドレナージ	PTGBD
経皮経肝門脈枝塞栓術	PTPE
経皮経肝門脈造影	PTP
経皮経肝門脈塞栓術	PTPE
経皮経管冠動脈形成術	PTCA
経皮経静脈的僧帽弁交連裂開術	PTMC
経皮的エタノール注入療法	PEIT
経皮的マイクロ波凝固療法	PMCT
経皮的冠状動脈血栓溶解療法	PTCR
経皮的吸収治療システム	TTS
経皮的血管拡張(術)	PTA
経皮的血管形成(術)	PTA
経皮的心肺補助装置	PCPS
経皮的腎結石超音波砕石術	PUL
経皮的腎砕石術	PNL、PCN、PCNL
経皮的腎瘻(術)	PNS
経皮的腎瘻造設術	PCN
経皮的炭酸ガス分圧	TcPCO$_2$
経皮的胆管ドレナージ	PTCD
経皮的電気の神経刺激	TENS
経皮内視鏡的胃瘻造設術	PEG
頸部	Cx
頸部リンパ節	CLN
頸部食道	Ce
頸部脊椎症	CS
頸部脊椎症性脊髄症	CSR
経腰大動脈造影	TLA
痙攣ショック療法	CST
痙攣性疾患	CD

け

和文	略語
外科、産婦人科	SGO
外科集中治療室	SICU
劇症肝炎	FH
劇症肝不全	FHF
血圧	Bp、BP
血液	B
血液一酸化炭素	BCO
血液ガス分析	BGA
血液型	BT
血液灌流	HP
血液吸着	DHP
血液凝固時間	CLT
血液神経関門	BNB
血液透析	HD
血液透析性水疱症	BDH
血液透析濾過	HDF
血液二酸化炭素	BCO_2
血液尿素窒素	BUN
血液脳関門	BBB
血液培養	BLC、BC
血液量	BV
血液濾過	HF
血管	BV
血管運動神経性浮腫	ANE
血管運動性鼻炎	VMR
血管拡張神経、血管拡張薬	VD
血管拡張物質	VDM
血管筋脂肪腫	AML
血管作働性腸管ポリペプチド	VIP
血管収縮率	VCR
血管周囲リンパ球浸潤	PLC
血管造影	AG、Angio
血管抵抗	VR
血管壁	VW
血管攣縮性狭心症	VSA
結核	TB
結核菌	TB
月経前症候群	PMS
月経量	MBL
月経歴	MH
結合織疾患	CTD
血漿	P
血漿吸着	PA
血漿交換	PE、PH、PP
血漿浸透圧	Posm
血漿蛋白分解	PPF
血漿鉄	PI
血漿鉄交代（率）	PIT（R）
血漿鉄消失率	PIDR
血漿プロトロンビン時間	PPT
血小板	PLT
血小板活性化因子	PAF
血小板凝集因子	PAP
血小板減少性紫斑〔病〕	TPP
血小板減少橈骨欠損症候群（常染色体性劣性遺伝）	TAR
血小板濃厚液	PC
血小板由来増殖因子	PDGF
血漿量	PV
血漿レニン活性	PRA
血漿レニン濃度	PRC
血清	S、BS
血清アミロイドA	SAA
血清肝炎	SH
血性胸水	Eh
血清クレアチニン	SCR
血清クレアチンキナーゼ	SCK
血清殺菌濃度	SBC
血清蛋白	SP
血清尿素窒素	SUN
血清ワッセルマン反応	SWR
結節性硬化症	TS
結節性紅斑	EN
結節性黒色腫	NM
結節性動脈周囲炎、（結節性）多発性動脈炎	PAN、PN
結節性皮膚アミロイドーシス	ACN
結節性皮膚ループスムチン症	NCLM
血栓性血小板減少性紫斑病	TTP
血栓性微小血管障害	TMA
血栓内膜摘除術	TEA
血中アルコール濃度	BAL、BAC
血中薬物濃度測定	TDA
結腸癌	Cca
血糖	BS、BG
血糖自己測定（患者による）	SMBG
腱移植	TG

牽引	tr、tx
牽引性網膜剥離	TRD
原因不明	CUD
原因不明の心筋症	MUO
原因不明の突然死	SUUD
原因不明熱	FUO
腱延長	EOT
限外濾過率	UFR
検眼鏡	Oph
肩関節周囲炎、五十肩	PSH
肩関節的装具	BFO
研究のための診断基準	RDC
限局性播種性エリテマトーデス	L-DLE
肩甲骨	Sc
言語療法	ST
現在症検査	PSE
検査結果に異常認めず	NAD
現実見当識訓練	RO
検出できない	ND
見当識検査	OT
見当識調査票	OI
検尿	UA
原発腫瘍の大きさ（TNM分類）	T
原発性アメーバ性髄膜脳炎	PAM
原発性開放隅角緑内障	POAG
原発性肝癌	PLC、
	PHC
原発性感情疾患	PAD
原発性硬化性胆管炎	PSC
原発性後天性鉄芽球性貧血	PASA
原発性視神経萎縮	POA
原発性心筋疾患	PMD
原発性全般てんかん	PGE
原発性胆汁性肝硬変	PBC、
	PBI
原発性脳内出血	PIH
原発性肺癌	L1
原発性肺高血圧症	PPH
原発性非定型肺炎	PAP
原発性副甲状腺機能亢進症	PHP、
	PHPT
原発性閉塞隅角緑内障	PCAG、
	PACG
原発性慢性肝炎	PCH
原発巣不明腺癌	ACUP

こ

原発不明癌	PUA、
	UPC
原発不明腫瘍	UPT
原発不明熱	PUE、
	PUO
現病歴	PI、HP
肩峰骨頭距離	AHI
肩峰鎖骨関節	ACJ、
	AC joiut
肩腕症候群	SAS

こ

コーネル健康調査士	CMI
ゴールドマン視野計	GP
高圧機械呼吸	HPMV
高圧酸素療法	HBO
	therapy、
	OHP
高圧浣腸	HE
高位脛骨骨切術	HTO
好塩基球	Bas
高温、高体温	HT
口蓋咽頭形成（術）	PPP
口蓋軟口蓋咽頭形成（術）	UPPP
口蓋裂	CP
光覚	PL、SL
抗核因子	ANF
抗核抗体	ANA
光覚なし	NLP、
	no pl
後下小脳動脈	PICA
硬化性萎縮性苔癬	LSA
硬化療法	ST
交感神経系	SNS
光凝固	LK、PC、
	PHC
抗凝固薬	AC
抗胸腺細胞グロブリン	ATG
口腔外科医	ORS
口腔気管の	OT
口腔内所見	OC
後脛骨筋	TP
合計特殊出生率	TFR
高血圧（症）	HBP、HT
高血圧性心血管疾患	HCVD

こ

和文	略語
高血圧性心疾患	HHD
高血糖性高浸透圧性非ケトン性昏睡	HHNC
抗血友病A因子	AHA
抗血友病因子、血液凝固Ⅷ因子、抗血友病ヒトグロブリン	AHF
抗原	Ag
抗原結合能	ab
抗原抗体反応	AAR
膠原病	CD
後交通動脈	P com（A）、PC
交叉反応物質	CRM
好酸球	Eo、Eos
好酸球性白血病	EL
好酸球増加を伴う肺浸潤	PIE
好酸球増多症候群	HES
抗酸菌	AFB
好酸球遊走因子	ECF
光刺激	PS
高脂血症	HL
後視床穿通動脈	PTPA
鉱質コルチコイド	MC
後十字靱帯	PCL
後縦靱帯骨化症	OPLL
後縦靱帯	PLL
抗出血因子	ABF
甲状腺ホルモン	TH
甲状腺ホルモン結合蛋白	TBG
甲状腺ヨウ素摂取率	TIU
甲状腺刺激ホルモン	TSH、TTH
甲状腺刺激ホルモン放出ホルモン	TRH
甲状腺刺激ホルモン放出因子	TRF
甲状腺刺激免疫グロブリン	TSI
高所性脳浮腫	HACE、HAPE
抗心筋抗体	AMA
口唇口蓋裂	CLP
口唇単純ヘルペス	HSL
高浸透圧性非ケトン性（糖尿病）	HONK
高浸透圧性非ケトン性高血糖昏睡	HONK
高浸透圧性非ケトン性昏睡	HNKC
後水晶体線維増殖（症）	RLF
抗膵島細胞抗体	ICA
抗ストレプトキナーゼ	ASK
抗生物質持続効力	PAE
抗生物質随伴下痢症	AAD
高性能液体クロマトグラフィー	HPLC
後前方向	PA
光線力学療法	PDT
（悪性腫瘍の）構造模型	SAT
拘束型心筋症	RCM
後側壁枝	PL
酵素免疫測定法	EIA
抗体	Ab
抗体依存性細胞障害	ADCC
抗体依存性細胞媒介性細胞傷害作用	ADCMC
抗体産生細胞	AFC
交代性共同性内斜視	ACCS
交代性斜視	ADS
交代性上斜位	DVD
交代性内斜視	ACS
後大脳動脈	PCA
抗体被覆細菌	ACB
抗体不全症候群、抗体欠損症候群	ADS
好中球	N、Neutro
好中球アルカリホスファターゼ	NAP
好中球絶対数	ANC
後頂	O
抗てんかん薬	AED
後天性心疾患	AHD
後天性嚢胞腎	ACKD
後天性免疫不全症候群	AIDS
後天性溶血性貧血	AHA
行動異常	BD
後頭横位（胎位）	OT
喉頭癌	KKK
喉頭気管麻酔	LTA
後頭骨後方	OP
後頭骨前方	OA
口頭指示	VO
後頭仙骨位（胎位）	OS
後頭動脈・後下小脳動脈	OA-PICA
後頭部の	O
行動療法	BT、CBT

こ

和文	略語
光毒性治療法	PTT
高度治療室	HCU
後囊下白内障	PSC
高濃度範囲	HAD
広背筋皮弁	LDMC
抗破傷風血清	ATS
広範囲知能人格検査	WRIPT
広汎性子宮全摘術	RTH
広汎性発達障害	PDD
紅斑性狼瘡、ループスエリテマトーデス	LE
高比重リポ蛋白	HDL
後鼻漏、鼻後方滴注(法)	PND
高頻度ジェット換気	HFJV
高頻度人工換気	HFV
高頻度振動換気	HFO、HFOV
後部硝子体剥離	PVD
後腹膜リンパ節郭清(術)	RND、RPLND、RLND
高分化型小球性悪性リンパ腫	WDLL
興奮性シナプス後電位	EPSP
後壁心筋梗塞	PMI
後房コンタクトレンズ	PCL
後房内レンズ	PCL
硬膜外血腫(エピドラ)	Epidura、EH、EDH
硬膜外麻酔	Epid
硬膜下血腫(サブドラ)	Subdura、SDH
硬膜下水腫	SDE
硬膜下出血	SDH
硬膜下腹腔短絡術	S-P shunt
肛門管	P
肛門性器間距離	AGD
肛門側不完全切除(組織学的)の記号	d(+)
肛門側不完全切除(肉眼的)の記号	D(+)
抗利尿性物質	ADS
抗利尿ホルモン(バソプレシン)	ADH
抗利尿ホルモン分泌異常症候群	SIADH
交流分析	TA
抗リン脂質抗体症候群	APS
抗リンパ球グロブリン	ALG
抗リンパ球血清	ALS
抗リンパ球抗体	ALA
高齢者、眼の見えない人、障害者	ABD
高レニン本態性高血圧症	HREH
語音聴取閾値	SRT
(人工)股関節全置換術	THA
股関節の屈曲、外転、外旋、伸展テスト	FABERE
股関節の屈曲、内転、内旋、伸展テスト	FADIRE
股関節表面全置換術	THARIES
股関節離断	HD
呼気	Exp
呼気気道陽圧	EPAP
呼気終末陽圧	PEEP
呼気肺活量	EVC
呼気閉塞指数	CVI
呼気量	VI
呼吸	br、R、resp
呼吸運動	RM
呼吸音	BS、RS
呼吸器合胞体ウイルス	RSV
呼吸器疾患集中治療室	RICU
呼吸窮迫症候群	RDS
呼吸ケア実施士	RCP
呼吸指数	RI
呼吸集中治療室	RCU
呼気終末炭酸ガス濃度	ETCO2
呼吸商	RQ
呼吸数	R、RR、f
呼吸性補正	RC
呼吸代謝	RM
呼吸中枢	RC
呼吸調節中枢	PC
呼吸調節率	RCI
呼吸停止	RC
呼吸不全	RF
呼吸療法	RT
国際疾病分類	ICD
国際単位	IU
国際標準化機構	ISO

こ

和文	略語
コクサッキーウイルス	Cox-V
黒色表皮症、黒色表皮腫	AN
黒内障性家族性白痴	AFI
午後	pm
個人歴	PH
午前	am
骨壊死	ON
骨関節症	OAP
骨形成不全	OI
骨形成不全症	OGI
骨髄	BM
骨髄異形成症候群	MDS、CMS
骨髄移植	BMT
骨髄炎	osteo
骨髄化生を伴う骨髄硬化症	MMA
骨髄性白血病	MLD
骨髄線維症	MF
骨髄増殖性疾患	MPD
骨髄転移	BMM
骨髄由来細胞	B-cell
骨折	Fx
骨(髄)転移	MAR、OSS
骨導	BC
骨軟化症	OM
骨肉腫	OS
骨年齢	BA
骨盤位	BEL
骨盤位外回転術	ECV
骨盤位分娩	Breech
骨盤出口横径	BI
骨盤動脈造影	PAG
骨盤内炎症性疾患	PID
骨盤内血管造影	PAG
ゴナドトロピン放出ホルモン	GnRH
ゴナドトロピン放出ホルモン作用薬	GnRHa
ゴナドトロピン放出因子	GRF
鼓膜	m flac、MT、TM
鼓膜切開術	paracen
固有筋層	pm
固有筋層までの癌(壁深達度)	mp癌
固有受容器神経筋促進法	PNF
コリンエステラーゼ	ChE
コルチゾンブドウ糖負荷試験	CGTT
コレシストキニン・パンクレオザイミン	CCK-PZ
コロニー刺激因子	CSF
コンカナバリンA	Con A
混合性結合組織病	MCTD
混合性中胚葉腫瘍	MMT
根治手術	rad op
コンジローマ	Con
コンタクトレンズ	CL
コンピュータ(補助)診断システム	CAD
コンピュータ断層撮影	CT
根本的頚部郭清術	RND

さ

和文	略語
再拡張性肺水腫	REP
細気管支	B
細気管支性間質性肺炎	BIP
細菌性心内膜炎	BE
サイクリックAMP	cAMP
最高酸濃度	MAC
最高酸分泌量	MAO
最高代謝率(寒冷時)	PMR
最終月経(期)	LMP、LPM、LR
最小光毒量	MPD
最小紅斑量	MED
最小侵襲手術	MIT
最小致死量	LFD、MFD
最小発育阻止濃度	MIC
臍静脈	UV
臍静脈カテーテル	UVC
再診	RTC、rtc
再生不良性貧血	AA
最大換気量、分時最大呼吸量	MBC、MVV
在胎期間に比して適当な大きさの児(適性発育児)	AGA
最大吸気圧	MIP、PIP
最大吸気量	IC
最大許容線量	MAD
最大駆出率	PER

さ

最大(収縮期)血圧	SBP
臍帯血幹細胞移植	CBSCT
最大呼気圧	MEP
最大呼気速度	PEFR、Vmax
最大呼気流量	MEF、PEF
最大刺激時酸分泌量	PAO
最大充満速度	PFR
最大出力音圧レベル	SSPL
最大短縮速度	Vmax
最大中間呼気速度	MMF
最大努力性呼気流量	FEFmax
最大拍動点	PMI
最大反復回復	RM
最大流速	PFR
最大膀胱許容量	MBC
左胃大網動脈	LGE
在宅(中心)静脈栄養法	HPN
在宅経管経腸栄養法	HEN
在宅酸素療法	HOT
在宅人工呼吸療法	HMV
在宅成分栄養経管栄養法	HEEH
左胃動脈	LGA
臍動脈	UA
臍動脈カテーテル	UAC
サイトメガロウイルス	CMV
サイトメガロウイルス感染症	CMV
再発性アフタ性口内炎	RAS
左頤部横位(胎位)	LMT
左頤部後位(胎位)	LMP
左頤部前位(体位)	LMA
臍ヘルニア・巨大舌・巨人症症候群	EMG syndrome
細胞異型度	CAT
細胞外液	ECF
細胞傷害試験	CT
細胞障害性Tリンパ球	CTL、Tc
細胞性免疫	CMI、CI
細胞性免疫不全症候群	CIDS
細胞接着分子	CAM
細胞内液(量)	ICF
細胞変性効果	CPE
細網内皮系	RES
細網肉腫	RCS
サイロキシン	T4
左回旋枝	LCX
左下腹部	LLQ
左眼	LE、Os
左眼眼圧	Tos
左冠状動脈	LCA
左眼視力	LV、V.s.
左冠動脈回旋枝	LCX
左冠動脈主幹部	LMT
左冠動脈前下行枝	LAD
左肝静脈	LHV
左肝動脈	LHA
左脚前枝ブロック	LAH
左脚ブロック	LBBB
作業関連疾患	WRD
作業療法	OCC th、OT
作業療法士	OT
左結腸動脈	LCA
左肩甲骨後位	LScP
左後頭横位(胎位)	OLT
左後頭後方位(胎位)	OLP
左後頭前方位(胎位)	OLA
鎖骨下静脈	SV
鎖骨下動脈	ASC、SCA
坐骨棘線	SP
坐骨棘と第2・3仙椎間	PSO
鎖骨上リンパ節	SCN
鎖骨中線	MCL
左軸偏位	LAD
左室1回仕事係数	LVSWI
左室1回仕事量	LVSW
左室拡張末期径	LVEDD
左室機能不全	LVD
左心室駆出時間	LVET
左室径	LVD
左室後壁	LVPW
左室収縮末期径	LVESD
左室造影	LVG
左室体積	LV mass
左室肥大	LVH
左室不全	LVF
左室補助装置	LVAD、LVAS

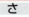

和文	略語
左室容量	LVV
左室流出路	LV out
左上大静脈	LSVC
左上大静脈遺残症	PLSVC
左上腹部	LUQ
左(肺)上葉	LUL
左心カテーテル法	LHC
左心形成不全	HPLH
左心形成不全症候群	HLHS
左腎結核症	NPS
左心室	LV
左心性単心室	DILV
左腎動脈	LA
左心バイパス	LHB
左心不全	LHF
左心房	LA
左(心)房圧	LAP
左前頭横位(胎位)	LFT
左前頭後位(胎位)	LFP
左前頭前位(胎位)	LFA
左総頚動脈	LCA
左側付属器摘出(術)	LSO
左鼠径ヘルニア	LIH
サッチ足	SACH
左内胸動脈	LIMA、LITA
左背後位(胎位)	LDP
左肺上葉切除	LUL
左背前位(胎位)	LDA
サブスタンスP	SP
左房肥大	LAH
坐薬	Supp
左右障害	R-L
左右短絡	L-R shunt
左右肺別換気	DLV
左葉外側区域(肝)	L
左葉内側区域(肝)	M
サラゾスルファピリジン(サラゾピリン)	SASP
サルコイドーシス	Sar
産科(学)	OB
産科集中治療室	OICU
産科真(的)結合線	CVO、OC
三環系抗うつ薬	TCA
残気率	RVI
残気量	RV
三枝病変	TVD
三尖弁	TV
三尖弁逸脱	TVP
三尖弁狭窄症	TS
三尖弁形成(術)	TVP
三尖弁前尖	ATL
三尖弁置換術	TVR
三尖弁閉鎖症	TA
三尖弁閉鎖不全	TR
三尖弁閉鎖不全症	TI
三尖弁弁輪形成術	TAP
酸素	O
酸素解離曲線	ODC
酸素消費量	OC、VO$_2$
酸素透過性ハードコンタクトレンズ	RGP
酸素分圧	PO$_2$
酸素飽和濃度	SO$_2$
残存腎機能	RRF
残尿測定	RUM
残尿率	RR
産婦人科	OB-GYN

し

和文	略語
死因	COD
視運動性眼振	OKAN、OKN
シェーグレン症候群	SS
シェーグレン病	SJS
シェーンライン・ヘノッホ紫斑病	SHP
シェーンライン・ヘノッホ紫斑病性腎炎	HSPN
シェーンライン・ヘノッホ症候群	SHS
シェッツ眼圧測定計	ST
紫外線	UV
痔核	Hemo
視覚アナログ尺度	VAS
視覚記憶スパン	VMS
視覚識別正確度	VDA
視覚性的刺激	VSS
視覚誘発電位	VEP
耳科学	Oto

し

和文	略語
自家骨髄移植	auto-BMT
自家造血幹細胞移植	auto-SCT
自家末梢血幹細胞移植	ABSCT、auto-PBSCT
弛緩骨盤底部	RPF
弛緩部	PF
時間肺活量	TVC
色素血管母斑症	PPV
色素指数	CI
色素性乾皮症	XP
色素性絨毛結節性滑膜炎	PVS
色素沈着, 浮腫, 多発神経障害症候群	PEP
子宮外妊娠	EUP、EP、GEU
子宮癌	Ut ca、UTC
子宮鏡下卵管内受精法	HIT
子宮筋腫	myoma
子宮頸管拡張および掻爬術	D&C
子宮頸癌	CC、ZK
子宮頸管乾燥スミア	CDS
子宮頸部上皮内新生物	CIN
子宮血流	UBF
子宮口	MM
子宮収縮	UC
子宮全摘術	TH
糸球体基底膜	GBM
糸球体腎炎	GN
子宮胎盤機能不全	UPI
子宮体部癌	KK
糸球体濾過値(率)	GFR
子宮単純全摘術	STH
子宮弛緩因子	URF
子宮内圧	IUP
子宮内胎児死亡	IUFD、FDIU
子宮内胎児発育不全(遅延)	IUGR
子宮内避妊器具	IUCD、IUD
子宮内膜	EM
子宮内膜癌	EMCa
子宮内膜細胞診	EMS
子宮内膜症	EM
子宮内容除去術	Aus、D&C
子宮内容総容積	TIuV
子宮卵管境界	UTJ
子宮卵管造影	HSG
磁気共鳴	MR
磁気共鳴画像診断装置	MRI
磁気共鳴血管造影法	MRA
磁気共鳴コンピュータ画像診断法	MR-CT
磁気共鳴膵胆管造影	MRCP
死腔換気量	VD
シクロホスファミド, アドリアマイシン, シスプラチン併用療法	CAE、CAP
シクロホスファミド, アドリアイシン, ビンクリスチン併用療法	CAV
シクロホスファミド, ドキソルビシン, ビンクリスチン, プレドニゾロン併用療法	CHOP
シクロホスファミド, アドリアマイシン, ビンクリスチン, プロカルバジン, プレドニゾロン, ブレオマイシン併用療法	COP-BLAM
シクロホスファミド, アドリアマイシン, フルオロウラシル併用療法	CAF
シクロホスファミド, エトポシド, プロカルバジン, プレドニゾロン併用療法	CEPP
シクロホスファミド, オンコビン, プレドニゾロンの併用療法	COP
シクロホスファミド, オンコビン, プロカルバジン, プレドニゾロン併用療法	COPP
シクロホスファミド, カルボプラチン併用療法	CP
シクロホスファミド, シスプラチン併用療法	CP
シクロホスファミド, ドキソルビシン, シスプラチン併用療法	CAP
シクロホスファミド, ビンクリスチン, プレドニゾロン併用療法	COP、CVP

し

和文	略語
シクロホスファミド、ドキソルビシン、ビンクリスチン、プレドニゾロン併用療法	CHCP
シクロホスファミド、ビンクリスチン、ドキソルビシン、ダカルバジン併用療法	CYVADIC
シクロホスファミド、ビンクリスチン、プロカルバジン、プレドニゾロン併用療法	CCPP、C-MOPP
シクロホスファミド、ビンクリスチン、メソトレキセート、メルファラン併用療法	CCMPA、DRI-V
シクロホスファミド、ビンクリスチン、メソトレキセート、メルファラン、ドキソルビシン併用療法	COMPA RDR
シクロホスファミド、メソトレキセート、フルオロウラシル併用療法	CMF
シクロホスファミド大量静注療法	IVCY
刺激後ペプシン分泌量	SPO
刺激生体反応	S-O-R
視交叉上核	SCN
自己(自家)	auto
自己愛性人格障害	NPD
自己乳房管理	SMC
自己評価うつ病尺度	SAD
自己評価不安尺度	SAS
自己免疫疾患	AID
自己免疫性肝炎	AIH
自己免疫性血小板減少性紫斑病	ATP
自己免疫性好中球減少症	AIN
自己免疫性プロゲステロン皮膚炎	AIPD
自己免疫性溶血性疾患	AHD
自己免疫性溶血性貧血	AIHA、AHA
自己免疫補体結合反応	AICF
視索上核	SON
自殺企図	SA、SMV
支持の精神療法	ST
指示票	WO
四肢麻痺	tetra
歯状核赤核淡蒼球ルイ体萎縮症	DRPLA
視床下部－下垂体－副腎系	HPA axis
視床(内側)出血	TH
視床腹外側核破壊術	VL thalamotomy
視神経	ON
指数弁	nd
ジスキネジアを伴わない	WD
シスプラチン、エトポシド、ブレオマイシン併用療法	BEP
シスプラチン、シクロホスファミド、アドリアマイシン併用療法	CISCA
シスプラチン、ダカルバジン、ビンデシン併用療法	CDV
シスプラチン、ビンクリスチン、アドリアマイシン、エトポシド併用療法	CODE
シスプラチン、フルオロウラシル併用療法	CF
シスプラチン、ブレオマイシン、ビンクリスチン併用療法	CBV
シスプラチン、ペプロマイシン併用療法	CP
シスプラチン、メソトレキセート、ビンブラスチン併用療法	CMV
耳性眼瞼反射	APR
指節間関節	IPJ、IP
指尖手掌間距離	TPD
自然腟分娩	SVD
自然流産	SpAb
持続陰圧呼吸	CNP
持続温熱腹膜灌流	CHPP
持続血液透析	CHD
持続血液濾過透析	CHDF
持続式携帯腹膜透析	CAPD
持続睡眠療法	DS
持続性甲状腺刺激物質	LATS
持続性全身性リンパ節腫脹	PGL
持続性部分てんかん	EPC
持続静脈血液透析	CVVHD
持続静脈内インスリン注入療法	CIII
持続他動運動	CPM
持続注入肝動脈血管造影	IHA
持続的強制換気	CMV
持続的血液濾過	CHF
持続的循環式腹膜透析	CCPD

し

持続的静脈－静脈血液濾過	CVVH
持続的動静脈血液濾過法	CAVH
持続脳室ドレナージ	CVD
持続皮下インスリン注入法	CSII
持続腹膜透析	CPD
持続陽圧換気法	CPPV
持続陽圧呼吸	CPAP、CPPB
肢帯型筋ジストロフィー	LG
膝下（下腿）	BK
膝蓋腱移行術	PTT
膝蓋腱支持装具	PTB
膝蓋腱反射	PSR、PTR、KJ
膝蓋大腿関節	PF joint、PFJ
膝蓋大腿部	PF
膝蓋跳動	TdP
膝蓋軟骨軟化症	CMP
（人工）膝関節全置換術	TKA
膝胸位	KCP
シックビル症候群	SBS
失語症	APH
膝内障	IDK
失認	AGN
湿疹	Ez
湿布、罨法	WD
自動運動	AE
自動音量調節	AGC、AVC
児頭骨盤不適合	CPD
自動体外除細動器	AED
自動腹膜灌流	APD
自動明聴調節	ARC
視能訓練士	ORT
自発眼振	SN
自発呼吸、自発換気	SV、SB、SR
自発呼吸補助換気	ASB
自発的手術の避妊	VSC
市販薬（カウンターごしに買える薬剤という意味）	OTC
耳鼻咽喉	ENT
耳鼻咽喉科学	ORL
指鼻試験	F to N
ジヒドロテストステロン	DHT
視標追跡検査	ETT
ジフテリア・破傷風トキソイド	DT
ジフテリア・百日咳・破傷風三種混合	DPT
自閉症ならびに関連コミュニケーション障害	TEACH
死亡	D
脂肪肝	FL
脂肪肝・腎症候群	FLKS
脂肪塞栓症候群	FES
脂肪負荷試験	FTT
視野	VF
斜位	Ob
シャイ・ドレーガー症候群	SDS
社会技能訓練	SST
社会遂行能面接基準	SPS
社会成熟指数	SQ
社会適合係数	SAI
社会不安障害	SAD
尺骨神経	UN
尺側手根屈筋	FCU
尺側手根屈筋腱	FCU
尺側手根伸筋	ECU
若年型糖尿病	JOD
若年性関節リウマチ	JRA
若年成人平均値	YAM
若年性成人型糖尿病	MODY
若年性糖尿病	JDM
若年性慢性骨髄性白血病	JCML
シャルコー・マリー・ツース病	CMT
シャント血流量	QS
種、分析種	Sp
縦隔	Med
縦隔腫瘍	MT
習慣性流産	HA
周期性四肢麻痺	PP
周期性方向交代性眼振	PAN
周産期集中治療部	PICU
収縮期雑音	SM
収縮気圧	PS
収縮時間	STI
（子宮）収縮ストレステスト	CST
収縮性心膜炎	PC
収縮末期容量	ESV

し

和文	略語
重症急性呼吸器症候群	SARS
重症筋無力症	MG
重症複合免疫不全症	SCID
重症複合免疫不全症候群	SCIS
就寝前	vds
修正右前斜位	MRAO
修正大血管転位	CTGA
集中治療医学	CCM
集中治療室	ICU
重度再生不良性貧血	SAA
十二指腸ファイバースコープ	FDS
十二指腸潰瘍	DG、DU、U-D
終板電位	EPP
十分量	Qs
周辺虹彩切除	PI
周辺虹彩前癒着	PAS
終末肝動脈枝	THA
絨毛癌	CC
絨毛上皮癌	chorio
絨毛羊膜炎	CAM
重要人物	VIP
主観的、客観的、評価、計画	SOAP
宿主対移植片反応	HVGR
手根管症候群	CTS
手根骨と中手骨の間	CM
手根中手間関節	CMJ、CM joint、CMC
樹枝状血管	bV
手術	OP
手術室	OR
手術室技師	ORT
手術部位感染	SSI
主訴	CC
出血時間	BT
出生時体重	B
術後	PO
術後性頰部膿疱	POWZ
術後性上顎嚢胞	POMC
術後日	POD
術前化学療法	ICT
術中心筋梗塞	PMI
術直後義肢装着法	IPSF、IPPF
手動弁	HM、mm
腫瘍移殖抗原	TTA
腫瘍壊死因子	TNF
腫瘍関連抗原	TAA
腫瘍関連表面抗原	TASA
腫瘍血管新生因子	TAF
腫瘍浸潤リンパ球	TIL
腫瘍随伴体液性高カルシウム血症	HHM
腫瘍成長因子	TGF
主要組織適合複合体	MHC
受容体生活酵素	RDE
主要体肺側副動脈	MAPCA
腫瘍特異抗原	TSA
腫瘍特異性移殖抗原	TSTA
腫瘍特異性表面抗原	TSSA
腫瘍マーカー	TM
純音聴力検査	PTA
循環血液量	CBV
循環血漿蛋白	TPP
純型肺動脈弁狭窄症	PPS
純粋運動性片麻痺	PMH
純赤血球性貧血	PRCA
上位運動ニューロン	UMN
上衣下出血	SHE
上衣腫	EP
消化管	GIT
消化管間質腫瘍	GIST
消化管喘々吻合	EEA
消化管ホルモン	GEP、GIH
上顎癌	OKK
上顎結節線	TM line
上顎洞	MS
上顎洞炎	empy
消化性潰瘍	PU
小顆粒	SGV
笑気	NO
上気道	URT
上気道感染症	URI、URTI
笑気麻酔	GO
条件刺激	CS
条件反射	CR
上行結腸	A

し

症候性原発性胆汁性肝硬変	s-PBC	小児科	PED
上行大動脈瘤	AAA、AA	小児期発症型広範性発達障害	COPDD
猩紅熱	SF	小児丘疹性末端皮膚炎、ジャノッティ皮膚炎	PAC
証拠に基づいた医療	EBM		
証拠に基づいた看護	EBN	小児型多嚢胞腎	CPKD
錠剤、タブレット	Tab	小児集中治療施設	PICU
詳細不明	NOS	小児統覚テスト	CAT
小細胞癌	SCC	小児慢性水疱症	CBDC
小細胞肺癌	SCLC	小児用人格調査表	PIC
小指外転筋	ADQ、ADM	小脳橋角	CPA
		小脳橋角部	CP angle
硝子体混濁	OCV	上皮小体	PTG
上室性期外収縮	SVC、SVPC	上皮小体機能亢進症	HPT
		上皮成長因子	EGF
上室性頻拍	SVT	上皮内癌	CIS、Tis
床上安静	BR	上部消化管（撮影）	UGI(S)、GI
上小脳動脈	SCA		
床上浴	BB	上部食道括約部	UES
上斜筋	SO	上部直腸	Ra
上斜視	HT	小胞体	ER
症状	Sx	小発作	PM
症状の訴え	C / O	漿膜下層	ss
掌蹠爪下黒色腫	PPSM	漿膜下層までの癌（壁深達度）	ss癌
掌蹠膿疱症	PPP	漿膜までの癌（壁深達度）	s癌
常染色体優性遺伝	AD	静脈	V
常染色体優性多発性囊胞腎	ADPKD	静脈（注射）	IV、iv
常染色体劣性遺伝	AR	静脈圧	VP
常染色体劣性多発性囊胞腎	ARPKD	静脈確保	KVO
上前腸骨棘	ASIS、ASS	静脈血	V、VB
		静脈血圧	VBP
上大静脈	SVC、VCS	静脈性腎盂造影	IP、IVP
		静脈性糖負荷試験	IGTT
上大静脈症候群	SVCS	静脈性尿路造影	IVU
上大静脈造影	SVCG	静脈洞	SV
静注用帯状疱疹免疫グロブリン	ZIG-v	静脈洞欠損症	SVD
		静脈動脈バイパス（法）	V-A
上腸間膜静脈	SMV	静脈内（の）	IV
上腸間膜動脈	SMA	静脈内注射	I.v.
上腸間膜動脈症候群	SMAS、SMAO	静脈弁不全	VI
		上矢状静脈洞	SSS
小腸大量切除術	SBR	上矢状静脈洞血栓（症）	SSST
小腸閉塞症	SBO	常用者、常習者	AD
上直腸動脈	SRA	小葉中心性肺気腫	CE
常同(性)行動	SB	上輪部角結膜炎	SLK
小児うつ病特性尺度	CDI	上腕囲	AC

323

し

和文	略語
上腕三頭筋腱反射	TJ、TTR
上腕神経叢神経症	BPN
上腕切断	AE amp
上腕動脈	BA
上腕二頭筋反射	BJ
食間に	zw d E
職業性頚肩腕症候群	OCD
食後	pc
職歴	OH
食前	a.c.
(毎)食前	vdE
褥瘡潰瘍	DU
食中毒	FP
食道	ES
食道胃管式エアウェイ	EGTA
食道胃接合部	EGJ
食道癌	EC、Eca、OK
食道静脈瘤形態の分類記号	F1-3
食道内圧	Pes
食道ファイバースコープ	EF
食道噴門接合部	E-C junction、ECJ
食道閉鎖式エアウェイ	EOA
所見なし、異常なし、苦痛(訴え)なし	OB
除細動	DF
初産	PP
所属リンパ節転移の程度 (TNM分類)	N
徐波睡眠	SWS
徐頻脈症候群	BTS
処方、処方箋	Rp、Rx
自律神経機能障害	ANSD
自律神経系	ANS
自律神経失調症テスト	OD test
自律訓練	AT
視力	VA
視力矯正不能	n.c.、nc
シルバーヘルスプラン	SHP
腎、尿管、膀胱(撮影)	KUB
心移植	HTX
腎移植	RTX
シングルフォトンエミッションCT	SPECT
心因性多飲症	CDW
腎盂腎炎	PN
腎盂尿細管移行部	PUJ
腎炎因子	NeF
腎横紋筋肉腫瘍様腫瘍	MRTK
心音	HS
心音図	PCG
人格因子	PF
人格障害	PD
人格評点スケール	PRS
心機図	MCG
心胸郭比	CTR
心筋梗塞	MI
心筋梗塞後症候群	PMI
心筋酸素消費量	MVO_2
心筋症	CM
心筋線維症	MF
神経	N
神経因性膀胱	NB
神経学的年齢	NA
神経活動電位	NAP
神経芽細胞腫	NB
神経筋接合部	NMJ
神経筋単位	NMU
神経系	NS
神経系肉芽腫性血管炎	GANS
神経血管圧迫症候群	NVC
神経血管減圧術	MVD
神経血管性	NV
神経原性筋萎縮	NMA
神経興奮性検査	NET
神経循環無力症	NCA
神経症	N
神経鞘腫	NN
心係数	CI
神経性、進行性筋委縮症	NPMA
神経性うつ病	ND
神経性子宮頚管粘液検査	CMT
神経性食思不振症	AN
神経性膀胱機能障害	NBD
神経線維腫症	NF
神経伝導速度	NCV
神経内科、神経学、神経学の	Neuro
神経難聴	ND
神経膠芽腫	GBMF

和文	略語	和文	略語
心血管造影	CAG	腎細胞癌	RCC
腎血管(動脈)性高血圧症	RVH、RVHT	深指屈筋	FDP
		心室拡張終期圧	VEDP
心血管造影法	ACG	心室拡張終期容積	VEDV
腎血管抵抗	RVR	腎疾患集中治療室	KICU
真結合線	CV、TC	心室前駆出期・駆出時間比	PEP/(V)ET
腎血流量	RBF		
腎血漿流量	RPF	心室興奮伝達時間	VAT
心原性ショック	CS、CGS	心室細動	Vf
心原性肺水腫	CPE	心室性期外収縮	PVC、VPB、VPC
(病気の)進行	PD		
人工気胸	AP		
人工肛門	Afta	心室性頻拍	VT
人工股関節置換術	THR	心室粗動	VF
人工呼吸器関連性肺炎	VAP	心室遅延電位	LP
人工膝関節置換術	TKR	心室中隔	IVS、VS
人工授精	AI	心室中隔欠損	ISD
人工心肺	CPB	心室中隔欠損症	VSD
人工心肺装置	PO	心室中隔穿孔	VSP
人工腎臓	AK	心室中隔破裂	VSR
進行性塊状線維症	PMF	心室中部閉塞症	MVO
進行性外眼筋麻痺	PEO	心室抑制心房同期型ペーシング	VDD
進行性核上性麻痺	PSP	心室瘤	VA
進行性核性眼筋麻痺	PNO	滲出性中耳炎	OME
進行性球麻痺	PBP	浸潤、癌浸潤度	INF
進行性筋ジストロフィー	PMD、DMP	浸潤癌	IC
		腎昇圧物質	RPS
進行性筋萎縮症	PMA	尋常性乾癬	PSO
進行性自律神経機能不全症	PAF	尋常性天疱瘡	PV
進行性神経性筋萎縮症	PNMA	尋常性疣贅	vv
進行性脊髄性筋萎縮症	PSMA	腎静脈	RV
進行性全身性強皮症	PSS	腎静脈圧	RVP
進行性対称性紅斑角皮症	PSE	腎静脈血レニン比	RVRR
進行性多巣性白質脳症	PML	腎静脈血栓症	RVT
進行性肥厚性間質性神経炎	PHIN	心身症	PSD
進行性風疹性全脳炎	PRP	腎髄質嚢胞性疾患	MCD
進行性麻痺	GP	腎性骨異栄養症	ROD
人工足関節置換術	TAR	腎性尿崩症	NDI
人工の肝機能補助	ALS	腎生検	RB
人工妊娠中絶	IA	新生児	NB
人工弁心内膜炎	PVE	新生児一過性頻呼吸症	TTNB、TTN
進行麻痺	PP		
人工流産	AA	新生児壊死性腸炎	NEC
腎後性腎不全	PRRF	新生児エリテマトーデス	NLE
深在性エリテマトーデス	LEP	新生児黄疸	NNJ、IN

し

新生児過量吸引症候群	MAS	腎動脈圧	RAP
新生児肝炎症候群	NHS	腎動脈狭窄	RAS
新生児行動評価	NBAS	腎動脈造影(法)	RAG
新生児高ビリルビン血症	IHB	心内膜炎	EC
新生児呼吸促迫症候群	IRDS	心内膜下心筋梗塞	SEMI
新生児室	NBN	心内膜床欠損症	ECD
新生児集中治療部	NICU	心内膜心筋線維症	EMF
新生児出血性疾患	HDN	心内膜線維弾性症	ECFE
新生児遷延性肺高血圧症	PPHN	腎尿細管性アシドーシス	RTA
新生児溶血性黄疸	MHN	腎尿細管性アルカローシス	RTA
新生児溶血性疾患	HDN	心囊貯留液	PE
真性早熟	TPP	心肺移植	HLTx
真性多血症	PV	心肺係数	HLR
真性腹圧性尿失禁	GSI	心肺血流量	CPBV
新生物	NG	心肺蘇生法	CPR
新鮮液状血漿	FP	心肺停止	CPA
振戦せん妄	DTs	心肺脳蘇生法	CCPR、
新鮮凍結血漿	FFP		CPCR
心尖拍動図	ACG	心肺補助装置	CPS
心尖部肥大型心筋症	APH	心拍応答型ペースメーカー	RRPM
新鮮保存血	WB-F	心拍再開	ROSC
振戦麻痺	PA	心拍出量	CO、Qt
腎造影	NG	心拍数	HR
心臓	HZ	真皮深層熱傷	DDB
心臓移植術	CTx	真皮浅層熱傷	SDB
心臓カテーテル法	CC	深部腱反射	DTR
心臓血管障害	CVA	深部腱反射亢進	DTR
心臓呼吸性の	CR	深部静脈血栓症	DVT
心臓集中治療部	CICU	人物画テスト	DAP
心断層エコー図	UCT	心不全	CF、HF
心臓超音波検査(心エコー図)	UCG	腎不全	RF
心臓突然死	SCA、	心弁膜疾患	VHD
	SDHD	心房-ヒス束時間	AH
心臓弁膜症	VDH		interval
診断	Dx、D	心房圧	PA
診断群別分類	DRG	心房細動	AF
診断群別包括払い	PPS	心房収縮期雑音	ASM
診断的腹腔洗浄	DPL	心房性ナトリウム利尿ペプチド	ANP
身長	Ht	心房性期外収縮	APC、
心停止	CA		PAB、
伸展	ext		PAC、
伸展下肢挙上テスト	SLR		APB
心電図	ECG、EK	心房性早期収縮	APS
伸展反射	SR	心房粗動	AF
新導入化学療法	NAC	心房中隔	IAS

和文	略語
心房中隔欠損	IAD
心房中隔欠損症	ASD
心房同期型心室ペーシング	VDT/I
心房抑制型心房ペーシング	AAI
心膜気腫、気心膜症	PPC
鍼麻酔	AA
腎明細胞肉腫	CCSK
唇裂	CL

す

和文	略語
膵管胆道合流異常	APBD
髄核ヘルニア	HNP
髄芽腫	MB
膵機能テスト	PFT
膵機能診断テスト	PFD
膵空腸吻合カテーテル	P-J catheter
髄質海綿腎	MSK
水晶体乳化吸引術	PEA
水晶体嚢外摘出術	ECCE
水晶体嚢内摘出術	ICCE
膵全摘出術	TP
膵臓癌	PK
錐体外路症候群	EPS
錐体路	PT
錐体路ニューロン	PTN
推定胎児体重	EFBW
水痘	chpx
水痘・帯状ヘルペスウイルス	VZV
水痘抗体価血清	ZIP
水痘抗体免疫グロブリン	ZIG
水痘帯状疱疹免疫グロブリン	VZIG
膵頭十二指腸切除術	PD
膵頭部癌	PKK
水痘免疫グロブリン	VIG
膵尾部切除術	DP
水平面	H
水疱性口〔内〕炎ウイルス	VSV
水疱性類天疱瘡	BP
髄膜腫	M
睡眠関連呼吸障害	SRRD
睡眠時無呼吸症候群	SAS
睡眠代謝率	SMR
睡眠脳波検査	PSG
頭蓋内圧	ICP
頭蓋内圧亢進	IICP、ICH
スタンフォード知能テスト	SIT
ステロイドホルモン	SH
ストーマ療法士	ET
ストレプトキナーゼ	SK
ストレプトマイシン	SM
スモン、亜急性脊髄視神経症	SMON
スルホニル尿素剤	SU
スワン・ガンツカテーテル	S-G、SGC

せ

和文	略語
声音振盪	VF
性格障害	CD
整形外科、整形外科医	Ortho
整形外科医	OS
生検	Bx
性行為感染症	STD
性交後試験	PCT
性行動中枢	SBC
星細胞腫	AST
青酸感受性因子	CSF
精子凝集試験	SAT
成熟度指数	MI
正常圧水頭症	NPH
正常下限	LLN
正常眼圧緑内障	NTG
正常血清	NS
正常色素性赤血球	NCE
正常自然満期産	NSFTD
正常所見	NCF
星状神経節ブロック	SB
正常赤血球	NBL、NRBC
正常値の最高	ULN
正常洞調律	NSR
正常範囲	NL、NR、WNL
精神（科）医	P
精神医学、精神科	Psy、P
精神医学の	PS
精神科救急チーム	PET
精神科集中管理室	PICU
精神科ソーシャルワーカー	PSW

せ

和文	略語
成人型多嚢胞症	APCD
成人型糖尿病	MOD
成人呼吸窮迫症候群	ARDS
精神障害の診断・統計便覧	DSM
精神情動疾患	PAD
精神神経医学	NP
精神神経学	PN
精神神経症の	PN
精神(発達)遅滞	MR
成人T細胞白血病	ATL
成人T細胞白血病ウイルス	ATLV
成人T細胞白血病(リンパ腫)	ATLL
成人T細胞白血病関連抗原	ATLA
成人T細胞リンパ腫	ATL
精神的うつ病	PD
成人発症型多嚢胞腎	APKD
成人発症型糖尿病	AOD
精神発達遅滞	MD
精神皮膚電流反射	PGR
精神病	P
精神病性進行麻痺	GPI
精神保健センター	MHC
精製ツベルクリン	PPD
精巣性女性化症候群	TFS
青壮年休止症候群	SMDS
声帯	VC
声帯共鳴	VR
生体腎移植	DST
生体リズムに基づく内服	RCR
正中頚嚢胞	MCC
成長期集中治療部	GCU
成長ホルモン	GH、STH
成長ホルモン分泌抑制ホルモン	GH-IH
成長ホルモン放出ホルモン	GRH
成長ホルモン放出因子	GRF
性同一性障害	GID
(血清値の)精度管理	QC
性病	VD
性病研究所梅毒検査法(アメリカ)、ガラス板法	VDRL
性病性リンパ肉芽腫	VLG
生物学的偽陽性(反応)	BFP(R)
生物(化)学的酸素要求量	BOD
生物学的半減期	Tb
成分栄養	ED
生命の質、生活の質	QOL
生命の尊厳	DOL
生命維持装置	LSS
製薬企業の医療品情報担当者	MR
生理学	Physiol
生理食塩水	NS、PSS
正量	QR
世界保健機関	WHO
赤芽球癆	PRCA
脊髄延髄脊髄反射	SBS
脊髄小脳変性症	SCD
脊髄髄膜瘤	MMC
脊髄性筋萎縮	SMA
脊髄性進行性筋萎縮症	SPMA
脊髄性痙性麻痺	SSP
脊髄前方固定	ASF
脊髄造影法(ミエロ)	Myelo、MLG
脊髄麻酔後頭痛	PSH
脊椎(の)	SP
脊椎骨端異形成(症)	SED
脊椎麻酔	Sp
赤点斑	P
舌下	SL
切開排膿	I&D
積極的の介助運動	AAE
赤血球(数)	RBC、E、ER
赤血球凝集反応	HAR
赤血球沈降速度	ESR
赤血球鉄代謝	RCIT
赤血球鉄利用率	RCU
赤血球濃厚液	CRC
赤血球容積	PCV、RCV
石けん水浣腸	SSE、SE
石けん清拭	SB
接合尿細管	CNT
切痕	DN
接触性膿疱性皮膚炎	CPD
接触皮膚炎	CD
絶対床上安静	CBR
切断	Amp
切迫性尿失禁	UI
切迫早産	PTL

切迫分娩	TPL	全腎血流量	TRBF、TRPF
切迫流産	TA		
線維化性肺疾患	FLD	全身性強直性間代性発作	GTCS
線維筋形成不全	FMD	全身性硬化症	SS
前腋窩線	AAL	全身性エリテマトーデス	SLE
遷延性可逆性虚血性神経脱落	PRIND	全身麻酔	GA
遷延性植物状態	PVS	全脊椎麻酔(法)	TSB
前額面	F	全赤血球鉄	TRI
全荷重	FWB	全赤血球量	TRCV
前下小脳動脈	AICA	全層植皮	FTSG
前下膵十二指腸動脈	AIPD	全層植皮術	FTG
腺癌、アデノカルチノーマ	ad-ca、AC	漸増抵抗運動	PRE
		漸増抵抗運動(10段階)	10 RM
全冠動脈血液量	TCF	戦争捕虜症候群	POW
前期破水	PROM	喘息性気管支炎	AB
前胸部横径	ACD	浅側頭動脈	STA
前胸壁	ACW	前大脳動脈	ACA
占拠性病変	SOL	選択的胃迷走神経切離術	SV
前駆出期	PEP	選択的近位迷走神経切断術	SPV、PCV
前屈	AF		
前脛骨筋	TA	選択的臓器動脈造影	SVA
前脛骨部色素斑	PPP	選択的肺胞気管支造影法	SAB
潜血	OB	選択的腹腔動脈造影	SCA
全血	WB	前庭眼反射	VOR
全血液量	TBV	前庭神経炎	VN
全血管抵抗	TVR	先天奇形	CM
全血球計算	CBC	先天性横隔膜ヘルニア	CDH
前交通動脈	A com、ACA	先天性肝線維症	CHF
		先天性筋ジストロフィー症	CMD
前交通動脈瘤	A com	先天性股関節脱臼	CDH、LCC
前広背筋	ALD		
前後径、後前頭径	OF	先天性骨髄性ポルフィリン症	CEP
仙骨	S	先天性再生不良性貧血	CHA
全骨髄除臓〔術〕	TPL	先天性心疾患	CHD
仙骨の、仙髄の	S	先天性心臓奇形	CMH
前後方向、背腹方向	A-P	先天性脊椎・骨端変形成症	SEDC
浅指屈筋	FDS	先天性赤血球産生異常性貧血	CDA
前十字靱帯	ACL	先天性大腿骨欠損	PFFD
前収縮期雑音	PSM	先天性多嚢胞性腎	CMK
前縦靱帯	ALL	先天性多発性関節拘縮症	AMC
洗浄赤血球	WRC	先天性胆道拡張症	CBD
線条体黒質変性症	SND	先天性胆道閉鎖症	CBA
全身炎症性反応症候群	SIRS	先天性内反足	CCF
全身血圧	SAP	先天性肺胞異形成	CAD
		先天性非進行性ミオパシー	CNM

せ

先天性皮膚欠損症	ACC
先天性風疹症候群	CRS
先天性副腎過形成	CAH
先天性副腎性器症候群	CAGS
先天性免疫不全症候群	CIDS
先天性リパーゼ欠損症	CPLD
前頭部の	F
前投薬	pre-medi
前頭葉	FL
前頭葉型痴呆	FLD、FD
全24時間尿量	TUV
全乳	VKM
全肺気量	TLC
全肺血管抵抗	TPR、TPVR
全肺静脈還流異常症	TAPVC
全肺容量	TLV
全般性強直性間代性痙攣	GTC
全般性不安障害	GAD
全般てんかん	GE
前鼻棘	ANS
前部虚血性視神経症	AION
前壁心筋梗塞	AMI
前房	AC
前房コンタクトレンズ	ACL
腺房細胞癌	ACC
前方切除術	AR
前房内レンズ	AC-IOL
全末梢(血管)抵抗	TSPR、TSVR、SVR、TPR
専門看護師	CNS
腺様嚢胞癌	ACC
前立腺癌	Ca-P、PC、PCa、PK
前立腺癌関連抗原	PAP
前立腺性酸性ホスファターゼ	PAP
前立腺痛	PD
前立腺特異抗原	PSA
前立腺肥大症	BPH
全流量	TF
前リンパ球性白血病	PLL
全リンパ節照射法	TNI
全リンパ組織照射(法)	TLI
ゼロ呼息終期圧呼吸	ZEEP
ゼロ人口成長	ZPG
前腕切断	BE amp

そ

ソーシャルワーカー	SW
ソーミーブレス	SOMI
総アンモニア窒素	TAN
躁うつ病	MD、MDI
造影剤	CM
増加	inc
総カロリー補給	RME
総肝動脈	CHA
早期胃癌	EGC
早期破水	EROM
総虚血時間	TIT
総頚動脈	CCA
造血幹細胞移植	HSCT
総血清ビリルビン	TSB
総血中好酸球数	TEC
総コレステロール	TC
総子宮容積	TIUV
総指伸筋	EDC
巣状糸球体硬化症	FGS
巣状増殖性ループス腎炎	FPLN
巣状肺気腫	FE
増殖型糖尿病網膜症	PDR
増殖細胞核(蛋白)抗原	PCNA
増殖硝子体網膜症	MVR、PVR
増殖性糸球体腎炎	PGN
相対危険度	RR
双胎間輸血症候群	TTTS
相対的腎機能	RF
総体表面積	TBSA
相対不応期	RRP
総胆管	CBD、CHD
総胆管空腸吻合	C-J stomy
総胆管結石	CBDS
総胆汁酸	TBA
総蛋白	TP
総腸骨動脈	CIA

た

和文	略語
早朝尿	EMU
総鉄結合能	TIBC
総動脈幹遺残	PTA
総動脈幹症	TA
総肺静脈還流異常症	TAPVD、TAPVR
早発性痴呆	DP
早発卵巣不全	POF
総ビリルビン	T-Bil、TB
僧帽弁	MV
僧帽弁(弁輪)形成術	MAP
僧帽弁逸脱症候群	MVP
僧帽弁逆流, 僧帽弁閉鎖不全	MR
僧帽弁狭搾症	MS
僧帽弁狭窄閉鎖不全	MSI、MSR
僧帽弁形成術	MVP
僧帽弁後尖	PML
僧帽弁口血流速波形	TMF
僧帽弁前尖	AML
僧帽弁前尖の収縮期前方運動	SAM
僧帽弁大動脈弁置換	MAVR
僧帽弁置換術	MVR
僧帽弁閉鎖症	MA
僧帽弁閉鎖不全	MI
総リンパ球数	TLC
側頭, 後頭, 頭頂葉連合野	TOP
側頭部の	T
側頭動脈炎	TA
側頭葉てんかん	TLE
足背動脈	DP
足白癬	TP
側方伸展型(大腸)腫瘍	LST
組織プラスミノゲンアクチベーター	t-PA
組織因子	TF
蘇生せず	DNR
蘇生後死亡	DAR
ソフトコンタクトレンズ	SCL
ソラレン紫外線療法	PUVA
ゾリンジャー・エリソン症候群	ZES
存続絨毛症	PTD

和文	略語
第1〜12胸椎	T1, T2, T3,…T12
第1〜7頚椎	C1〜7
第1骨盤位(胎位)	LST
第1骨盤位第1分類(胎位)	LSA
第1骨盤位第2分類(胎位)	LSP
第1頭位(胎位)	LOT
第1頭位第1分類(胎位)	LOA
第1頭位第2分類(胎位)	LOP
第1〜5腰椎	L1、L2、…L5
第2骨盤位(胎位)	RST
第2骨盤位第1分類(胎位)	RSA
第2骨盤位第2分類(胎位)	RSP
第2大動脈音	A2
第2頭位(胎位)	ROT
第2頭位第1分類(胎位)	ROA
第2頭位第2分類(胎位)	ROP
第2肋間胸骨右縁	2R
第3肋間胸骨左縁	3L/3LSB
第4肋間胸骨左縁	4L/4LSB
体位性縮瞳反応	PMR
体位ドレナージ	PD
体位変換	PC
退院	ENT、Disc、DS
大うつ病	MD
大横径(児頭)	BPD
体温	BT、T
体温, 脈拍, 呼吸	TPR
体外式心肺補助	ECLHA
体外式肺補助	ECLA
体外式膜型人工肺	ECMO
体外受精	IVF
体外受精卵卵管内移植	PROST、ZIFT
体外受精胚移植	IVF-ET
体外循環	ECC
体外衝撃波結石破砕療法	ESWL
体外腎砕石術	ECSWL

た

体外心マッサージ	ECM	大腿骨長	FL
体外的微小発破砕石術	EML	大腿四頭筋セッティング運動	QSE
大感情障害	MAD	大腿静脈	FV
大気圧	PB	大腿切断	AK amp
大胸筋皮弁	PMM-C flap	大腿動脈	FA
		代替補完医療	CAM
大血管転位（症）	TGV	大腸癌	CK、Colon-Ca
大後頭三叉神経症候群	GOTS		
対光反射	LR	大腸菌	E coli、EC
胎児エコー	FE		
胎児仮死	FD	大腸直腸癌	CRC
胎児監視装置	EFM	大腸内視鏡検査	FCS
胎児胞郭横径	FTD	大腸ファイバースコープ	CF、CFS
胎児躯幹面積	FTA	胎動	FM
胎児呼吸様運動	FBM	耐糖能異常	IGT
胎児循環遺残	PFC	大動脈	Ao
胎児心音	FHS、FHT	大動脈冠動脈バイパス術	A-C bypass、ACBG
胎児心音図	FPCG		
胎児心電図	FECG	大動脈冠動脈移植術	ACG
胎児振動音刺激試験	VAST	大動脈弓遮断	IAA
胎児心拍	FHB	大動脈弓症候群、大動脈炎症症候群	AAS
胎児心拍陣痛図	CTG		
胎児心拍数	FHR	大動脈駆出音	AES
胎児心拍動	FHM	大動脈縮窄複合	COAC
胎児性アルコール症候群	FAS	大動脈後壁	AoPW
胎児性細胞癌	ECC	大動脈三角	AT
胎児先進部	PP	大動脈縮窄（症）	COA、CoA、CA
胎児大腿骨長	FFL		
胎児胎盤不均衡	FPD	大動脈前壁	AoAW
代謝当量（代謝率）	MET	大動脈大腿動脈バイパス術	AFB
体重	Wt	大動脈腸骨動脈閉塞症	AIOD
対称性緊張性頚反射	STNR	大動脈内バルーンパンピング	IABP
帯状疱疹	HZ	大動脈肺動脈窓	AP window
帯状疱疹ウイルス	HZV		
帯状疱疹後神経痛	PHN	大動脈肺動脈中隔欠損	APW
大静脈	VC	大動脈肺動脈中隔欠損症	APSD
大静脈肺動脈吻合術	CPS	大動脈弁	AV、AoV
耐性、抵抗力	R	大動脈弁狭窄および閉鎖不全症	ASI、ASR
体性感覚誘発電位	SEP		
大泉門	AF	大動脈弁狭窄症	AS
大腿－大腿動脈バイパス	F-F bypass	大動脈弁形成術	AVP
		大動脈弁疾患	AVD
大腿頚骨角、膝外側角	FTA	大動脈弁上狭窄症候群	SASS
大腿骨頚部骨折	FNF	大動脈弁置換術	AVR

和文	略語	和文	略語
大動脈弁閉鎖不全症	AR、AI		VOD
大動脈弁輪拡張症	AAE	多臓器不全症候群	MODS
体内総水分(量)	TBW	直ちに、至急	stat
胎嚢	GS	多段階運動試験	GXT
大脳誘発電位	CEP	脱臼	Dis
胎盤アルカリホスファターゼ	PL	脱臼、転位	LX
胎盤機能不全症候群	PDS	多動機能亢進	hyperactivity
胎盤着床部絨毛性腫瘍	PSTT	多嚢胞化萎縮腎	ACDK
体表熱傷	BSB	多嚢胞腎	PKD、
体表面積	BSA		PCK
大便	F	多嚢胞性卵巣	PCD、
胎便吸引症候群	MAS		PCO
大発作	GM	多嚢胞性卵巣症候群	PCOS
対麻痺	Para	多発梗塞性痴呆	MID
代理ミュンヒハウゼン症候群	MSBP	多発神経炎	PRN
大量化学療法	HDT	多発性筋炎	PM
体力指数	PFI	多発性梗塞性痴呆	DMIT
ダウノマイシン、キロサイド、プレドニン併用療法	DCP	多発性硬化症	MS
		多発性骨髄腫	MM
ダウノマイシン、ビンクリスチン、プレドニゾロン併用療法	DVP	多発性骨端骨異形成症	MED
		多発性先天異常	MCA
ダウノルビシン、シタラビン、メルカプトプリン、プレドニゾロン併用療法	DCMP	多発性動脈炎	PA
		多発性内分泌腺腫	MEN、MEA
ダウン症候群	DS	多発性嚢胞腎	PCKD
ダカルバジン、ニムスチン、ビンクリスチン併用療法	DAV	ダブルプロダクト	PRP
		ダブルルーメンカテーテル	DLC
ダカルバジン、ニムスチン、ビンクリスチン、ペプロマイシン併用療法	DAVP	痰	sp
		単位	U
		単一臍帯動脈	SUA
多関門集積スキャン	MUGA	短胃動脈	SGA
タキソテール、シスプラチン併用療法	DP	単右心室	SRV
		単回使用医療器材、ディスポ器材	SUD
多形核(好中球性)白血病	PMN		
多形日光疹	PLE	段階別式患者ケア	PPC
多形滲出性紅斑	EEM	短下肢ギプス包帯	SLC
多系統萎縮症	MS、MSA	短下肢装具	SLB、AFO
多血小板血漿	PRP		
多源性心房性頻脈	MAT	胆管癌	CC
多重人格障害	MPD	胆管癌の十二指腸側胆管断端の癌浸潤(組織学的)の程度を示す記号	dw0-3
打診音	PT		
多腺性自己免疫(症候群)	PGA		
多臓器機能不全	MOSF	胆管癌の十二指腸側胆管断端の癌浸潤(肉眼的)の程度を示す記号	DW0-3
他臓器転移	OTH		
多臓器不全	MOF、		

た

和文	略語
胆管細胞癌	CCC
胆管胆汁	A bile
短期記憶	STM
単球	Mo
単球性白血病	MoL
単極性うつ病	uMDD
炭酸ガス分圧	PCO$_2$
短時間増強感覚指数テスト	SISI test
短縮携帯型精神状態質問表	SPMSQ
単純型糖尿病性網膜症	SDR
単純頭蓋撮影法	PCG
単純部分発作	SPS
単純ヘルペス性脳炎	HSE
単純疱疹(ヘルペス)	HS
単純疱疹(ヘルペス)ウイルス	HSV
短小指屈筋	FDM
単心室	SV
単心房	SA
胆膵管鏡	CPS
胆石症	GS
胆石仙痛	BC
断層撮影	tomo
断層心エコー図	2DE
端側	E-S
端々	E-E
胆道癌の十二指腸浸潤程度(組織学的)の記号	d0-3
胆道癌の十二指腸浸潤程度(肉眼的)の記号	D0-3
短橈側手根伸筋	ECRB
胆道閉鎖(症)	BA
胆嚢	GB
胆嚢癌	GBK
胆嚢造影検査	GB exam
胆嚢胆汁	B bile
胆嚢胆石	GBS
胆嚢動脈	CA
蛋白栄養代謝障害	PCM
蛋白エネルギー栄養失調症	PEM
蛋白結合ヨウ素	PBI
単発性骨嚢腫	SBC
短波長紫外線	UVC
ダンピング症候群	DS
短母指外転筋	APB
短母指屈筋	FPB
短母指伸筋	EPB

ち

和文	略語
チアノーゼ性心疾患	CHD
チアノーゼ性先天性心疾患	CCHD
チェーンストークス呼吸	CSB
遅延型アレルギー	DTH
遅延型アレルギー反応	LAR
遅延型過敏症反応	DH
遅延型皮膚過敏症	DCH
知覚神経伝導速度	SCV
知覚騒音レベル	PNL
地球医療再検討方策	LMRP
恥骨上膀胱穿刺術	SPA
致死量	LD
腟鏡の異常所見	ACF
腟式子宮全摘出(術)	TVH、VTH
腟式子宮摘出術	VH
腟上皮内癌	VAIN
腟スメア指数	SI
窒素酸化物	NOx
腟トリコモナス	TV
腟内診	VE
腟内洗浄	VI
腟内容塗布	VS
腟部びらん	PE
知能指数	IQ
遅発型喘息反応	LAR
遅発ジスキネジア	TD
遅発性ウイルス感染症候群	SVI
遅発性外傷性脳内血腫	DTICH
遅発性虚血性神経脱落症状	DIND
注意欠陥障害	ADD
注意欠陥多動障害	AD-HD
中央材料室	CSR
中肝静脈	MHV
肘関節離断	ED
中間層皮膚移植、分層植皮	STSG
中結腸静脈	VCM
中結腸動脈	MCA
中鎖トリグリセリド	MCT
中鎖脂肪酸ミルク	MCT milk

ち

和文	略語
中耳炎	OM
注射	inj
中手骨指節骨間関節	MP、MPJ、MP joint、MCP、MCPJ
中心静脈	CV
中心静脈圧	CVP
中心静脈栄養	IVH、TPN、CV
中心静脈カテーテル	CVC
中心動脈圧	CAP
虫垂	AP
虫垂炎	app
虫垂切除術	AP
中枢型睡眠時無呼吸症候群	CSAS
中枢興奮状態	CES
中枢神経管欠損	NTD
中枢神経系	CNS、ZNS
中枢神経系白血病	CNS-leukemia
中枢性協調障害	ZKS
中枢性尿崩症	CDI
中性脂肪(トリグリセリド)	NF、TG
中足指節関節	MTP joint、MTPJ
中大脳動脈	MCA
中直腸動脈	MRA
中毒性ショック症候群毒素	TSST
中毒性表皮壊死症	TEN
中毒単位	TU
中毒様症候群	TSLS
中波長紫外線	UVB
治癒過程期(胃潰瘍)	Stage H
腸炎ビブリオ	VP
超音波	US
超音波ガイド下経尿道的レーザー前立腺切除(術)	TULIP
超音波検査	US
超音波砕石術	USL
超音波水晶体乳化吸引術	PEA、KPE
超音波断層法	UST
超音波内視鏡検査法	EUS
超音波ネブライザー	USN
聴覚性電気眼球運動図	AOG
聴覚誘発電位	AEP
聴覚誘発反応	AER
長下肢ギプス包帯	LLC
長下肢装具	KAFO、LLB、SKA orthosis
腸管出血性大腸菌	EHEC
腸間膜動脈閉塞症	MAO
長期間救命処置	PLS
長期記憶	LTM
長期血液透析	CHD
長期酸素療法	LTOT
長期床上安静	CBS
蝶形骨洞炎、蝶骨洞炎	S-s
超高比重リポ蛋白	VHDL
腸骨前上棘・果部間距離	SMD
腸雑音	BS
長指屈筋	FDL
腸重積症	INVAGI
長掌筋	PL
朝食前	a.j.
聴神経腫	AN
聴神経腫瘍	AT
聴診と打診	A&P
聴性脳幹反応(聴覚脳幹反応)	BEAR、ABR
調整粉乳	PM
調節環境治療法	CET
調節機械換気	CMV
調節呼吸	CR
腸チフス	TA
超低カロリー食	VLCD
超低比重リポ蛋白	VLDL
長橈側手根伸筋	ECRL
長波長紫外線	UVA
腸閉塞	IO
長母指外転筋	APL

ち

和文	略語
長母指屈筋	FPL
長母指伸筋	EPL
長母趾伸筋	EHL
超未熟児	ELBW
聴力損失、難聴	HL
直視下レーザー前立腺切除術	VLAP
直視下僧帽弁交連切開術	OMC
直視下大動脈弁交連切開術	OAC
直接型ビリルビン	DB
直接凝集妊娠試験	DAPT
直線加速器	linac
直腸S状部	Rs
直腸チューブ	RT
直腸癌	R ca、RK
直腸脱	RP
直流除細動	DC shock
治療	Tx
治療、処置	Tr
治療可能比	TR
治療後TMN分類	Y-TMN
治療指数	TI
治療増強因子	TGF
治療のレーザー角膜切除術	PTK
治療の患者クラブ	TPC
治療の血漿交換	TPE
治療の流産	TAB
治療必要数	NNT
治療薬物モニタリング	TDM
チロシン結合淡白	TBP
沈殿物	Ppt
陳旧性結核	OT
陳旧性心筋梗塞	OMI
陳旧性脳血管障害	OVA
沈降率	Sed rate

つ、て

和文	略語
頭囲	HC
椎間板ヘルニア	HID、PID
椎間板ヘルニア症候群	HDS
椎間板ヘルニア髄核脱出	NPH
椎骨下小脳動脈分岐部動脈瘤	VA-PICA
椎骨動脈	VA
椎骨動脈造影(法)	VAG
椎骨脳底動脈	VBA
椎骨脳底動脈循環不全	VBI
対麻痺	Para
通常型間質性肺炎	UIP
通常体重	USWT
頭痛	HA
頭痛、不眠、うつ	HID
頭殿長	CRL
ツベルクリン反応	TR
手足口病	HFMD
低悪性度腫瘍	LPM
低位前方切除術	LAR
定位脳手術	Stereo
帝王切開	CS
帝王切開による出産	CD
低眼圧緑内障	LTG
低灌流充血	LPH
低吸収濃度域	LDA
低血圧	LBP
低在横定位	OT
低酸素性虚血性脳症	HIE
低子宮頚部帝王切開(術)	LCCS
定時の服薬、24時間療法	RTC
低出生体重児	LBW、LBWI
低進行性インスリン依存性糖尿病	SPIDDM
低心拍出量症候群	LCOS、LOS
低比重リポ蛋白	LDL
低分子蛋白	LMWP
テイラー不安検査(顕在性不安尺度)	MAS
停留睾丸	UDT
定量の冠状動脈造影(法)	QCA
定量の骨塩量測定法	QCT
定量噴霧吸入器	MDI
低レニン血症性低アルドステロン症	SHH
デオキシリボ核酸	DNA
デキサメサゾン抑制試験	DST
デキサメサゾン、高用シタラビン、シスプラチン併用療法	DHAP
適性発育(出生体重)児	AFD

日本語	略語
適用されない、不必要な	NA
デジタル減算(サブトラクション)血管造影法	DSA
デシベル	dB
鉄	Fe
鉄欠乏性貧血	IDA
テトラサイクリン	TC
テトラサイクリン系抗生物質	TCs
テトロドトキシン	TTX
デヒドロ酢酸	DHA
デュシュンヌ型筋ジストロフィー	DMD
デュビン・ジョンソン症候群	D-J syndrome
転移性腎細胞癌	MRC
転移性肺癌	L2
てんかん	Ep、Epi
てんかん重積状態	SE
てんかん大発作	GMS
点眼液	ED
電気眼位図	EOG
電気眼振図	ENG
電気ショック療法	ES
電撃療法	ECT
伝染性海綿上脳症	TSE
伝染性単核球症	IM
伝染性軟属腫	MC
点状表層角膜炎	SPK
点滴	DI
点滴静注腎盂造影	DIP
点滴静注胆管造影法	DIC
点滴静脈内注射	DIV
伝導収縮解離	EMD
点鼻	NB

と

トイレ歩行可	BRP
トータルヘルスプロモーションプラン	THP
ドーパ(ジヒドロキシフェニルアラニン)	DOPA
頭蓋咽頭腫	CRP
頭蓋内血腫	ICH
頭蓋内腫瘍	ICT
洞回復時間	SNRT
頭蓋癆	CT
動悸	pal
同期式間欠的強制呼吸	SIMV
凍結乾燥豚真皮	LPDS
洞結節	SAN、SN
洞結節不全症候群	SSS
糖原病	GSD
瞳孔間距離	PD
統合失調症、シゾ	S、SZ
統合失調症家族歴	SFH
統合失調症残存状態	SRS
統合失調症反応	SR
糖鎖抗原19-9	CA19-9
糖質コルチコイド	GC
同種の	allo
同種骨髄移植	allo-BMT
同種造血幹細胞移植	allo-SCT
同種末梢血幹細胞移植	allo-PBSCT
動静脈の	A-V
動静脈奇形	AVM
動静脈吻合	AVA
動静脈瘻	AVF
洞徐脈	SB
橈側手根屈筋	FCR
橈側手根屈筋腱	FCR
動態撮影	Kymo
到着時心肺停止	CPAA、CPAOA
到着時死亡	DOA
頭頂部の	P
洞調律	SR
疼痛性チック	TD
糖尿病	DM
糖尿病性ケトアシドーシス	DKA
糖尿病性筋萎縮症	DA
糖尿病性糸球体硬化症	DGS
糖尿病性神経症	DN
糖尿病性網膜症	RET、DIAB、DR、DMR
糖尿病母体児	IDM
洞〔性〕頻拍(脈)	ST
頭部外傷	HI
頭部外傷後遺症	PTB

と

和文	略語
洞房ブロック	SA block、SAB
洞房伝導時間	SACT
動脈	A
動脈圧	PA、ABP、AP
動脈管	DA
動脈管開存症	PDA
動脈血	a
動脈血ガス	ABG
動脈血酸素分圧	PaO_2
動脈血酸素飽和度	SaO_2
(パルスオキシメーターによる)動脈血酸素飽和度	SpO_2
動脈血栓症	AT
動脈血炭酸ガス分圧	$PaCO_2$
動脈血中ケトン体比	AKBR
動脈血肺胞気窒素ガス分圧差	$a\text{-}ADN_2$
動脈硬化症	As
動脈硬化性心血管疾患	ASCVD
動脈硬化性疾患	ASHD、AHD
動脈硬化性腎炎	ASN
動脈周囲炎	PA
動脈静脈バイパス	VAB
動脈造影	AG
動脈内	IA
動脈閉塞性疾患	AOD
動脈瘤様骨嚢腫、動脈瘤様骨腫	ABC
透明帯精子注入法	SUZI
同名半盲	HH
ドキソルビシン、タキソテール併用療法	AT
ドキソルビシン、ビンクリスチン、プレドニゾロン併用療法	AdVP
ドキソルビシン、ロムスチン、フルオロウラシル併用療法	ACF
特異的赤血球粘着試験	SRCA
特記すべき疾患なし	NAD
特殊限外濾過法	ECUM
読書年齢	RdA
毒素、抗毒素	TA、TAT
毒素性ショック症候群	TSS
特発性間質性肺炎	IIP
特発性起立性低血圧症	IOH
特発性血小板減少性紫斑病	ITP
特発性呼吸窮迫	IRD
特発性呼吸窮迫症候群	IRDS
特(自)発性細菌性腹膜炎	SBP
特発性心拡大	ICM
特発性心筋疾患	IDM
特発性新生児呼吸障害	IRDNI
特発性全般てんかん	IGE
特発性大腿骨頭壊死	INFH、ION
特発性ネフローゼ症候群	INS
特発性肺ヘモジデリン沈着症	IPH
特発性肺高血圧症	EPH
特発性肺線維症	IPF
特発性肥大型大動脈弁下狭窄症	IHSS
特発性プラズマ細胞性リンパ腺炎	IPL
特発性門脈圧亢進症	IPH
匿名酒害者会	AA
徒手筋力テスト	MMT
ドセタキセル	TXT
突然死	DIE
突発性出血性壊死	SHN
突発性難聴	SD
突発性発疹	ES
ドナーリンパ球輸注	DLT
ドパミン	DA
塗布剤	Lin
トブラマイシン	TOB
トムゼン現象	T
トラコーマ封入体結膜炎	TRIC
ドラッグデリバリーシステム	DDS
トランスファーRNA、転移リボ核酸	tRNA
トリニトログリセリン	TNG
トリヨードサイロニン	T3
努力性吸気肺活量	FIV
努力性吸気流量	FIFx
努力性呼気肺活量	FEV
努力性呼気流量	FEFx
努力性肺活量	FVC
トレッドミル〔運動〕負荷試験	TET

トレポネーマ	Trep
トレポネーマパリダム補体結合テスト、TPCFテスト	TPCF
トロンビン凝固時間	TCT、TT
トロンボポエチン	TPO
鈍縁枝	OM

な

ナースコール	NC
内因性急死	SUD
内頚動脈	ICA、IC
内頚動脈後交通動脈	IC-PC
内頚動脈後交通動脈瘤	ICPC
内視鏡	E
内視鏡下胆道ドレナージ	EBD
内視鏡的逆行性括約筋切開術	ERS
内視鏡的逆行性膵管造影	ERP
内視鏡的逆行性大腸挿入法	ERBIM
内視鏡的逆行性胆管膵管造影	ERCP
内視鏡的逆行性胆管造影	ERC
内視鏡的逆行性胆管内瘻術	ERBE
内視鏡的逆行性胆道ドレナージ	ERBD
内視鏡的逆行性胆嚢胆管ドレナージ	ERGBD
内視鏡的経鼻膵管ドレナージ	ENPD
内視鏡的経鼻膵胆管ドレナージ	ENPBD
内視鏡的経鼻胆管ドレナージ	ENBD
内視鏡的経鼻胆嚢ドレナージ	ENGBO
内視鏡的硬化(薬剤注入)療法	EIS、Sclero
内視鏡的静脈瘤結紮術	EVL
内視鏡的食道静脈瘤硬化療法	Evs
内視鏡的膵石破砕術	EPL
内視鏡的膵胆管造影法	EPCG
内視鏡的超音波カラー・ドプラー法	ECDUS
内視鏡的乳頭括約筋切開術	EST
内視鏡的乳頭切開術	EPT
内視鏡的乳頭バルーン拡張	EPBP
内視鏡的粘膜切除術	EMR
内耳道	IAM
内斜視	ET、ST
内旋	IR
内臓幼虫移行症	VLM

に

内側側副靭帯	MCL
内側半月	MM
内腸骨動脈	IIA
内転、内反	ADD、Add
内毒素	ET
内反尖足	TEV
内用	ad.us.int.
ナチュラルキラー細胞	NK cell
ナトリウム	Na
ナトリウム-カリウムポンプ	Na-K pump
生ワクチン	LV
軟膏	Ug、Ung
軟骨肉腫	CS
難聴	HOH
軟部腫瘍	SPT

に

肉眼の癌口側断端	OW
肉眼の肝転移の程度の分類	H0〜3
肉眼の腹膜播種性転移の程度の分類	P0〜3
肉眼の肛門側断端癌浸潤の有無	AW (＋),(−) (anal wedge ＋,−)
ニコチン酸アデニンジヌクレオチド	NAD
二次救命処置	ALS
二次循環救命処置	ACLS
二次性全般化てんかん	SGE
二段脈	big
日常生活動作	ADL
日光角化症	AK
日光蕁麻疹	SoU
日数不当重量児	LFD infant
日本骨髄バンク	JMDP
日本昏睡スケール	JCS
日本脳炎	JE
二点識別テスト	TPD test
二頭筋反射	BTR

に

日本語	略語
ニトラゼパム	NZP
ニトログリセリン	NG、NTG
ニューモシスチス肺炎	PCP
ニューヨーク心臓協会心機能分類	NYHA
ニューロレプト麻酔	NLA
入院	Adm
入院と退院	A&D
乳癌（マンマ）	MMK
乳酸脱水素酵素	LDH
乳酸蓄積閾値	OBLA
乳児壊死性脳脊髄障害	INE
乳児自閉症	IA
乳児重症ミオクローヌスてんかん	SME、SMEI
乳児突然死症候群	SIDS
乳汁漏出・無月経症候群	AGS
乳糖	SL
乳頭筋	PM
乳頭腫、パピローマ	Pap
乳頭状新生血管	NYD
乳腺癌	PAC
乳房撮影法、マンモグラフィー	MMG
乳房自己検査法	SBE
乳房自己検診	BSE
乳房腫瘍	BT
乳房生検	BB
乳幼児突発性危急事態	ALTE
尿	Hr
尿/血漿濃度比	U/P
尿ウロビリノーゲン	UU
尿管腎盂結合部	UPJ
尿管膀胱結合部	UVJ
尿細管間質性腎炎	TIN
尿細管基底膜	TBM
尿細管腔液	TF
尿細管最大輸送量	Tm
尿細管糖再吸収極量	TmG
尿細管排泄率	TRFR
尿細管無機リン再吸収量	TRP
尿酸	U、UA
尿生殖器の	GU
尿潜血	UB
尿素	U
尿素窒素	UN
尿蛋白	UP
尿中ナトリウム排泄率	FENa
尿糖	US
尿道造影法	UG
尿道膀胱造影法	UCG
尿崩症	DI
尿量	UO、UQ、UV
尿路	UT
尿路感染症	UTI
尿路奇形	UTM
尿路結石	UTS
二卵性双生児	DZ
任意の量	qp
妊娠	preg、Sgt、SS
妊娠高血圧（症）	PIH、PAH、HIP
妊娠週数	GA
妊娠性掻痒性丘疹	PPP
妊娠性掻痒性蕁麻疹様丘疹兼局面症	PUPPP
妊娠性疱疹、妊娠性ヘルペス	HG
妊娠糖尿病	GDM
妊娠末期骨盤位外回転術	LECV
認知療法	CT

ね、の

熱傷指数	BI
熱性痙攣	FC
熱帯性痙性不全対麻痺	TSP
熱帯性肺好酸球増多症	TPE
ネフローゼ症候群	NS
年	Yr
捻髪音	crep
粘膜下	sm
粘膜下腫瘍	SMT
粘膜下層までの癌（壁深達度）	sm癌
粘膜下鼻中隔切除（術）	SMR
粘膜関連リンパ組織	MALT
粘膜筋板	mm
粘膜上皮内	ep
粘膜性潰瘍性大腸炎	MUC
粘膜層の癌（壁深達度）	m癌
粘膜皮膚眼症候群	MCOS

和文	略語
脳幹反応	BER
脳肝腎症候群	CHRS
脳灌流圧	CPP
脳器質症候群	OBS
脳血液量	CBV
脳血管造影	CAG
脳血管疾患	CVD
脳血管障害	CVA
脳血管性痴呆	VD
脳血栓	CT
脳血流量	CBF
脳梗塞	CI
脳酸素代謝率	CMRO₂
脳死	BD
脳室圧	VP
脳室撮影	VG
脳室周囲白質軟化症	PVL
脳室上衣下出血	SEH
脳室心房シャント	VAS
脳室心房短絡術	V-A shunt
脳室内出血	IVH
脳室腹腔短絡術	V-P shunt
脳出血	HC
脳腫瘍	BT
脳障害なし	NBD
脳神経	CN
脳性小児麻痺	CP
脳性麻痺	CP
脳静脈造影	CVG
脳脊髄液	CFS、CSF
脳脊髄膜炎	CSM
脳組織圧	BTP
脳卒中	Apo
脳代謝率	CMR
脳底動脈	BA
脳底動脈頂点動脈瘤	BA top
脳転移	BRA
能動抵抗運動	ARE
脳内出血	ICH
脳波	EEG
脳波聴力検査	EEG audiometry
脳ブドウ糖代謝率	CMR glu
脳閉塞症	CE
脳閉塞性血栓血管炎	CTO
囊胞性線維症	CF
囊胞様黄斑浮腫	CME
脳梁	CC
ノルアドレナリン	NA
ノルエピネフリン	NE
ノンストレステスト	NST
ノンレム睡眠、徐波睡眠	NREM、NREM-sleep

は

和文	略語
パーキンソン症候群	PKN
パーキンソン認知症	PD
パーキンソン認知症症候群	PDC
パーキンソン病	PD
肺移植	LTX
胚移植	ET
梅毒	VDS
バイパップ、二相性陽圧呼吸	BiPAP
肺炎	Pn
肺芽異形成神経上皮腫瘍	DNT
肺拡散能力	DL
肺活量	VC
背下部	LB
肺癌	LC
肺癌治療効果の組織学的判定基準を示す記号	Ef0-3
肺気腫	PE
肺機能	PF
肺機能検査	LFT、PFT
配偶者間人工授精	AIH
肺結核	PP
肺血管造影	PAG
肺血管抵抗	PVR
肺血管閉塞性病変	PVOD
敗血症性肺水腫	SPE
肺血流量	PBF、PBV

は

和文	略語
肺高血圧(症)	PAH、PH、PHT
胚細胞腫	G
肺シャント率	QS/QT
肺塞栓症	PE
肺疾患	PD
肺静脈	PV
肺静脈うっ血	PVC
肺静脈還流異常	APVC
肺静脈閉塞	PVO
肺性心	CP
排泄性尿路造影	XU
肺中葉	ML
肺動脈	PA
肺動脈(弁)狭窄症	PS
肺動脈圧	PAP
肺動脈拡張期圧	PADP
肺動脈拡張終期圧	PAEDP
肺動脈血栓塞栓(症)	PTE
肺動脈血流量	QPA
肺動脈絞扼術	PAB
肺動脈閉鎖症	PA
肺動脈弁	PV
肺動脈弁開放速度	PVOV
肺動脈弁逆流(症)	PR
肺動脈弁狭窄兼閉鎖不全症	PSR
肺動脈弁置換術	PTR
肺動脈弁閉鎖不全(症)	PR、PI
肺動脈楔入圧	PAWP、PCWP
梅毒	L
梅毒血清反応	STS
梅毒性心疾患	LHD
梅毒トレポネーマ	TP
梅毒トレポネーマ血球凝集反応	TPHA
梅毒トレポネーマ・パリダム感作血球凝集テスト	TPHA
肺内ガス混合指数	PMI
排尿後残尿量	PVR
排尿時膀胱造影	VCG、MCG
排尿時膀胱尿道造影(法)	VUG
排尿量	Vv
背腹方向	DV
背部の	D
排便、便通	BM
肺胞気-動脈血酸素分圧差	A-aDO$_2$
肺胞気酸素濃度	F$_A$O$_2$
肺胞気炭酸ガス濃度	F$_A$CO$_2$
肺胞上皮癌	ACC
肺胞毛細管ブロック症候群	AC
肺毛細血管	PC
排卵誘発ホルモン	OIH
ハウスダスト	HD
破壊性脊椎関節症	DSA
白色上皮	W
白内障	Cat
剥離性間質性肺炎	DIP
白蠟病	VWF
播種状掌蹠孔角化症	PPPD
播種性血管内凝固症候群	DIC
播種性紅斑性狼瘡	LED
破傷風免疫グロブリン	TIG
破水	ROM
パスタ(泥膏)〔剤〕	Past
バソトシン	VT
バソプレシン	VP
発育異常緑内障	DG
発育性股関節脱臼	DDH
発育遅延児	SGA
発育良好	WD
はっきりした異常なし	NAA
白血球(数)	WBC
白血球エステラーゼテスト	LET
白血球除去赤血球	LPRC
白血球接着不全症	LAD
白血球破壊性血管炎	LCV
白血球分類	CD
抜糸	SR、DSO
発達指数	DQ
発痛物質	PPS
鼻-胆囊チューブ	N-B
鼻ポリープ	NP
パニック障害、恐怖症候群	PD
バニリルマンデル酸	VMA
母親	Mo
パパニコロー試験	Pap test
パパニコロー染色法	PAP

ひ

和文	略語
パパニコロー標本	Pap smear
ハプトグロビン	Hp
ハミルトンうつ病評価尺度	HDS、HAM-D
パラアミノ馬尿酸	PAH
パラアミノ馬尿酸塩の尿細管排泄極量	TmPAH
パラノイア	Pa
バリウム	Ba
バリウム注腸検査	BE
バルーンカテーテル閉塞下肝動脈造影	BOHA
バルーンカテーテル閉塞下肺血管造影	BOPA
バルーン心房中隔裂開術	BAS
バルーン閉塞下動注法	BOAI
反回神経	RLN
半規管機能低下	CP
パンクレオザイミン・セクレチン試験	PS test
バンコマイシン耐性腸球菌	VRE
バンコマイシン低感受性黄色ブドウ球菌	VISA
瘢痕期（胃潰瘍）	Stage S
反射	ref
反射性交感神経性ジストロフィー	RSD
伴性遺伝性魚鱗癬	XLI
伴性劣性遺伝	SR
汎小葉型肺気腫	PE
半側顔面痙攣	HFS
ハンチントン舞踏病	HC
汎動脈炎	PA
反応・ショック間隔	R-S
反応性リンパ細網細胞増成（症）	RLH
反応率	RR
晩発性小脳皮質萎縮症	LCCA
晩発性皮膚ポルフィリン症	PCT
反復時間	TI
反復性緊張障害	RSI
ハンフリー自動視野計灌流吸引チップ	Hu
半分、半分の	ss
汎網膜光凝固	PRP

ひ

和文	略語
非A非B肝炎	NANB、NANBH
ヒアルロン酸	HA
非アレルギー性好酸球増多性鼻炎症候群	NARES
ピークフロー、最大流量	PF
鼻咽頭癌	NPC
皮下（注射）	Hypo-、SC、sc
非開胸心マッサージ	CCM、CCCC
非潰瘍性消化不良	NUD
皮下トンネル感染	TI
皮下（第3度）熱傷	DB
皮下の	sub-Q、subcu-、subcut
非観血的整復	CR
非器質性発育不良症候群	NFTT
被虐待児症候群	BCS
非経口の栄養補給、静脈栄養	PN
非痙攣性てんかん	NCE
非ケトン性高浸透圧性昏睡	NHC
肥厚性幽門狭窄症	HPS
非硬変症性門脈線維症	NCPF
非細菌性咽頭炎	NBP
非細菌性血栓性心内膜炎	NBTE
微細脳損傷（症候群）	MBD
ピシバニール	PIC
肘反射	EJ
比重	SG
微小血管障害性溶血性貧血	MHA
微小残存病変（腫瘍）	MRD
微小浸潤癌	MIC
微小変化群	LN、MC
微小変化型ネフローゼ症候群	MCNS
微小脳障害	MBD
微小発破砕石術	MEL
微小変化型ネフローゼ症候群	MLNS
脾静脈	SV
非心原性胸痛	NCCP
非心原性浮腫	NCE

ひ

和文⇒略語

日本語	略語
ヒス−心室時間	HV interval
ヒス束心電図	HBE
ヒステリー	Hy
非ステロイド系抗炎症薬	NSAID
鼻洗	NS
肥大型硬髄膜炎	CHP
肥大型心筋症	HCM
肥大型閉塞性心筋症	HOCM
非対称性緊張性頚反射	ATNR
非対称性心室中隔肥大	ASH
左の	S
ビタミン	Vit
ビタミンB	VB
ビタミンC	VC
ビタミンK非存在下誘導蛋白	PIVKA
左	L
左耳	AS
非蛋白性窒素	NPN
非チアノーゼ性先天性心疾患	NCCHD
鼻中隔矯正術	SMR
鼻中弯曲症	DSN
非直視下僧帽弁交連切開術	CMC
ピック病	PD
必須アミノ酸	EAA
必要ある時	Sos
非定型抗酸菌	AAFB
非定型抗酸菌症	AM
非定型精神病	ATP
非定形性白血病	DMPS
脾摘痕重症感染症	OPSI
脾動脈	SA
非特異性反応性肝炎	NSRH
ヒト絨毛性ゴナドトロピン	HCG、hCG
ヒト絨毛性乳腺刺激ホルモン	hCS
ヒト赤血球濃厚液	MAP
ヒト胎盤性ラクトゲン	hPL
ヒトT細胞白血病ウイルス	HTLV
ヒトT細胞リンパ行性ウイルス1型	HTLV-1
ヒト乳頭腫ウイルス	HPV
ヒトにおけるメンデル遺伝	MIM
ヒト白血球抗原	HLA
ヒト閉経期尿性ゴナドトロピン	hMG
ヒト免疫不全性ウイルス、エイズ	HIV
泌尿器科、泌尿器科学	Uro
非配偶者間人工授精	AID
非必須アミノ酸	NEAA
皮膚移植	SG
皮膚エリテマトーデス	CLE
皮膚筋炎	DM
皮膚結節性動脈周囲炎	PNC
皮膚試験	ST
皮膚転移	SKI
皮膚T細胞性リンパ腫	CTCL
皮膚電気活動	EDA
皮膚良性リンパ腺腫症	LABC、LBC
鼻閉	NO、NV
非閉塞性肥大型心筋症	HNCM
非抱合ビリルビン	UB
非ホジキンリンパ腫	NHL
肥満指数	BMI
肥満性低換気症候群	OHS
びまん性間質性線維化肺炎	DIFP
びまん性気管支拡張症	DBE
びまん性糸球体腎炎	DGN
びまん性軸索損傷	DAI
びまん性増殖性ループス腎炎	DOLN
びまん性増殖性糸球体腎炎	DPGN
びまん性転移性骨髄膜癌腫症	DMLC
びまん性肺疾患	DPD
びまん性肺胞障害	DAD
びまん性汎細気管支炎	DPB
びまん性表層角結膜炎	KSD
非免疫性胎児水腫	NIHF
百日咳毒素	PTX
百万分量単位中の絶対数	ppm
ヒュー・ジョーンズ分類	H-J
病原性大腸菌	EPEC
表在性黒色腫	SSM
標準(模擬)患者	SP
標準化死亡比	SMR
標準誤差	SE
標準失語症検査	SLTA
標準代謝率	SMR
標準注射針ゲージ	SWG
標準偏差	SD
表皮脂質	SSL

和文	略語
表皮水疱症	EB
表皮熱傷	EB
病歴要約	SR
日和見感染症	OI
びらん	Er
ピルビン酸脱水素酵素(欠損症)	PDHC
ビルロートⅡ法	B-Ⅱ
ビルロートⅠ法	B-Ⅰ
頻脈	tachy

ふ

和文	略語
ファイバー気管支鏡検査	FBS
ファロー3徴症	Tri/F
ファロー4徴症	TF
不安神経症	AN
不安定狭心症	UA(P)
不安定ヘモグロビン症	UHD
不安定膀胱	USB
部位不明出血	BUO
フィブリン(/フィブリノーゲン)分解産物	FDP
フィラデルフィア染色体	Ph⁺, Ph1
フェイススケール	FS
フェニトイン	PHT
フェニルケトン尿症	PKU
フェノールスルホンフタレイン(PSP排泄)試験	PSP (test)
フェノバルビタール	PB
フォークト-小柳-原田病	VKH
不応性貧血	RA
フォン・ウィルブランド病	VW
不快指数	DI
不完全右脚ブロック	IRBBB
不完全左脚ブロック	ILBBB
腹圧性尿失禁	SUI
腹囲	AC、ac、AG
腹会陰式直腸切除術	APR
腹腔鏡下総胆管切石術	LCL
腹腔鏡下胆嚢摘出術(ラパコレ)	LC、LSC、LSCT
腹腔鏡下レーザー胆嚢摘出術	LLC
腹腔鏡検査	Lapa (ro)
腹腔鏡補助下子宮摘出術	LAVH
腹腔鏡補助下大腸切除術	LAC
腹腔―静脈短絡術	P-V shunt
腹腔神経叢ブロック	CPB
腹腔動脈	CA
腹腔内の	IP
副交感神経系	PNS、PSNS
副甲状腺ホルモン	PTH
副甲状腺機能低下―アジソン―モニリア症候群	HAM syndrome
副甲状腺全摘出術	PTX
複合免疫不全	CID
伏在静脈バイパス移植	SVBG
複雑部分てんかん重積発作	CPSE
複雑部分発作	CPS
腹式子宮全摘出術	TAH
腹式子宮単純全摘術	ATH
腹式子宮摘出術	AH
副腎髄質	AdM
副腎性器症候群	AGS
副腎脊髄神経障害	AMN
副腎白質ジストロフィ	ALD
副腎皮質	ADC、AC
副腎皮質ステロイド	GCS
副腎皮質癌	ACC
副腎皮質機能不全	ACI
副腎皮質刺激ホルモン	ACTH
副腎皮質刺激ホルモン放出ホルモン	CRH
副腎皮質腺腫、アルドステロン産生腫瘍	APA
副腎を摘出した	Adrex、ADS
腹水	AF
副鼻腔炎	Empy
腹部、腹部の	abd
腹部外傷スコア	ATS
腹周囲/殿囲比	W/H
腹部食道	Ea
腹部前後径	APD
腹部大動脈瘤	AAA

ふ

和文	略語
腹部皮弁	AF
腹壁反射	BDR
腹膜	P
腹膜機能検査	PET
腹膜転移	PER
腹膜透析	PD
福山型先天性筋ジストロフィー	FCMD
服用	Zn
浮腫、蛋白尿、高血圧(妊娠中毒症)	EPH
婦人科(ギネ)	GYN
不随意運動	IVM
不随伴の臨床所見	ACF
不正性器出血	DUB
不整脈	CA
不全型(分類困難な)膠原病	UCTD
付属器	Ad
物理学的半減期	Tp
不適例	UCF
ブドウ球菌	Staph
ブドウ球菌性中毒性表皮壊死性融解症	S-TEN
ブドウ球菌性腸毒素F	SEF
ブドウ球菌性熱傷様皮膚症候群	SSSS
不当軽量児	SFD
不当重量児	LFD
不当低体重児	SFD infant
ブドウ糖	Glu、glu
ブドウ糖インスリン負荷試験	GITT
ブドウ糖負荷試験	GTT
舞踏病-有棘赤血球症	CA
部分	P
部分荷重	PWB
部分寛解	PR
部分的回腸バイパス術	PIB
部分的心肺補助装置	PCPS
部分的肺静脈還流異常	PAPVC、PAPVR
部分的脾動脈塞栓術	PSE
部分てんかん	PE
部分トロンボプラスチン時間	PTT
部分肺静脈還流異常	PAPVD
不変、特記事項なし、特別に変化のないこと	NC
不飽和鉄結合能	UIBC
フムサルファレイン試験	BSP test
プライマリヘルスケア	PHC
ブラロック・タウシッヒ短絡術	B-T shunt
ブランド-ホワイト-ガーランド症候群	BWG
フリクテン性角膜結膜炎	PKC
振子様回転検査	PRT
フルオロウラシル、アドリアマイシン、シクロホルファミド併用療法	FAC
フルオロウラシル、アドリアマイシン、マイトマイシンC併用療法	FAM
フルオロウラシル、アドリアマイシン、メトトレキセート併用療法	FAM
フルオロウラシル、エピルビシン、マイトマイシンC併用療法	FEM
フルオロウラシル、シクロホスファミド、マイトマイシン、トヨマイシン併用療法	FAMT
フルオロウラシル、シスプラチン併用療法	FP
フルクトサミン	FA
ブレオマイシン、イホスファミド、シスプラチン併用療法	BIP
ブレオマイシン、エンドキサン、6-MP、プレドニン併用療法	BENP
ブレオマイシン、オンコビン、ナツラン、プレドニゾロン併用療法	BONP
ブレオマイシン、シクロホスファミド、アクチノマイシンD併用療法	BCD
ブレオマイシン、ビンクリスチン、シクロホスファミド、プレドニゾロン併用療法	BVCP
ブレオマイシン、ビンクリスチン、マイトマイシンC、シスプラチン併用療法	BOMP

プレドニゾロン	PDN、PSL	閉塞肝静脈圧	WHVP
		閉塞性黄疸	OJ
プレドニゾロンブドウ糖負荷試験	PGTT	閉塞性気管支閉気管支炎	BBO
プロゲステロン	OYL	閉塞性気道障害	OAD
プロスタグランジン	PG	閉塞性血栓(性)脈管炎	TO、TAO
プロスタグランジンE1	PGE1	閉塞性細気管支炎	BO
プロトロンビン時間	PT	閉塞性細気管支炎器質化肺炎	BOOP
プロトンポンプ阻害薬	PPI	閉塞性睡眠時無呼吸症候群	OSAS
プロラクチン	PL、PRL	閉塞性動脈硬化症	ASO
プロラクチン放出因子	PRF	ペースメーカー	PM
プロラクチン放出抑制ホルモン	PIH	ペースメーカー植え込み術	PMI
プロラクチン放出抑制因子	PIF	ベータ遮断薬	BB
プロラクチン抑制因子	PIF	ベクトル心電図	VCG
吻合部ポリープ状肥厚性胃炎	SPHG	ベタメサゾン	Bm
分時換気量	MV、VE	ベッカー型進行性筋ジストロフィー	BMD
分枝鎖アミノ酸	BCAA	ペニシリン	PC
文章完成法	SCT	ペニシリンG	PCG
分腎機能比	SFR	ペニシリンV	PCV
分層植皮術	STG	（フェノキシメチルペニシリン）	
分娩後出血	PPH	ペニシリン結合蛋白	PBP
分娩予定日	CDC、EDC、TC	ヘノッホ・シェーンライン紫斑病	HSP
		ヘマトクリット値	Ht
噴門部	C	ヘモグロビン(血色素)	Hb
分類不能腫瘍	uc	ヘモグロビンA1c	HbA1c
		ヘリコバクターピロリ	HP
		ヘルツ	Hz
ヘア・アン症候群	HAIR-An syndrome	ヘルパーTリンパ球	Th
		ベル麻痺	BP
平滑筋細胞	SMC	ベロ毒素産生性大腸菌	VTEC
平均血圧	MABP、MBP	便	kot
		変形性関節疾患	DJD
平均循環時間	MTT	変形性関節症	OA
平均身体投与量	ABD	変形性筋ジストニー	DND
平均腎血流量	MRBF	変形性脊椎症	SD
平均赤血球ヘモグロビン(血色素)濃度	MCHC	ベンス・ジョーンズ蛋白	BJP
		ベンス・ジョーンズ尿蛋白	BJP
平均赤血球ヘモグロビン(血色素)量	MCH	変性	DEG
		変性関節炎	DA
平均赤血球容積	MCV	片側痙攣片麻痺てんかん	HHE
平均肺動脈圧	mPAP	片側性肺門リンパ節腫大	UHL
閉経後出血	PMB	片側肺換気	ILV
閉経後症候群	PMS	便通正常	BOR
閉経後卵巣腫大	PMPO	扁桃周囲膿瘍	PTA
米国病院医療評価機構	JCAHO	扁桃腺、小脳扁桃	AM
閉鎖密封療法	ODT		

へ

扁桃摘出（術）とアデノイド切除（術）	T＆A
扁平円柱上皮境界	SCJ
扁平上皮	S
扁平上皮癌	SCC、sq

ほ

縫合（単数）	sut
縫合（複数）	sutt
膀胱	UB
膀胱鏡	CS
膀胱頸部狭窄症	BNC
膀胱腫瘍	BT
膀胱造影	CG
膀胱内圧測定	CMG
膀胱尿管逆流現象	VUR
膀胱尿管結合部	VUJ
膀胱尿道造影法	CUG
膀胱留置カテーテル	BT
傍糸球体装置	JGA
房室	A-V、AV
房室回帰性頻拍	AVRT
房室管孔欠損	AVCD
房室結節	AV node、AVN
房室伝導時間	PQ
房室ブロック	AV block
房室弁	AVV
放射受容体測定	RRA
放射状角膜切開術	RK
放射性アレルギー吸着試験	RAST
放射性ヨード	RAI
放射性ヨード摂取試験	RAIU
放射性乳頭周囲血管炎	RPC
放射性免疫吸着試験	RIST
放射線医学	Radiol
放射線化学療法	CRT
放射線学的診断	Rad DX
放射線効果	RR
放射線全身照射	TBI
放射線治療学	TR
放射線治療計画	RTP
放射線免疫沈降法	RIP
放射線誘発肝疾患	RILvD
放射線誘発肺疾患	RILD
放射線療法	RT
放出ホルモン	RH
胞状奇胎	Mole
傍正中橋網様体	PPRF
包帯交換	DC
乏突起膠腫	OLG
ボールマンの胃癌分類	Borr Ⅰ〜Ⅳ
飽和の	satd
飽和回復法	SR
保健師	PHN
ホジキン病	HD
ポジトロン断層シンチグラフィー	PET
母指外転筋	ADP
補助機械換気	AMV
補助呼吸法	AR
補助人工心臓	VAS、VAD
ボストン失語診断検査	BDAE
補体	C
補体結合反応	CF
母体搬送	MT
補体レセプター	CR
ボタロー管切断術	PDA-division
勃起障害	ED
発作の、痙攣の	parox
発作性寒冷ヘモグロビン（血色素）尿症	PCH
発作性上室性頻拍	PST、PSVT
発作性心室性頻拍	PVT
発作性心房細動	PAF
発作性心房性頻拍	PAT
発作性頻脈	PT
発作性夜間ヘモグロビン（血色素）尿症	PNH
発作性夜間呼吸困難	PND
発作頻度	SF
発赤所見	RC sign
母乳	MM
骨と関節	B＆J
母斑細胞母斑	NCN
ホモバニリン酸	HVA
ポリープ	Po

ポリオ後症候群	PPS	末梢静脈栄養	PVN
ポリメラーゼ連鎖反応	PCR	末梢挿入中心静脈カテーテル	PICC
ホルモン補充療法	HRT	末先端部黒子型黒色腫	ALM
本態性高血圧症	EH	末端感覚	TS
本態性腎出血	ERB	松葉杖歩行	CW
本態性不応性鉄芽球性貧血	IRSA	麻痺性イレウス	CI
		麻痺量	PD
		丸山ワクチン	SSM
ま		マロリーワイス症候群	M-W syndrome
毎朝	Qm		
マイクロ波凝固療法	MCT	満期産生存児	TBLU
マイコプラズマ肺炎	MPP	満期出産、出生児	TBLC
毎時	qh	満期正常経腟分娩	FTNVD
毎週	Qw	満期正常自然分娩	FTNSD
毎食後	ndE	満期正常分娩、満期産	FTND、TND
毎分呼吸数	BPM、bpm		
		慢性アルコール性膵炎	CAP
毎分心拍数	BPM、bpm	慢性萎縮性胃炎	CAG
		慢性咽頭炎	PC
毎夜	Qn	慢性円板状エリテマトーデス	CDLE
膜性ループス腎炎	MLN	慢性炎症性脱髄性多発根ニューロパチー（神経症）	CIDP
膜性糸球体腎炎	MGN		
膜性腎症	MN	慢性潰瘍性大腸炎	CUC
膜性増殖性糸球体腎炎	MPGN	慢性活動性肝炎	CAH
マグネシウム	Mg	慢性活動性肝疾患	CALD
マクロファージコロニー刺激因子	M-CSF	慢性化膿性中耳炎	OMPC
		慢性化膿性副鼻腔炎	Sppc
麻疹、風疹ワクチン	MR	慢性過敏性症候群	CHS
麻疹・流行性耳下腺炎・風疹混合ワクチン	MMR	慢性顆粒球性白血病	CGL
		慢性感染性心内膜炎	CBE
麻酔後の回復	PAR	慢性肝炎	CH
麻酔後回復ユニット	PARU	慢性肝疾患	CLD
麻酔後回復室	PACU	慢性肝性脳症	CHE
末期胃癌	AGC	慢性冠動脈不全	CCI
末期腎不全	ESRD、ESRF	慢性期	CP
		慢性気管支炎	CB
マックバーニー圧痛点	McB	慢性器質性脳症候群	COBS
末梢血幹細胞移植	PBSCT	慢性気道閉塞	CAO
末梢血管疾患	PVD	慢性光線過敏性皮膚炎	CPD
末梢血管抵抗	PVR	慢性光線皮膚炎	CAD
末梢血白血球	PWBC	慢性喉頭炎	LC
末梢血リンパ球	PBL	慢性好中球性白血病	CNL
末梢神経	PN	慢性後天性真性赤血球系無形成症	CAPRCA
末梢神経系	PNS		
末梢神経障害	PNP		
末梢静脈圧	PVP		

慢性硬膜下血腫	CSH、CSDH
慢性呼吸器疾患	CRD
慢性呼吸不全	CRF
慢性骨髄性白血病	CML
慢性骨髄増殖性疾患	CMPD
慢性骨髄単球性白血病	CHMOL、CMMoL、CMML
慢性細菌性前立腺炎	CBP
慢性糸球体腎炎	CG、CGN
慢性持続性肝炎	CPH
慢性腎盂腎炎	CPN、CP
慢性進行性外眼筋麻痺	CPEO
慢性進行性多発性関節炎	PCE
慢性進行性ミエロパチー	CPM
慢性腎疾患	CRD
慢性心不全	CHF
慢性腎不全	CRF
慢性膵炎	CP
慢性精神分裂病(統合失調症)	CS
慢性脊髄性筋萎縮症	CSMA
慢性増殖性糸球体腎炎	CPGN
慢性代謝性アシドーシス	CMA
慢性単球性白血病	CMoL
慢性胆道閉塞症	COBT
慢性動脈閉塞	CAO
慢性特発性再発性多発神経症	CIRPN
慢性特発性腸管仮性閉塞症	CIIP
慢性肉芽腫症	CGD
慢性尿細管間質性腎炎	CTN
慢性の	chr
慢性脳血管疾患	CCVD
慢性脳症候群	CBS
慢性肺気腫	CPE
慢性肺疾患	CLD
慢性肺性心	CCP
慢性白血病	CL
慢性非化膿性破壊性胆管炎	CNSDC
慢性非活動性肝炎	CIH
慢性非細菌性前立腺炎	CNP
慢性非特異性肺疾患	CNSLD
慢性疲労症候群	CFS
慢性疲労免疫異常症候群	CFIDS
慢性皮膚エリテマトーデス	CCLE
慢性皮膚粘膜カンジダ症	CMCC
慢性副鼻腔炎	CS
慢性腹膜透析	CPD
慢性閉塞性気管支炎	COB
慢性閉塞性気道疾患	COAD
慢性閉塞性肺疾患	COPD、COLD
慢性有結石胆囊炎	CCC
慢性溶血性貧血	CHA
慢性リンパ性白血病	CLL

み、む

ミオクローヌスてんかん	ME
右	R
右下肢	RLE
右耳	AD
短い胎児心拍数基線細変動	STV
未熟児	PI
未熟児の持続性呼吸障害	PPDP
未熟児慢性肺機能不全	CPIP
未熟児網膜症	ROP
水	aq.
未然型乳児突然死症候群	nearmiss
	SIDS
ミネソタ多面的人格検査	MMPI
未分化型リンパ性リンパ腫	PDLL
未分化癌	ud
未分化神経外胚葉(性)腫瘍	PNET
ミミズ腫れ様所見	RWM
脈圧	PP
脈管膜毛細管性糸球体腎炎	MCGN
脈拍	P
脈拍数	PR
脈絡膜剝離	CD
ミュンスター式果部荷重下腿義足	KBN
無βリポ蛋白症	ABL
無影響量	NEL、NOEL
無菌室	LAFR
無菌性壊死	AN
無菌溶液	SS
無血管性大腿骨頭壊死症	ANF
無呼吸指数	AI
ムコ多糖体(沈着)症	MPS

無腫瘍期	TFI
無症候性キャリア	AC、ASC
無症候性細菌尿	ABU
無症候性心筋虚血	SMI
無条件刺激	UCS
無条件反射	UCR
無毒性量	NOAEL
無抑制収縮	UIC

め

メープルシロップ尿症	MSUD
メサンギウム性増殖性糸球体腎炎	MPGN
メサンギウム性増殖性糸球体腎炎	MPN
メチシリン耐性黄色ブドウ球菌	MRSA
メッツ(安静時の酸素摂取量 = 1 MET)	METS
メトトレキサート(メソトレキセート)	MTX
メトトレキセート、アクチノマイシンD、エトポシド、ロイコボリン併用療法	EMA-CC
メニエール症候群	MS
メニエール病	MD
メラス型ミトコンドリア脳筋症	MELAS
メラニン細胞刺激ホルモン	MSH
メラノトロピン放出抑制ホルモン	MIH
免疫芽球性リンパ腺症	IBL
免疫芽球性肉腫	IBS
免疫グロブリン	Ig
免疫グロブリンA	IgA
免疫グロブリンG	IgG
免疫グロブリンM	IgM
免疫性胎児水腫	IHF
免疫反応性インスリン	IRI
免疫不全症候群	IDS
免疫抑制薬	ISD
免荷	NWB

も

毛細血管	c
毛細血管拡張性運動失調	AT
毛細管浸透圧	COP
毛細血管瘤	MA
毛状細胞性白血病	HCL
網状赤血球	Ret
盲腸	C
網膜黄斑	YS
網膜芽細胞腫	RB
網膜色素上皮	RPE
網膜色素変性症	Pig deg
網膜静脈分枝閉塞症	BRVO
網膜神経線維束	RNFL
網膜中心静脈閉塞症	CRVO
網膜電図	ERG
網膜剥離	RD
網膜中心動脈閉塞症	CRAO
網様体	RB
毛様体	CB
沐浴	TB
モザイク	M
モズリー性格検査	MPI
モノアミン酸化酵素	MAO
問題思考型診療録	POMR
問題思考型システム	POS
門脈	VP
門脈圧亢進症	PHT
門脈下大静脈吻合(術)	PCS
門脈肝炎	PH
門脈血栓症	PVT
門脈血流量	PVF
門脈臍部	UP
門脈静脈	PV
門脈大静脈吻合	PCA

や、ゆ

夜間陰茎勃起(現象)	NPT
薬剤性大腸炎	DIC
薬剤誘発性過敏性腎炎	DIHN
矢状面	S
矢田部・ギルフォード性格検査	Y-G test
有核細胞数	NCC
有効肝血流量	EHBF
有効半減期	Teff
有効不応期	ERP
有効量	ED
夕食前	a.p.
有熱時	ad.feb.

ゆ

幽門狭窄症	PS
幽門形成術	PP
幽門側胃切除	DPG
幽門輪温存膵頭十二指腸切除術	PPPD、PpPD
幽門輪保存胃切除術	PPG
遊離脂肪酸	FFA、UFA
輸血	BT、BTF
輸血関連移殖片対宿主病	TA-GVHD
輸血関連性肺障害	TRALI
輸血後肝炎	PTH
癒着	ADH
緩やかな胎児心拍数基線細変動	LTV

よ

陽圧換気	PPV
陽圧呼吸	PPB
（自動）陽陰圧呼吸装置	PNPV
陽陰圧呼吸法	PNPB
溶液	Sol
溶血性尿毒症症候群	HUS
溶血性貧血	HA
葉状魚鱗癬	LI
羊水	AF
羊水過量吸引症候群	MAAS
羊水塞栓症	AFE
羊水量	AFV
陽性支持反射	PSR
陽性反応の中度	PVP
容積	Vol
腰仙部、腰仙椎、腰仙髄	L-S
溶存酸素	Do
腰椎	L、LW
腰椎の、腰髄の	
腰椎クモ膜下腔－腹腔短絡術	L-P shunt
腰椎穿刺（ルンバール）	LP
腰椎椎間板ヘルニア	LDH
腰痛	LBP
腰動脈	LA
腰部脊柱管狭窄症	LSCS
羊膜索症候群	ABS
用量	DOS
溶連菌感染後急性糸球体腎炎	PSAGN
抑うつなきうつ病	DSD
抑制性シナプス後電位	IPSP
予後判定栄養指標	PNI
予備吸気量	IRV

ら

来院時心肺停止	DOA
ライ症候群	RS
ラ音	rh
裸眼視力	Nv
ラジオアイソトープ（放射性同位元素）	RI
ラジオアイソトープ脳槽造影	RI
ラジオイムノアッセイ（放射免疫測定法）	RIA
ラムゼイ・ハント症候群	RHS
卵円孔	FO
卵円孔開存	PFO
卵円窓	OW
卵管采周囲癒着	PFA
卵管周囲癒着	PTA
卵管内胚移殖	TEST
卵管内胚細胞移植	GIFT
乱視	AS
乱視矯正角膜切開（術）	AK
卵実質内精子注入法、顕微受精	ICSI
卵巣過剰刺激症候群	OHSS
卵巣癌	Ova Ca、OVC
卵巣包囊腫瘍	YST
卵胞刺激ホルモン	FSH
卵胞刺激ホルモン放出ホルモン	FSHRH

り、る

リード・スタンバーグ細胞	RS
リーメンビューゲル（先天性股関節脱臼治療用装具）	RB
リウマチ因子	RAfactor、RF
リウマチ性疾患	RD
リウマチ性心疾患	RHD
リウマチ性多発筋痛	PMR
リウマチ熱	RF
理学的検査、身体検査	PE

理学療法	PT
理学療法士	PT
リコール(髄液)	Liq
離脱症候群	Wd-syndrome
立体撮影	stereo
リハビリテーション	Rehabili
リファンピシン	RFP
リポプロテインリパーゼ	LPL
リボ核酸	RNA
リボ核蛋白	RNP
リポ蛋白	Lp
リポ蛋白X	LpX
隆起性皮膚線維肉腫	DFSP
流行性角結膜炎	EKC
流行性肝炎	IH
流行性出血熱	EHF
流産	AB、SA
硫酸亜鉛混濁試験	ZST
両眼視力	BV
両眼同時認知	SP、sP
両脚ブロック	BBBB
両耳音の大きさバランス検査	ABLB test
両室肥大	CVH、BVH
良性潰瘍	bU
良性筋痛性脳脊髄炎	ME
良性呼吸窮迫症	BRD
良性小児てんかん	BCECT
良性上皮腫瘍	BET
良性頭蓋内圧亢進	BIH
良性単クローン性免疫グロブリン症	BMG
良性乳房疾患	BBD
良性発作性体位性眩暈	BPPV
両側	Bil、bil
両側肺門リンパ節腫脹	BHL
両側卵管卵巣摘出術	BSO
両大血管右室起始	DORV
両大血管左室起始	DOLV
量不足	QNS
両卵管結紮術	BTL
緑内障	GL、Gla
リン	P

れ

臨界閉鎖圧	CCP
リン酸排泄係数	PEI
リン脂質	PL
臨時	ex
淋疾後尿道炎	PGU
臨床検討会	CC
臨床心理士	CP
臨床痴呆評価尺度	CDR
臨床病理討論会	CPC
リンパ管内マッサージによる間質液吸収促進	MLD
リンパ球	Lym
リンパ球刺激テスト	LST
リンパ球性間質性肺炎	LIP
リンパ球性白血病	LL
リンパ球性脈絡髄膜炎	LCM
リンパ球増多症	LDGL
リンパ上皮性病変	LEL
リンパ性白血病ウイルス	LLV
リンパ節	L/N、LN
リンパ節症関連ウイルス	LAV
リンパ節転移	LYM
リンパ増殖性疾患	LPD
リンパ肉芽腫	LGV
リンパ肉腫	LS
淋病	VDG
ルーY型腸吻合(術)	R-Y
ループス腎炎	LN

れ

レイノー症候群	RS
レイノー病	RD
レーザー角膜内切削形成(術)	LASIK、Lasik
レーザー屈折矯正角膜切除術	PRK
レーザー線維柱帯形成術	LTP
レートプレッシャープロダクト(心拍数×収縮期血圧)	RPP
歴年齢	CA
レギュラーインスリン	RI
劣性遺伝性ジストニー	RD
劣性栄養障害性表皮水疱症	RDEB
レニン-アンギオテンシン-アルドステロン系	RAA

れ

レム睡眠	REM、REM-sleep
連合弁膜症	CVD
レンサ球菌	Strept
連続トロンビン時間	STT
連続波ドプラー	CWD

ろ、わ

ローン・ギャノング・レバイン症候群	LGL
労作性狭心症	AA、EA
労作性呼吸困難	DOE
老視	Pr
老人性円板状黄斑変性症	SDMD
老人性角化症	SK
老人性脳疾患	SBD
老人斑	Sp
老年うつ病スケール	GDS
老年性記憶障害	AAMI
老年痴呆	SD
老年の老人(性)の	S
濾過率	FF
ロゼット形成細胞	RFC
肋間腔	ICS
肋間の	IC
肋骨	C
論理療法	RET
ワーファリン	WF
話声域	SR
ワッセルマン反応	Wa-R、WR
ワレンベルグ症候群	WS

看護・医学 略語・用語ガイドブック
2016年1月5日　第1版第1刷発行

監修者	飯田恭子（いいだやすこ）
発行人	中村雅彦
発行所	株式会社サイオ出版
	〒101-0054
	東京都千代田区神田錦町 3-6　錦町スクウェアビル3階
	TEL 03-3518-9434　FAX 03-3518-9435
カバーデザイン	Anjelico
カバーイラスト	前田まみ
DTP	株式会社メデューム
印刷・製本	株式会社朝陽会

ISBN 978-4-907176-45-7　ⓒ Scio Publishers Inc.
●ショメイ：カンゴイガクリャクゴヨウゴガイドブック
乱丁本、落丁本はお取り替えします。

JCOPY ＜(社)出版者著作権管理機構　委託出版物＞

本書の無断複写は著作権法上での例外を除き禁じられています。複写する場合は、そのつど事前に、(社)出版者著作権管理機構（電話 03-3513-6969、FAX 03-3513-6979、e-mail: info@jcopy.or.jp）の許諾を得てください。

本書の無断転載、複製、頒布、公衆送信、翻訳、翻案などを禁じます。本書に掲載する著作物の複製権、翻訳権、上映権、譲渡権、公衆送信権、通信可能化権は、株式会社サイオ出版が管理します。本書を代行業者など第三者に依頼し、スキャニングやデジタル化することは、個人や家庭内利用であっても、著作権上、認められておりません。